CULTURE
OF DEATH

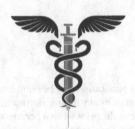

The Age of "Do Harm" Medicine

WESLEY J. SMITH

Encounter Books
New York

First American edition published in 2000 by Encounter Books. First paperback edition published in 2002 by Encounter Books, an activity of Encounter for Culture and Education, Inc., a nonprofit, tax exempt corporation. Encounter Books website address: www.encounterbooks.com

Manufactured in the United States and printed on acid-free paper. The paper used in this publication meets the minimum requirements of ANSI/NISO Z39.48-1992 (R 1997) (*Permanence of Paper*).

SECOND PAPERBACK EDITION

Interior page design and composition: BooksByBruce.com

LIBRARY OF CONGRESS CATALOGING-IN-PUBLICATION DATA:
Smith, Wesley J., author.
Culture of death : the age of "do harm" medicine / Wesley J. Smith. — 2nd edition.
  p. ; cm.
ISBN 978-1-59403-855-6 (pbk. : alk. paper) — ISBN 978-1-59403-856-3 (ebook)
I. Title.
[DNLM: 1. Withholding Treatment—ethics. 2. Bioethical Issues. 3. Euthanasia—ethics. 4. Tissue and Organ Procurement—ethics. 5. Value of Life. WB 60]
R724
174.20973—dc23
2015028083

OTHER BOOKS BY WESLEY J. SMITH

The Lawyer Book: A Nuts and Bolts Guide to Client Survival

The Doctor Book: A Nuts and Bolts Guide to Patient Power

The Senior Citizens' Handbook: A Nuts and Bolts Approach to More Comfortable Living

Winning the Insurance Game (co-authored with Ralph Nader)

The Frugal Shopper (co-authored with Ralph Nader)

Collision Course: The Truth about Airline Safety (co-authored with Ralph Nader)

No Contest: Corporate Lawyers and the Perversion of Justice in America (co-authored with Ralph Nader)

Forced Exit: Euthanasia, Assisted Suicide, and the New Duty to Die

Culture of Death: The Assault on Medical Ethics in America

Power over Pain: How to Get the Pain Control You Need (co-authored with Eric M. Chevlen, MD)

Consumer's Guide to a Brave New World

A Rat Is a Pig Is a Dog Is a Boy: The Human Cost of the Animal Rights Movement

The War on Humans

To Ralph Nader, friend, mentor, visionary, great American.

ACKNOWLEDGMENTS

No author writes a book in a vacuum. All of us who struggle to find the right words, sentences, and paragraphs—whether writing nonfiction, as here, or fiction—are assisted invaluably in our work by sources, colleagues, editors, friends, and family.

I want to thank everyone who willingly shared their ideas, perspectives, and experiences with me, whether in the original version of this book and/or this revised edition—many knowing that I would be critical of their viewpoints. (Please forgive me if I have left anyone out.) These include George A. Agich, Marshall Bedder, James L. Bernat, William J. Burke, Ira Byock, Arthur Caplan, Eric Chevlen, Tom A. Coburn, Carl Cohen, Diane Coleman, Marion Danis, Vincent Fortanasce, Roland Foster, Renée C. Fox, Jeffrey I. Frank, Michael Franzblau, Lisa Gigliotti, Carol Gill, Frederick K. Goodwin, Kathy S. Guillermo, Gregory Hamilton, Kathy Hamilton, John Hardwig, Nat Hentoff, William Hurlbut, Dianne Nutwell Irving, Jennifer Lahl, Albert R. Jonsen, Leon R. Kass, John Keown, David Kilgour, C. Everett Koop, Kit Costello, George Krausz, Richard D. Lamm, Herbert London, Tom Lorentzen, Joanne Lynn, John Morse Luce, Nettie Mayersohn, Alice Mailhot, Mary Meehan, Diane Meier, Gilbert Meilaender, Steve Miles, William Newsom, Mark O'Brien, Adrian R. Morrison, D. S. Oderberg, F. Barbara Orlans, Robert D. Orr, Edmund D. Pellegrino, Mark Pickup, David Prentice, Tom Regan, Sharon M. Russell, Barbara Sarantitis, Dame Cecily Saunders, Cary Savitch, Bobby Schindler, Amil E. Shamoo, Vera Hassner Sharav, D. Alan Shewmon, Janie Siess, Dick Sobsey, Edward Taub, Nancy Valko, Robert M. Veatch, Gregor Wolbring, Sidney Wolfe, and Stuart J. Youngner. Also, thanks to those people who were so helpful but asked to remain anonymous.

A hearty appreciation to my wonderful friends and colleagues who do such good and important work combating assisted suicide and medical utilitarianism with the Patients Rights Council: Rita Marker, Mike Marker, Kathi Hamlon, Robert Hiltner, Jason Negri, and Nancy Minto. You have profoundly influenced my life in ways I can never repay.

My heartfelt appreciation to all my pals and colleagues at the Discovery Institute, for the faith they have shown in my work and support over these many years: Bruce Chapman, Steve Buri, Steve Meyer, John West, Richard Sternberg, Rob Crowther, David Klinghoffer, Ann K. Gauger, Jay Richards, Janine Dixon, and the rest of the gang.

I want to thank everyone at Encounter Books, especially my publishers past and present, Peter Collier (who also did a splendid job editing the original work) and Roger Kimball, as well as Katherine Wong. Thanks too for the great edit of this revised edition, Dave Baker at Super Copy Editors.

Finally, my deepest love and gratitude to friends and family who put up with me with such patience and eye-rolling good cheer, especially: Dean and Gerda Koontz; Mark and LaRee Pickup; Rita and Mike Marker; John and Kathi Hamlon; William and Erica Hurlbut; Tom Lorentzen; Susan Lauffer; Daniel and Jennifer Lahl; Bruce and Valerie Schooley; Bradford William Short; Richard and Leann Doerflinger; David and Diane Prentice; Bobby Schindler; my priest, Fr. John Karcher, and Matushka Eva; and James and Patricia Shinn. My love to the Saunders family, South Carolina, Connecticut, New York, Rhode Island, and Florida Branches: Jerry and Barbara; Jim and Vickie; Jennifer; Jeremiah and Sara and their children, Patrick, Connor, and Aidan; Stephen and Leslie; Rebecca and Jonathan Shulman; Eric; and Joshua. Undying devotion to my beautiful mother, Leona Smith—still going strong—and most of all, to the joy of my life and the source of so much love and laughter, Debra J. Saunders, wife and total sweetheart.

TABLE OF CONTENTS

PREFACE

This book had its genesis when the former editor of Encounter Books, Peter Collier, approached me to write about the modern bioethics movement. Immediately intrigued by the idea, I initially thought *Culture of Death* would be a "policy" book. But as I entered the subject of bioethics more deeply, it became quite personal. I should have known that it would be. Bioethics, as philosopher Leon Kass told me at the time, is about "ultimates," by which he meant the meaning of life, the challenges of mortality, the rights and responsibilities that flow from being a member of the human family. How we deal with these ultimates defines who we are, both as individuals and as a people.

It is a bit jaw-dropping to consider how prophetic this book turned out to be. More than fifteen years have passed since the first edition, during which time the trends and themes about which I warned have accelerated. For example, in the original version I spent many pages cautioning about how dehydrating cognitively disabled patients to death by removing their feeding tubes was becoming normalized and a matter of clinical routine. In those years, people were often shocked at the very prospect. Then, Terri Schiavo burst into the headlines. In the aftermath, not only are people aware that we cause these cruelly slow deaths, but if polls are to be believed, most support so doing. Indeed, in the wake of the Schiavo imbroglio, the resistance to dehydrating helpless patients has all but collapsed. And what was once the ceiling has now become the floor as the bioethics discourse now debates withholding spoon-feeding from people with advanced-stage dementia—even if they willingly eat—if the patient so instructed in an advance directive.

The first edition of *Culture of Death* also warned against the growing euthanasia movement that threatened the soul of Hippocratic medicine. When the book was published in early 2001, the discussion about assisted suicide and euthanasia was mostly a caveat of what I thought was likely to come. At that time, only one jurisdiction in the world—Oregon—had explicitly legalized assisted suicide (although the Netherlands had decriminalized the practice and allowed death doctors to go unpunished if "guidelines" were followed). And, while the first edition of this book discussed the assisted suicide campaign of Jack Kevorkian with much concern, by the time the book hit the bookstores, he was safely imprisoned for murder.

Today, Kevorkian is dead, but the moral values and practices he so zealously espoused certainly didn't succumb with him. Indeed, it is tempting to conclude that we are becoming a Jack Kevorkian world. Not only has the Netherlands formally legalized lethal injection euthanasia, but so too has Luxembourg. In 2002, Belgium instituted an even more radical regime of doctor-administered death than practiced by the Dutch—and the country subsequently embraced euthanasia with a deadly ardor that even surprised me. Meanwhile, Switzerland allows "suicide tourism"—in essence turning the land of the Alps into Jack Kevorkian as a country—to where many hundreds of suicidal people have taken a one-way trip to die in legal suicide clinics.

Worse is yet to come. Just before this revised edition's completion, Canada's Supreme Court imposed a very broad euthanasia license across the country as a Charter right in the wake of Quebec legalizing lethal injections as a form of end-of-life care known in the law as "aid in dying." Euthanasia will also soon be legally administered in Colombia; the country's parliament recently effectuated an old Supreme Court ruling.

The line against doctor-prescribed death has mostly held in the United States—despite scores of legalization attempts, including an unsuccessful 2012 voter referendum in Massachusetts. But that may be changing. Oregon legalized assisted suicide by a referendum in 1994. It took a long time for the next domino to fall, but Washington State and Vermont legalized assisted suicide in 2008 and 2013, respectively. The American assisted suicide movement, bounteously funded and supported by a boosting media, went into overdrive in 2015, a year in which more than half the states saw legislation introduced to legalize assisted suicide. That effort succeeded in California, capping more than twenty years of intense efforts in the Golden State, from where activists hope their agenda will sweep the country.

There is better news on the organ transplantation ethics front. In the first edition, I worried that the dead donor rule—which requires that vital organs only be removed from those who had died—was under threat. It was and still is. But at least on that flank the moral line has held. While advocacy for "redefining death" and allowing people to be killed for their organs has intensified, as we will discuss, organ transplant medicine remains—for the most part—an ethical and moral enterprise.

The same goes for (what I call) "futile care theory" (FCT), against which I spent much effort inveighing in the first edition. Medical futility—which allows doctors to refuse wanted life-sustaining treatments—remains a cogent threat, but it has not yet become normalized in most jurisdictions. Still, that is not for lack of bioethicists trying, and so the issue remains a matter of intense discussion and concern in these updated pages.

This brings me to describing the major differences between the original and revised editions. With so much having happened in the last fifteen years in bioethics and public policies around health care—most especially the passage of the Affordable Care Act—I had to make some significant changes from the original text to keep up with the times. Yet I also had to prevent bloating to keep the book intellectually digestible for the popular audience for which it is intended. That turned out to be a far more involved process than I thought it would be when I first undertook the updating project.

Readers of the original edition will find two major changes. The most sweeping is the deletion of the entire chapter on the ethical questions surrounding animal research, despite much positive reaction about its content in the years since the book was released. It isn't that the issues raised were not, and are not, important. Quite the opposite: I believe the ethics and moralities surrounding the human/animal relationship are so ethically portentous and crucial to human thriving that I wrote an entire book, *A Rat Is a Pig Is a Dog Is a Boy: The Human Cost of the Animal Rights Movement*, on the subject.[1] Since that book dealt in far more detail with the issues raised in the animal research chapter, among many other matters, it seemed superfluous to retain the original material here.

I have replaced the animal chapter with a discussion on what I call "biological colonialism." The exploitation of human body parts and functions—particularly gestation—is becoming a big business, sparking a cultural whirlwind. The new material explores the contentious debate over paying for organs—with special attention paid to the international black market in kidneys—and decries how women, particularly the destitute in developing countries, are used as "gestational carriers." In short, I believe that the bodies of the world's poor are being exploited by the well-off and powerful in much the same way that the original colonialists did to weak nations' natural resources.

For many of the same reasons, I also omitted the original section on embryonic stem cell research and human cloning. Those issues similarly remain important. Indeed, in the years after this book's publication, embryonic stem cell research became, for a time, one of the country's most contentious political and moral issues. That being so, I believed I could not do justice to—nor adequately describe—the intricate controversies involving our fast-emerging biotechnologies in one section of a general chapter, like in the first edition. Indeed, as with animal issues, I believed these issues to be so important I wrote an entire book about them—*Consumer's Guide to a Brave New World*[2]—to which I refer interested readers.

I have replaced the stem cell discussion in the original book with an exploration of a related but distinct futuristic social movement gaining a lot of steam in the last few years. Known generally as "transhumanism," this materialistic quasi-religion challenges traditional Judeo/Christian moral principles about the intrinsic dignity and importance of human life, as it pursues policies it hopes will culminate in our recreation into a "post human" species. While I was unable to give the subject the full attention it requires, I hope the reader finds the discussion sufficiently provocative to stimulate further exploration.

Before we begin, a few words about the general approach I took to upgrading and revising a book fifteen years on the shelves: *Culture of Death* is not an "issues" book so much as one based on themes. I maintained that approach in this edition. That made the revision more challenging to me as a writer because I couldn't simply append new stories and cases like so many Lego© pieces onto old chapters. In other words, it wouldn't do to simply add new assisted suicide cases onto "the euthanasia chapter," as the issues involving doctor-administered death are discussed across most of the book. This structure thus presented me with the creative challenge of weaving new material into the existing themes in a way that I hope is both seamless and edifying to the reader.

But that required difficult choices. I could have deleted all the older material and replaced it with newer stories and issues bearing on the same themes. Or I could have kept all the old material, adding in only a few updates. I chose a middle ground, removing significant sections of dated material but maintaining sufficient original text to show the continuity between what I foresaw then, what has happened since, and the reasons for my even greater alarm about where we seem to be heading now. I hope I have integrated the old and the new in a way that illuminates how we didn't "just arrive" at our current peril but were brought intentionally to this place step by intentional step.

That noted, here are the most prominent changes readers will find in this new edition, beyond simple updating of case studies:

- Detailed material about the Terri Schiavo controversy;
- Updated text across several chapters on assisted suicide and euthanasia, including a discussion of the new horrors out of Belgium and reference to the late Brittany Maynard, who became a media-driven celebrity at the end of 2014 for committing assisted suicide;
- Continued and updated discussion of futile care theory;
- A more detailed focus on advance medical directives and a brief discussion of a new form of advance health care planning known as the POLST (physician's order for life-sustaining treatment);
- Updating the question of health care rationing;
- A discussion of the impact the Affordable Care Act—also known as Obamacare—could have on bioethics;
- A greater discussion of the abortion question while omitting the issue of partial-birth abortion because a federal law was enacted that banned the procedure; and
- New discussion of the question of medical conscience protections and the threat of what I call "medical martyrdom" to health care professionals.

My primary purpose in writing this book has not changed since its original iteration: to alert readers to the subversive impact of bioethics and other ideological agendas on the fundamental moral principles that have long governed the practice of medicine specifically and our society's values and mores generally. In so doing, I hope to help make these crucial debates about medical ethics and health care public policy accessible to those beyond the so-called expert caste that not only dominates these deliberations but also threatens to transform our health care system into a sclerotic technocracy. Thus, I invite those who will be directly affected by these matters—in other words, each and every reader—to enter into these debates with the understanding that the decisions we make in the next decade about issues such as euthanasia, medical rationing, end-of-life care, and organ transplant ethics—just to name a few—will determine both the future of Western medicine and—dare I say it—the continuing morality of our society.

The hour is late. The cause is urgent. The risks are real. As a greater writer than I once put it, ask not for whom the bell tolls, it tolls for thee.

WESLEY J. SMITH
Castro Valley, California
June 5, 2015

INTRODUCTION (TO ORIGINAL VERSION)

This book is the product of two years' worth of intensive research and writing, but its genesis goes back much further than that. Since 1993, I have been an anti-euthanasia activist, during which time I have researched, written, appeared on national television and radio, lectured, and engaged in behind-the-scenes activism, fighting not only the euthanasia agenda but also the incursion of what I generally refer to as "related issues" into modern medical practice. My last book, *Forced Exit: The Slippery Slope from Assisted Suicide to Legalized Murder* [the title was revised in a subsequent edition to *Forced Exit: Euthanasia, Assisted Suicide and the New Duty to Die*] dealt primarily with assisted suicide and euthanasia, as the title indicates. With this book, I explore related issues, many of which I believe are as dangerous and urgent as—if not more than—the ongoing public policy wrestling match over euthanasia.

Assisted suicide is just the tip of the iceberg of what has come to be known as the "medical culture of death." Unbeknownst to most Americans, a small cadre of influential health care policymakers are working energetically and unceasingly to transform medical practice and the laws of health care away from the "do no harm" model established by the great Greek physician Hippocrates and toward a stark utilitarian model that would legitimize not only medical discrimination against the weakest and most vulnerable among us but also, in some cases, their active killing. To make matters worse, the first time many people become aware of what is happening to modern medicine is when they or loved ones experience a health care crisis and suddenly come face-to-face with the monster that they did not even know was lurking in their very midst.

Why are the ethics of our health care system so threatened? Some of it, no doubt, has to do with the times in which we live, in which objective truths are passé and the very concept of right and wrong itself is under assault. But make no mistake—more is at work than just societal drift or passive cultural evolution. The challenges to ethical medical practice and morality explored in this book are promulgated and promoted with great gusto by a cadre of so-called "experts," a genre of moral philosophers, academics, lawyers, physicians, and other members of the medical intelligentsia known generically as "bioethicists."

How does one become a bioethicist? It isn't hard. A bioethicist is as a bioethicist does—no tests have to be passed, no qualifications met. Indeed, practitioners are not licensed, as are other professionals such as attorneys, physicians, real estate agents, or, for that matter, hairdressers. And while more than thirty universities offer degrees in bioethics, there are no standards of education or excellence that apply universally. A Catholic priest can be a bioethicist just as easily as an atheistic college professor. Health care professionals, such as nurses or community ombudsmen, can be appointed to hospital ethics committees, take a few training courses, and then self-identify as bioethicists. Indeed, by writing and lecturing extensively over the last eight years on bioethical issues, including assisted suicide and moves to permit doctors to unilaterally remove wanted medical treatment from dying and disabled people, I could say that I am a bioethicist, too—but I won't.

Being designated a bioethicist in and of itself is of relatively little import. The title does not give one influence within the bioethics movement or the ability to sway society onto or away from the bioethics path. That is to say, there is a very big difference between *being a bioethicist* and the *ideology of mainstream bioethics*, the tenets of which will be described in the first chapter. It is the adherents to the ideology of bioethics—led by a relatively small "insider" group of elite practitioners—who are the *bioethicists* that hold a steadily increasing sway over the laws of public health, the application of medical ethics, and the protocols that govern hospital care. It is their agenda against which this book primarily warns.

As I began my research for this book, I had no idea the depth of the task that awaited me. Yes, I knew that matters were going badly akilter, but I really had little insight into how far bioethics has already helped push the practice of medicine away from the ideals and beliefs that most "regular" people count on to protect them when they or loved ones grow seriously ill or disabled. Indeed, the more I learned about the present being crafted by bioethicists and the future the mainstream movement seeks to create, the more I felt as if I had fallen through Alice's looking glass into a Salvador Dalí painting. Our culture is fast devolving into a society in which killing is beneficence, suicide is "rational," natural death is undignified, and caring properly and compassionately for people who are elderly, prematurely born, disabled, despairing, or dying is a "burden" that wastes emotional and financial resources. Perhaps most worrying: Bioethicists are constructing a system in which the rights of people in the medical system will be based on an explicit hierarchy of human life.

Culture of Death will tell the story of how these nihilistic attitudes are dismantling traditional medical ethics and endangering weak and vulnerable patients. The book will detail how bioethicists have generally abandoned the sanctity of human life ethic that proclaims the equal inherent moral worth of all human beings. Most do not believe in the Hippocratic Oath. Indeed, believers in what I call bioethics ideology reject the very notion that there is anything "special" per se about being a human being. Rather, they assert that being human is a relative thing and what matters morally is whether a "being" is entitled to membership in the "moral community," which, as we shall see, each individual must earn by possessing "relevant characteristics"—usually a minimum level of cognitive functioning—that bioethicists claim give rise to significant moral standing, including the right to life.

In the surrealist world of bioethics philosophy, those with sufficient cognitive qualifications to achieve membership in the moral community are often called "persons." Ironically, many bioethicists assert that persons may include "entities" that are not human. For example, animals are said by some bioethicists to qualify for personhood, which would give these beasts greater moral worth than some humans.

The influence of bioethics is pervasive. From their positions in the academy, in medical and bioethics think tanks, in law schools, and as editors of elite medical journals, financed by grants, honoraria, and book royalties, bioethicists are changing the very face of American health care. Here are just a few examples—a preview of coming attractions, if you will—of some of the topics I will detail later in these pages:

- Dr. Marcia Angell, editor of the *New England Journal of Medicine*, has editorialized that the definition of death be expanded to include a diagnosis of permanent unconsciousness or that other policies be implemented with the stated purpose of requiring that unconscious people be dehydrated to death—even if their families object.

- A peer reviewed article in the *Lancet,* one of the world's most famous medical journals, took this idea one step further, opining that unconscious people should be lethally injected to allow their organs to be harvested. This is not an isolated notion. The idea of permitting disabled people to be killed for their organs is gaining steam among many members of the organ transplant community.
- Peter Singer, an internationally renowned philosopher from Australia with a worldwide following, has declared that parents should have twenty-eight days in which to decide whether to keep or kill their newborn children. Rather than becoming a pariah, as one would expect of an infanticide advocate, he was appointed to a prestigious, tenured professorship at Princeton University.
- Daniel Callahan, one of the country's most influential bioethicists, has called for a harsh system of medical rationing in which research into the cures and causes of disease would be drastically reduced and health care resources diverted from medical treatment into public education programs intended to convince—and, if necessary, coerce—people into healthy lifestyles.
- Some bioethicists want to create a market for the sale and purchase of human organs. Others promote the creation of suicide clinics. A few have even proclaimed a "duty to die" upon reaching old age or becoming a financial or emotional burden.

That such discriminatory policies are ardently advocated in the world's most respected medical and academic journals would be enough cause for alarm. But bioethics is about much more than intellectual theory. Many bioethics agenda items have already imbedded themselves into the bedrock of law.

The 1999 Montana Supreme Court's decision in *James H. Armstrong, MD v. The State of Montana* is just one example. The state had passed a law requiring that only doctors perform abortions, which the court invalidated based on the Montana Constitution and *Roe v. Wade.* That should have been the extent of the decision. But rather than limit the ruling to the case at hand, a 6-2 majority decided to use the cultural flashpoint of abortion as a pretext for imposing a radical and audacious philosophical imperative on the people of Montana, unwarranted by specific facts of the case and unnecessary to its prudent adjudication. As a consequence, the ruling's extraordinary legal implications extend far beyond abortion, opening a Pandora's box of expansive litigation in Montana for years to come and threatening the right of Montana to effectively regulate the practice of medicine through the rule of law.

The scope of the majority ruling is almost unlimited: "The Montana Constitution broadly guarantees each individual the right to make medical judgments affecting her or his bodily integrity and health in partnership with a chosen health care provider free from government interference." This is far more alarming than it may appear at first reading. As the two justices who objected to this aspect of the ruling, Karla M. Gray and Chief Justice J. A. Turnage, rightfully worried, the ruling's broad breadth and radical scope strongly suggests that "the Legislature has no role at all in matters relating to health care to be provided to the people of Montana" and "sweeps so broadly as to encompass and decide such issues as the right to physician-assisted suicide and other important health and medical-related issues which simply were not litigated in this case."

If, indeed, almost anything goes medically in Montana, so long as a patient wants it and a health care professional is willing to do it—a reasonable interpretation considering the expansive language and philosophical thrust of the majority's decision—then it could be construed to permit a doctor to amputate a patient's healthy limbs upon request when the patient wants it removed to satisfy a neurotic obsession (a macabre surgery that has actually occurred in England); allow patients to ask doctors to kill them for organ donation purposes; permit infanticide of disabled infants at the request of caregivers or parents; or allow people to be experimented upon in dangerous ways that are currently illegal. Indeed, the court's ruling is so broad, it decreed that only "a compelling interest ... to preserve the safety, health and welfare of a particular class of patients or the general public from a medically-acknowledged bona fide health risk" warrants state involvement in medical decision making. In other words, regardless of the individual or societal consequences, absent extraordinary exigencies, such as preventing a plague, virtually anything may be allowable in Montana if it can be construed to involve obtaining "medical care from a chosen health care provider." That's an astonishing result from a little-noticed ruling overturning a law that would have simply required doctors to perform all abortions.

How did the court justify such an encompassing decision? Yes, the court looked to *Roe v. Wade* and a smattering of other cases. But the primary authorities that the majority decision relied upon for the broader context of its ruling were philosophical treatises. Indeed, the most frequently cited authority was not a statute, a law case, or even a legal essay but a philosophical discourse on the modern meaning of the "sanctity of human life" contained in a book—*Life's Dominion: An Argument about Abortion, Euthanasia, and Individual Freedom*—written by the attorney/bioethicist Ronald Dworkin in 1993. Dworkin's thesis: A true adherence to the sanctity of life ethic requires that all be permitted to "decide for ourselves" about abortion and euthanasia and that such decisions be accepted by society and tolerated by those who disagree; otherwise society is "totalitarian." The majority opinion cited *Life's Dominion* so frequently and applied its reasoning so enthusiastically that the Ronald Dworkin's philosophy may now be the court-mandated health care public policy of the entire state of Montana without a single vote even being cast—quite a triumph for a philosopher who is little known outside the world of the academy and another step down the road toward the new medicine of mainstream bioethics.

As this book will demonstrate, bioethicists and their allies are pushing the laws of the nation and the public discourse increasingly toward accepting killing and death as a legitimate answer to life's difficulties. This is leading to a rising human toll:

- Oregon, which has legalized assisted suicide, decreed that the act is a form of "comfort care" that must be paid for by Medicaid; this in a state that denies some curative treatments under the state's Medicaid health rationing scheme.
- *Desired* medical treatment is refused in hospitals and nursing homes around the country to patients who are dying or disabled, with the intent that the patients die. This abandonment is justified as ethical under a new theoretical construct known as futile care theory (FCT), which proclaims the right of doctors (and health care executives) to refuse wanted care based on their subjective views of the value of their patients' lives.
- Doctors, nurses, and other hospital staff in hospitals and nursing homes often pressure family members of stroke victims,

demented patients, and other cognitively disabled people to permit their brain-damaged relatives to be dehydrated to death by removing tube-supplied food and water.

- In New York, a man who smothered his wife with a plastic bag after her purported assisted suicide attempt failed, and who then covered up the crime with a falsified death certificate and a quick cremation, was given a mere two-week jail sentence.
- In Canada, Robert Latimer was convicted of murdering his twelve-year-old daughter by asphyxiation because she had cerebral palsy. Instead of receiving significant punishment, he was embraced by a majority of Canadians as a "loving father," resulting in his "mandatory" ten-year sentence being reduced to one year by a judge who labeled the girl's murder "altruistic." Latimer remains free on appeal nearly ten years after his daughter's killing.
- In England, the parents of an infant born with Down syndrome and the treating doctor who intentionally allowed the baby to starve to death were acquitted of all criminal wrongdoing.
- In the United States, the requirements of the Nuremberg Code to protect human beings in medical experiments are routinely violated without legal consequence. Indeed, thanks to the advocacy of "animal rights" activists, animals often receive greater protection in medical research than do people.

This growing indifference to the value of human life within the health care system and courts should be big news. Yet most people are but dimly aware of what is happening. There are several reasons for this. Popular culture promotes many of these practices as a positive, thereby camouflaging the evil that is taking place. Nonjudgmentalism reigns supreme as the growing relativism of our culture increasingly incapacitates people from "imposing their own beliefs on others" by making well-honed moral judgments. The mainstream media neither cover these important issues adequately (or sometimes even at all) nor place them in a proper and understandable context when they do. Thus, while stories involving death culture issues sometimes make the news, they are generally covered as if they have occurred in isolation. The overarching themes that would alert the populace to the bigger picture are generally ignored, and the dots remain unconnected. In this sense, we are like the proverbial frog slowly being boiled to death, unaware that the water is getting hot and that destruction is fast approaching.

A prime purpose of this book is to cast a bright light on the rising steam of the not-yet-boiling pot. Also, by focusing greater attention on the culture of death, I hope to help lead our society away from the immoral path we are on and toward a more profound commitment to the sanctity of human life, not necessarily in the spiritual sense but as a societal commitment that each and every one of us are moral equals. Just as we should not discriminate against each other on the basis of race, religion, nationality, or gender, neither should we cast aside people in the health care system because they are disabled, elderly, brain-damaged, or dying, these latter forms of invidious discrimination being mainstays of the culture of death movement.

Although I quote many philosophy treatises, this is not a philosophy book. And while I explore many laws and ethics protocols, this book does not get bogged down in specific policy proposals. Nor, I hasten to add, am I under the illusion that I can change the minds of the inbred denizens of the ivory tower who move bioethics forward in their never-ending discourse in academic journals and books, and at symposia; most are far too committed to their cause for that. Rather, this is a book primarily about how bad ideas lead to harmful consequences that hurt real people, inviting the people of the general public into the important debates that are already occurring beneath—or, better stated, above—the radar, debates that will not only determine the future of their health care but also the very morality of the society their children will inherit.

One last note before we get under way. In these pages, I take no position on whether abortion should be legal or illegal. I know this will frustrate some of my readers, but I am convinced it is the right thing to do to best accomplish my objectives. Abortion is the black hole of public discourse from which little light escapes. Were I to discuss the issue in depth, any publicity this book eventually receives would likely focus on that issue and divert attention away from the many important bioethics policies upon which this book seeks to shine the bright light. Moreover, many articulate and thoughtful voices already address abortion from both sides of the issue, and nothing I have to say would add substantially to that which has already been written. Finally, *Roe v. Wade* has settled for the foreseeable future whether abortion will or will not be a legal right. Thus anything I might write, either for or against abortion, would be quite superfluous and beside the point of what I hope to achieve in this writing.

That is not to say that *Roe v. Wade* is irrelevant. In a way, this book can be said to begin at the exact point where *Roe* leaves off. The people endangered by the culture of death policies about which I write (e.g., born people) are protected under *Roe v. Wade* but endangered by policies and protocols with which this book is filled. Indeed, whether one is pro-life or pro-choice, it is my sincere hope that the book's readers will agree with me that, regarding born people, each and every one of us should be treated as an unqualified equal in the health care system. None of us is expendable. No one should be abandoned to death because he or she fails to pass the muster established by the few elite academics and philosophers who, for the last thirty years, have taken upon themselves the power to decide when a life is not worthy to be lived.

WESLEY J. SMITH
Oakland, California
March 2000

CHAPTER 1

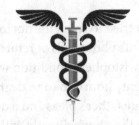

HARSH MEDICINE

"My mother's doctor is refusing to give her antibiotics," the woman caller told me in an urgent voice.

"Why is he refusing to prescribe antibiotics?" I asked.

"He says that she's ninety-two and an infection will kill her sooner or later. So it might as well be this infection."

As disturbing as this call was, as outrageous the doctor's behavior, I wasn't particularly surprised. I have been receiving such desperate communications with increasing frequency for the past two decades. Not every day, not every week, but with sufficient regularity—increasing in volume since this book was originally published—to become very alarmed about the state and ethics of American medicine, and its impact on culture.

Among the more disturbing calls I received came from John Campbell, whose teenage son, Christopher, had been unconscious for three weeks because of brain damage sustained in an auto accident. The boy had just been released from the hospital intensive care unit when he developed a 105-degree fever in the hospital's "step-down unit." Campbell asked the nurses to cool his fever. They replied that they needed a doctor's orders. Campbell asked them to obtain it, but Christopher's physician was out of town and the on-call doctor said no. "It was an evening of hell," Campbell says. "My son's life meant less than hospital protocol. When the doctor refused to order treatment, the nurses said that there was nothing they could do."

Campbell desperately tried to reach the doctor on call personally, but he refused to take Campbell's phone calls or return his increasingly urgent messages. Meanwhile, Christopher's condition worsened steadily, rising over a period of some twenty hours, to 107.6 degrees. Finally, the nurses, caught between a desperate father's pleas and a doctor's steadfast refusal to treat, put Campbell on the phone directly with the doctor.

Campbell demanded that his son's fever be treated immediately. The doctor refused. When Campbell grew more insistent, the doctor actually laughed. The boy was unconscious. His life was effectively over. What was the point?

"By this time," Campbell recalls with much emotion, "my son's eyes were black, as if he had been in a fight. He was utterly still. He was burning up. The back of his neck was so hot you couldn't keep your hand on it. I said to the doctor, 'This is not a joke! This is my son. His life is at stake. His temperature is over 107 and you *are* going to do something about it.'" The doctor, hearing the angry determination in Campbell's voice and perhaps fearing legal consequences if Christopher died untreated, finally acquiesced.

Christopher's temperature subsided. Soon thereafter he was moved to a rehabilitation center for therapy and began a slow recovery. Today he lives at home with his parents, where he is learning to walk with assistance. When not in rehabilitation, Christopher works at a local youth center where he feeds animals and counsels at-risk teenagers. Oh yes, Christopher is very glad to be alive, as are his parents and the many troubled people he helps every day.[3]

As I have spent more than twenty years traveling the country (and internationally) speaking about assisted suicide and other issues involving the ethics of modern medicine, as people react to my appearances on talk radio, television programs, and to my newspaper and magazine columns, with multiplying frequency I hear similar medical horror stories. People are afraid. They are deeply worried about what is happening to medicine: the potential impact of the Affordable Care Act (ACA, also known as Obamacare), doctors pressured by HMOs to reduce levels of care, hospital nursing staffs cut to the bone, the sickest and most disabled abandoned to inadequate care, elderly people dying in filthy nursing homes or in agony because their doctors fail to prescribe proper pain control.[4] There have even been reported instances of desperate patients in hospitals calling 911 because they were unable to access needed medical attention.[5]

These anecdotes are symptoms of a disintegrating value system in health care that disdains the sickest and most disabled among us as having lives that are not worth living; that views expensive medical treatments for such people as a waste of valuable resources; indeed, that accepts their demise—or increasingly, even their killing—as a legitimate answer to the difficulties caused by their serious illnesses and disabilities. In short, the ethics of health care are devolving into a stark utilitarianism that is quickly transforming the "do no harm" tradition of medicine that has for millennia been the cornerstone—and hope—of medicine.

At the same time, medical economics are exerting a gravitational pull into the moral abyss. For example, when Arizona's Medicaid program—the state/federal health insurance for the poor—ran into significant money problems, it canceled organ transplant surgeries for 98 percent of those eligible for the procedure.[6] As this book will explain—sometimes in painful detail—with medical technology growing ever more sophisticated and expensive, while the viability of the old sanctity/equality of life ethic comes under increased cultural pressure, these kinds of controversies are going to become increasingly common and the divisions they sow among us more deep and viscerally felt.

THE NEW HIGH PRIESTS

We have not entered this era of potential medical authoritarianism by chance. We were steered into it by an elite group of moral philosophers, academics, doctors, lawyers, and members of the medical intelligentsia—known generically as bioethicists—who have dedicated themselves over the last four decades to bending public and professional discourse about medical ethics and the broader issues of health care public policy to their desires. They are the cultural aggressors, as the mainstream view in the field is openly hostile to the traditional moral values and ethical traditions of our society.

Medical ethics focuses on the behavior of doctors in their professional lives vis-à-vis their patients. Bioethics focuses on the relationship between medicine, health, and *society*. This last element allows bioethics to pursue policies that go far beyond the well-being of the individual and to presume a moral expertise of breathtaking ambition and hubris. Many view themselves, quite literally, as the forgers of "the framework for moral judgment and decision making"[7] who will create "the moral principles" that determine how "we are to live and act," a "wisdom" they perceive as "specially appropriate to the medical sciences and medical arts."[8] Indeed, some claim that "bioethics goes beyond the codes of ethics of the various professional practices concerned. It implies new thinking on changes in society, or even *global equilibria*"[9] (my emphasis). Not bad for a school of thought that has only existed for about forty years.

Bioethicists typically see their work as integrating "medical ethics and universal morality" beyond "a few general principles" toward the determination of "the meaning of the good life."[10] It is "both a discipline and a public discourse, about the uses of science and technology" and the "values about human life ... with a view toward the formation of public policy and a teachable curriculum."[11] Put more simply, bioethics seeks to create the morality of medicine, define the meaning of health and wellness, and determine when life loses its value (or has less value than other lives) toward the end of forging the public policies and influencing the individual choices that will establish a new medical and moral order. More than a set of tenuous speculations, bioethics in recent years has ossified into an orthodoxy and perhaps even an ideology.

Many bioethicists rejected this claim after the publication of this book's first edition. They act in good faith, these objectors contended. The "quality of life" ethic will create a better world. Besides, they argued, bioethics is not monolithic.[12] After all, practitioners have widely divergent opinions about these issues and controversies—ranging from assisted suicide to cloning to the definition of "health"—with which bioethics discourse grapples. Moreover, many adherents claim, bioethics doesn't have an end goal. It is more akin to a conversation among professional colleagues, a *process* that merely seeks consensus about the most pressing moral and medical issues of our time.

If that were ever true, I contend that it is true no longer. Bioethics, at least of the kind without a modifier (conservative bioethics,

Christian bioethics, etc.) may not be a monolith—a claim I never made. Disagreements certainly exist within the field. But they are more akin—with some exceptions—to the arguing of people who agree on fundamentals but disagree on details—sort of like Catholics bickering with Lutherans.

Most bioethicists recoil at their depiction as "true believers" subject to orthodox precepts and the emotional zeal generated by intensely felt ideology. Their self-view is that of the ultimate rational analyzer of moral problems who, were pipe smoking still fashionable, would sit back, pipe firmly in mouth, acting as dispassionate "mediators" between the extremes of medical technology and the perceived need for limits.[13]

But that is self-deception. Once bioethics moved away from ivory tower rumination to actively influence public policy and medical protocols, by definition the field became goal oriented. Indeed, University of Southern California professor of law and medicine Alexander M. Capron noted that from its inception, "bioethical analysis has been linked to action."[14] If dialogue is linked to action, at the very least that implies an intended direction, if not a desired destination. Even bioethics historian Albert R. Jonsen, a bioethicist himself, calls bioethics a "social movement."[15] Has there been any social movement that was not predicated, at least to some degree, in ideology? Moreover, bioethics pioneer Daniel Callahan, cofounder of the bioethics think tank the Hastings Center, has admitted that "the final factor of great importance" in bioethics gaining societal respect was the "emergence ideologically of a form of bioethics that dovetailed nicely with the reigning political liberalism of the educated classes in America."[16] Thus, mainstream bioethics is explicitly ideological, reflecting the values and beliefs of the cultural elite.

I asked the venerable author, medical ethicist, and physician Leon R. Kass, MD, whether he shares my opinion. Kass told me, "With due allowances for exceptions, I think there is a lot to be said for that view. There are disagreements about this policy or that, but as to how you do bioethics, what counts as a relevant piece of evidence, what kinds of arguments are appropriate to make, there is a fair amount of homogeneity. If you don't hone to that view, you are considered an outsider."[17]

The noted sociologist Renée C. Fox, a close observer of bioethics from its inception, told me in a similar vein, "I would call it an inadvertent orthodoxy. You could even call it ideology, depending on how you define the term." Fox added, "I do think bioethics has gotten institutionalized. It is being taught in every medical school in this country. The training people receive and the content of the curriculum of the short courses as well as the masters' and doctoral programs, can be quite formulaic. In that sense, I think you could talk properly about orthodoxy." And while Fox told me that she does not believe (nor do I) that all bioethicists share the same "doctrinaire values and beliefs," she noted, "If you are referencing that, again and again, bioethical reasoning, deliberation, and maybe even outcomes take certain forms, that may be correct."[18]

British philosophy professor David S. Oderberg and Australian Supreme Court barrister Jacqueline A. Laing agree, writing, "It is plain that bioethics has been dominated by a certain way of doing moral philosophy," what they call an "establishment view."[19] In this regard, Fox and her co-author, Judith P. Swazey, president of the College of the Atlantic in Bar Harbor, Maine, have written, "Bioethics is prone to reify its own logic and to formulate absolutist, self-confirming principles and insights," as bioethicists "have established themselves, and their approach to matters of right and wrong, as the 'dominant force' in the field."[20] Those are pretty good descriptions of the mind-set of ideologues.

Sociologist Howard L. Kaye, PhD, author of *The Social Meaning of Modern Biology*,[21] believes that this bioethics establishment view conceives of itself "less as an attempt to arrive at an ethical regulation of biomedical developments" and more as a system in which "biology [is] transforming ethics." Kaye observes that many bioethicists "believe fervently that there needs to be a radical transformation in how we live and how we think based on new biological knowledge because our values, our ethical principles, our self conception are based on outmoded religious ideas or philosophical ideas that they think have been discredited."[22] If Kaye is correct—and there is abundant evidence that he is—the ultimate bioethics agenda is startlingly radical: dismantling the values and mores of our culture and forging a new ethical consensus in its own self-created image. There's a word for such a breathtaking agenda: ideology.

Adding heft to my claim was the adverse reaction within the field generally to the appointment of Leon Kass by President George W. Bush to head the relatively conservative President's Council on Bioethics in 2001. Never had a bioethics council received such a high profile. Moreover, as a prominent ethics professor at the University of Chicago and elsewhere, no one questioned Kass's academic or intellectual credentials. But rather than being pleased that the field's prominence had been recognized by the president of the United States, the attacks on Kass from prominent bioethicists and policy advocates flew fast and furious.

Liberal science writer Chris Mooney interviewed several prominent bioethicists for his piece "Irrationalist in Chief," published in the *American Prospect*, which concluded that Kass brings "a sixteenth-century sensibility to guide us through twenty-first-century [bioethical] conundrums."[23] In a similar vein, bioethicist James Hughes castigated Kass as a "bio-Luddite," while cloning-advocate Gregory E. Pence branded him as a "false prophet of doom."

The torrent of criticism jumped the shark when (then) University of Pennsylvania bioethics professor and editor in chief of the *American Journal of Bioethics* Glenn McGee editorially attacked Kass for advocating the moral concept of intrinsic human dignity into ongoing bioethical debates:

> It has become the era of Leon Kass, brought back to scholarly life by a call from President George W. Bush. It was a call to become a Presidential bioethics advisor [as head of the President's Council] in the service of putting a stop to embryonic stem cell research, and if possible, putting a stop to a number of other scientific and clinical projects objectionable to the far right wing of the Republican Party, and in particular, Southern Baptists.[24]

Bioethicists pride themselves on rational discourse, but this was rank diatribe from the head of an influential bioethics journal. Kass is Jewish, not Southern Baptist (and for that matter, neither is former President Bush nor, as far as I know, were any council members.) Claiming his approach to be in the service of the "far right" of the Republican Party did an injustice to Kass's nuanced and meticulous approach to bioethics. Moreover, demonstrating how politicized bioethics has become, McGee and his equally chagrined colleagues would have surely cheered if Kass had worked to "put a stop" to clinical projects held to be "objectionable" by the far left of the Democratic Party.

Why is this important? "Bioethics is a phenomenon of great social importance that extends far beyond medicine"[25] and, as Dr. Kaye noted, many leading bioethicists are generally dismissive of Western values and traditions and indeed seek to dismantle them. That would be of little consequence if the movement were relegated to the cultural fringe. But mainstream bioethicists are among society's most influential members. They serve on influential federal and state government public policy commissions, influencing the evolution of public policy. They are public advocates influencing popular views. They write health policy legislation. They consult in medical controversies at the clinical level, often influencing life and death decisions. They testify as expert witnesses in court cases and submit "friend of the court" briefs in legal cases of major significance. They appear on television and in the print media as "expert" commentators. Behind the scenes, they advise politicians from the local level all the way to the federal bureaucracies and, indeed, the president of the United States.

Every medical school teaches bioethics to every student, significantly influencing the attitudes of our doctors of tomorrow toward the health care system generally and their future patients specifically. Bioethics instruction is also provided to other university and postgraduate students studying to become lawyers, business executives, government policy makers, nurses, and educators. For those who wish to make a career in bioethics, many of our leading universities provide postgraduate degrees in the field, with graduates becoming consultants to nursing homes, HMOs, hospital organ procurement centers, and as scholars in think tanks.

Moreover, the influence of bioethicists has grown in the years since this book's first edition. Bioethics is now an international movement, its advocacy pursued in virtually every developed country.

I was certainly not the first critic of the movement. Years before I entered the fray, the late philosopher and theologian Richard John Neuhaus succinctly described this oozing of bioethics into every nook and cranny of the West's institutions when he wrote: "Thousands of ethicists and bioethicists, as they are called, professionally guide the unthinkable on its passage through the debatable on its way to becoming the justifiable, until it is finally established as the unexceptional."[26]

It is worth reflecting upon what has become unexceptional in contemporary medicine and public policy since Neuhaus wrote those words in 1988. Then, most people would have found it unthinkable to dehydrate cognitively devastated people to death by removing their feeding tubes.

It might even have been criminal. Today, due in large part to vigorous advocacy by bioethicists, which in turn led to court cases[27] and then to new laws permitting the practice, withholding "artificial nutrition and hydration" has become routine—and not just for those diagnosed as unconscious.

In 1988, assisted suicide was illegal in every country. Today, euthanasia is administered to an ever-widening cohort in the Netherlands, Belgium, and Luxembourg. It is legal in Quebec and was transformed by the Canadian Supreme Court into a Charter right in 2015. In the USA, assisted suicide has been legalized by statute in California, Oregon, Washington, and Vermont—with new legislative proposals pouring forth with the start of every state legislative session.

It was once unthinkable to procure organs from someone in a persistent vegetative state. Although that is not being done—yet—some of the most mainstream bioethicists and physicians in the organ transplant community dispassionately debate doing just that, in essence advocacy to permit killing for organs.[28]

Ironically, the medical ethics, public policies, and philosophical beliefs that mainstream bioethics espouses are being imposed on a public that does not share many of the underlying values upon which they are based. This results in a distinct and oppressive disconnection between the medical protocols and public policies forged by bioethics advocacy and the people impacted directly by them. Kass explains: "There is a kind of condescension toward the views of the general public [within bioethics] and a considerable divide about core moral views. The American people, as a whole, are a religiously affiliated or God believing people and it is on the basis of the wisdom of these traditions that they express their fears about the threats to sanctity of human life and to human dignity." Kass further warns: "There is the very real danger that what constitutes a 'meaningful life' among the intellectual elite [who make up much of the bioethics establishment] will be imposed on the people as the only standard by which the value of human life is measured."[29]

John Keown, former University of Cambridge law professor and current Rose F. Kennedy Professor of Christian Ethics at Georgetown University's Kennedy Institute of Ethics, accurately identifies this fundamental conflict:

Traditional common morality, as its name suggests, comprises ethical principles common to civilized cultures. The notion that that there are certain objective principles which societies must respect if they are to quality as civilized, has been expressed in the West in the Hippocratic Oath in Judeo-Christian morality, the prohibition against killing the innocent, and in the common law.... [But] much of modern bioethics is clearly subversive of this tradition of common morality. Rather than promoting respect for universal human values and rights, it systematically seeks to subvert them. In modern bioethics, nothing is, in itself, either valuable or inviolable, except utility.

Much damage has already been done. Indeed, society is only vaguely aware of the extent to which their most basic presumptions about health care have been undermined.

CREATING A HIERARCHY OF HUMAN LIFE

"The traditional Western ethic," a *California Medicine* editorial opined in 1970, "has always placed great emphasis on the intrinsic worth and equal value of every human life." This "sanctity of life ethic," the editorial continued, has been "the basis for most or our laws and much of our social policy" as well as "the keystone of Western medicine.... This tradition ethic is being eroded at its core and may eventually be abandoned.... Hard choices will have to be made ... that will of necessity violate and ultimately destroy the traditional Western ethic with all that portends. It will become necessary and acceptable to place relative rather than absolute values on such things as human lives."[30]

These chilling words were prescient. In the nearly fifty years since, that is exactly what has happened. Rather than believing in inherent human equality, most contemporary bioethicists measure the value of human life subjectively. Instead of embracing the human community—which means all of us—most bioethicists are concerned with the "moral community," which in theory and often in practice excludes some of us. For most bioethicists, human rights—assuming they exist; not all believe in them—are not inalienable but must be earned based on criteria *they* created—and, as we shall see, may include animals. Thus, equality ceases to be a universal vision.

If these words seem harsh, consider the thinking of an influential philosopher, the late Joseph Fletcher, whose ideas had enormous impact on the West in the second half of the twentieth century. Fletcher is most famous for creating "situational ethics," which emphasizes "cutting loose from moral rules" and "reasoned choice as basic to morality."[31] Applied to medical ethics and health care, situational ethics—along with Fletcher's writing and pronounced persuasive skills—made him, in Albert R. Jonsen's term, "the patriarch of bioethics."[32]

Fletcher was a radical utilitarian whose stated goal was to maximize happiness and minimize suffering. That sounds good in the abstract, but once he had freed himself from "moral rules," Fletcher developed a worldview that was paradoxically both anarchic and totalitarian. Thus, in the name of human freedom, he enthusiastically endorsed the wildest ideas, such as the manufacture of chimeras (part human, part animal) through genetic engineering.[33] Yet individuals *per se* actually counted for little in his thinking, and those he perceived as interfering with the general pursuit of happiness were expendable.

Early on, Fletcher dismissed the traditional medical "reverence for life," sniffing that "nobody in his right mind regards life as sacrosanct." Developing his thesis from the then newly crafted right to abortion, Fletcher distinguished "human life" from what he called "personal life." "What is critical," he wrote in 1973, "is personal status, not merely human status." He created a list of "criteria or indicators" that he hoped could be used to divide society between those individuals who possessed "human-hood" and those who did not—between "truly human beings" whom he saw as deserving of great moral concern and the "subpersonal," or humans he deemed of scant consequence.[34] He used the terms "human-hood" and "truly human" not as biological descriptions but as subjective terms to connote moral value.

The immediate problem facing Fletcher and those contemporaries who agreed with him was to devise a method for culling the human herd to prove that "we mean business."[35] Toward that end, Fletcher proposed a formula to gauge the quality of a human life "for the purposes of bio-medical ethics."[36] These included a list of fifteen "criteria or indicators,"[37] among which were:

- Minimum intelligence (score too low and one is deemed "mere biological life");
- Self-awareness ("essential to the role of personality");
- Self-control (i.e., if someone is not control of him or herself, "the individual is not a person");

- A sense of futurity ("subhuman animals do not look forward in time");
- Memory ("It is this trait alone that makes man ... a cultural instead of instinctive being");
- Concern for others ("The absence of this ambience is a clinical indication of psychopathology");
- Communication ("Disconnection from others, if it is irreparable, is dehumanization"); and
- Neocortical function ("In the absence of the synthesizing function of the cerebral cortex, the person is non existent. Such persons are objects, not subjects").

Fletcher also fashioned five "negative" points that he believed indicated true humanhood. For example, he claimed that man is not "anti-artificial." To the "anything goes" Fletcher, "to oppose technology is self-hatred." Thus, "a baby made artificially by deliberate and careful contrivance, would be *more human* than one resulting from sexual roulette—the reproductive mode of subhuman species" (my emphasis).[38] Fletcher also dismissed the notion of innate human rights: "The idea behind this is that such things are objective, pre-existent phenomena, not contingent on biological or social relativities."[39] In other words, Thomas Jefferson was all wet.

To understand how dangerous that thought of bioethics' "patriarch" really is, one need only read Fletcher's 1975 essay, "Being Happy, Being Human,"[40] in which he describes participating in a panel discussion of the treatment of babies born with serious birth defects. A physician who cared for a profoundly mentally retarded boy reported that while he possessed a very low IQ, the lad was clearly happy and clearly a human being. Fletcher coldly dismissed the human worth of this defenseless child—and that of many other developmentally disabled people: "Idiots are not, never were, and never will be in any degree responsible [because they cannot understand consequences of action]. Idiots, that is to say, are not human. The problem they pose is not lack of sufficient mind but of any mind at all. No matter how euphoric their behavior might be, they are outside the pale of human integrity. Indeed, sustained and 'plateau' euphoria is itself prima facie clinical evidence of mindlessness."[41]

Such a provocation had a purpose: to gain support for the notion that killing "idiots" could, depending on the facts of each individual case, be ethical and right—decisions that Fletcher described as a merely "clinical" matter.[42] In the case of disabled infants, he wrote elsewhere that killing should simply be considered "postnatal abortion."[43] As I will describe later, calls within bioethics to permit infanticide have proliferated in the years subsequent to Fletcher's advocacy.

Not every bioethicist agrees with all of Fletcher's ideas. Nor will every radical policy Fletcher promoted eventually become culturally or medically acceptable—although many of them, such as dehydrating to death cognitively disabled people, which Fletcher proposed as early as 1974,[44] already have. But it is particularly telling that Fletcher was not dismissed by the fledgling bioethics movement as some fanatic kook when he advocated infanticide, "research on living fetuses outside the womb,"[45] combining human and animal DNA,[46] and dehumanizing cognitively disabled people. In fact, his ideas received immediate respect, allowing them to travel from the realm of the unthinkable, to borrow Richard John Neuhaus's terminology, into the debatable, from whence many have become justifiable. Some are now unexceptional.

That is not to say that there was no intellectual resistance within the early bioethics movement to the steady growth of this sort of secularist, radically utilitarian thinking. A strong countermovement led by theologian Paul Ramsey provided a significant challenge to the Fletcher school for many years.

Ramsey believed that people owed each other a duty of fidelity based upon "covenant responsibilities" based in "justice, fairness, righteousness, faithfulness, canons of loyalty, the sanctity of life, *hesed, agapé* [steadfast love], or charity." This meant, according to Ramsey, that there is "sacredness and in 'bodily life' from which flow our mutual duties to care for each other, including the most weak and vulnerable among us."[47]

Where Fletcher's approach was a bioethical version of anything goes, Ramsey stood firmly against the idea that the ends justify the means. Where Fletcher sought to create invidious divisions among people based on purported humanhood criteria, Ramsey explicitly rejected the entire approach as immoral: "Fletcher is simply a sign of the times," Ramsey worried, as he asserted that creating criteria to judge how people should be treated in health care is wrong because it was to "play God as God plays God."[48] "To use such indices in the practice of medicine is a grave mistake," Ramsey warned, because it would lead to inequality and "add injustice to injury and fate."[49]

Gilbert Meilaender, the theologian and ethicist who has been a part of this struggle for decades, characterized this internal struggle for the soul of bioethics as a three-decade war. To make a long story short, the amoral Fletcher school (my term) prevailed over traditional moralists such as Ramsey, illustrated by the sad fact that few of Ramsey's books remain in print while most of Fletcher's books and articles are readily obtainable. In the end, Fletcher, not Ramsey, became the "patriarch" of modern bioethics. It is Fletcher's views that predominate within the field. Fletcher, not Ramsey, was the one who "articulated where bioethics was heading well before the more fainthearted were prepared to develop the full consequences of their views."[50]

Once Fletcher secured a beachhead, it was only a matter of time before someone like Peter Singer would stage his much-publicized landing in bioethics. If this were a movie, Singer's appearance would be entitled "Son of Fletcher." Beginning in the mid-1970s, Singer rose quickly in prominence to become one of the world's most influential contemporary utilitarian bioethicist/moral philosophers. But being the radical that he is, Singer took Fletcher's original formula and extended it to even more subversive ends. Where Fletcher sought to determine who had moral value strictly for the benefit of humans, Singer expanded the "moral community" into the world of animals.

Singer contended that being human in and of itself is irrelevant to moral status; what counts is whether a "being" is a "person." Toward creating a formula to make this determination, Singer simplified Fletcher's multi-point formula to "two crucial characteristics" that earn human being or animal the status of "person" (e.g., "rationality and self consciousness").[51] Species membership is irrelevant, Singer claimed. Indeed, he asserted that some *animals* are persons, including "whales, dolphins, monkeys, dogs, cats, pigs, seals, bears, cattle, sheep, and so on, perhaps even to the point which it may include all mammals."[52] On the other hand, some humans would not qualify, including newborn human infants (whether disabled or not), people with advanced Alzheimer's disease or other severe cognitive disabilities—since Singer claimed they are not self-conscious or rational—along with other nonpersons that exhibit similar relevant characteristics (e.g., clams or sardines).

Yes, Singer explicitly made a moral comparison between some people and fish, writing, "Since neither a newborn infant nor a fish is a person the wrongness of killing such beings is not as great as the wrongness of killing a person."[53] Thus, to Singer, a newborn infant is the moral equivalent of a mackerel and an advanced Alzheimer's patient is comparable to a pigeon. As we shall see later in the book, Singer, like Fletcher, asserted that his theories justify infanticide and non-voluntary euthanasia of cognitively disabled people.

In another world and time, Singer's advocacy would make him an intellectual outcast. He actually is in bad standing in Germany and Austria, where he cannot speak without generating angry protests from people who consider his opinions Nazi-like.[54] But many in academia and bioethics embrace him, or at least respect his intellectualism (and perhaps admire his radicalism). Far from being a fringe character, Singer is invited to present at seminars, symposia, and philosophy association conventions throughout the world. His 1979 book, *Practical Ethics*, which unabashedly advocates infanticide and euthanasia, and also decries "discrimination" based on species (a bizarre notion Singer labels "speciesism"), has become a standard text in many college philosophy departments. Singer is so mainstream that he even wrote the essay on ethics for the *Encyclopedia Britannica*. Most disturbingly, in 1999, he became a permanent member of the Princeton University faculty, where he is the Ira W. DeCamp Professor of Bioethics, a prestigious, tenured academic chair at the university's Center for Human Values.

The person/nonperson moral distinction is generally accepted throughout bioethics and increasingly applied to animals, as Singer has advocated. Writing in the influential *Kennedy Institute of Ethics Journal*, British academic John Harris, the Sir David Alliance Professor of Bioethics and Director of the Institute of Medicine, Law, and Bioethics at the University of Manchester, England, defines a person as "a creature capable of valuing its own existence," which he opines could include people, animals, extraterrestrials, and machines but does not include some humans, including infants "during the neonatal period." To Harris, only the lives of persons are morally important. It is not wrong to kill nonpersons or fail to save their lives:

> [T]o kill or to fail to sustain the life of a person is to deprive that individual of something that they value. On the other hand, to kill or to fail to sustain the life of a nonperson, in that it cannot deprive that

individual of anything that he, she, or it could conceivably value, does that individual no harm. It takes from such individuals nothing that they would prefer not to have taken from them.... Nonpersons and potential persons cannot be wronged in this way [killing them against their will] because death would not deprive them of anything they can value. If they cannot wish to live, they cannot have that wish frustrated by being killed.[55]

Similarly, Georgetown University's Tom L. Beauchamp, co-author of *The Principles of Bioethics*, similarly asserts in the *Kennedy Institute of Ethics Journal* that personhood and nonpersonhood designations may soon inform us whether we can use people as objects of exploitation in the ways that are presently restricted to our treatment of animals: "Because many humans *lack* properties of personhood or are less than full persons, they are thereby rendered equal or inferior in moral standing to some nonhumans. If this conclusion is defensible"—and Beauchamp clearly thinks it is—"we will need to rethink our traditional view that these unlucky humans cannot be treated in the same ways we treat relevantly similar nonhumans. For example, they might be aggressively used as human research subjects and sources of organs."[56]

Making instrumental use of humans denigrated as having lesser value based on their capacities is definitely on the bioethics table. In 2010, British bioethicist Alasdair Cochrane eloquently identified the stakes in the debate over whether "intrinsic dignity" is an inherent human characteristic: "Under this conception, the possession of dignity by humans signifies that they have an inherent moral worth. In other words, because human beings possess dignity we cannot do what we like to them, but instead have direct moral obligations toward them. Indeed, this understanding of dignity is also usually considered to serve as the grounding of human rights. As Article 1 of the Universal Declaration of Human Rights states, 'All human beings are born free and equal in dignity and rights.'"[57] He also stated: "If all individual human beings possess dignity, then they should not be viewed simply as resources that we can treat however we please. To take an example, it may be that we could achieve rapid and significant progress in medical science if we were to conduct wide-ranging experiments on groups of human beings. However, because human beings have dignity, so it is argued, this means that they possess a particular quality that grounds certain obligations and rights."[58]

Despite understanding the stakes, Cochrane took the familiar bioethics line, calling for an "undignified bioethics" that views humanhood per se as morally irrelevant and arguing that the ways we treat our fellow humans should depend on each individual's perceived "moral status"—such as personhood. "Simply stipulating that all and only human beings possess this inherent moral worth because they have dignity is arbitrary and unhelpful," he wrote.[59] Hardly arbitrary, given the stakes and the deep traditions behind this view. Unhelpful, perhaps—it impedes using vulnerable humans as lab rats, prevents raising fetuses for harvest, and argues against other utilitarian horrors—real and proposed—that are the subject of this book.

Not all bioethicists are as candid as Fletcher, Singer, Harris, Beauchamp, and Cochrane. The late Ronald Dworkin, an influential law professor and author whose effect on the Montana Supreme Court I mentioned earlier, argued in his book *Life's Dominion* that killing the weak and helpless can actually be a method of *upholding* the inherent value of human life.[60] Dworkin claimed that the argument between those who support abortion or euthanasia and those who oppose these practices isn't even an argument about whether the sanctity of life is a sound principle. Everyone agrees that it is, he claims: "We disagree so deeply because we all take so seriously a value that unites us as human beings—the sanctity or inviolability of every stage of every human life. Our sharp divisions signal the complexity of the value and markedly different ways that different cultures, different groups, and different people, equally committed to it, interpret its meaning."[61]

Yet, in Dworkin's hands, the meaning of the "sanctity of life" is left to each person to determine individually. Thus, Dworkin says, having an abortion is not denying life's sanctity to the human fetus but upholding life's sanctity for the woman who doesn't want a baby. "It may be more frustrating to life's miracle when an adult's ambitions, talents, training and expectations are wasted because of an unforeseen or unwanted pregnancy than when a fetus dies before any significant investment of that kind has been made."[62] Regardless of where one stands in the great pro-life/pro-choice cultural divide, to assert that having an abortion is somehow to embrace "the inviolability of *every* stage of *every* human life," as Dworkin does, is simply ludicrous.

Dworkin similarly asserts that euthanasia isn't actually a rejection of the sanctity of life but an embracing of it: "People who want an early, peaceful death for themselves are not rejecting or denigrating the sanctity of life. On the contrary, they believe that a quicker death shows more respect for life than a protracted one." Active killing of people promoted, without a hint of irony, as an embrace of life's sanctity is to suck all meaning from language. For Dworkin, the "sanctity of life" is not a principle but a mere contingency, defined essentially by where a person stands in his or her life at any given moment. Such a porous concept is incapable of protecting the weak and vulnerable from medical discrimination or killing, and that—as with the distinction between human beings based on personhood criteria—is exactly the point.

Dworkin repeatedly confused feelings with morality, arguing that since the deaths of some people cause more grief and sense of tragedy than do the deaths of other people, it is somehow justifiable to view the inviolability of individual human lives in relative terms: "Most people's sense of that [death-caused] tragedy, if it were rendered as a graph relating the degree of tragedy to the age at which death occurs, would slope upward from birth to some point in late childhood or early adolescence, then follow a flat line until at least very early middle age, and then slope down again toward extreme old age.... [Thus] The death of an adolescent girl is worse than the death of an infant girl because the adolescent's death frustrates the investments she and others have made in her life."[63]

Determining the value of life with such an emotional yardstick is a quixotic enterprise. One could just as easily argue that the newborn's life is more valuable because it is all potential—a blank slate—while the adolescent has already acquired a character and experiences that limit her range. Such opinions are at best an underwriter's version of morality and not worth the time it takes to make them.

EUTHANIZING HIPPOCRATES

"To regard life as sacred," Leon Kass wrote, "means that it should not be violated, opposed, or destroyed, and that positively, it should be protected, defended and preserved."[64] These precepts are especially important in medicine, considering the power accorded physicians to cut, drug, and manipulate the bodies of their patients. Meilaender summarized the obligation as a positive obligation of physicians to "be committed to the bodily life of their patients."[65] A robust belief in the equality/sanctity of human life takes these prescriptions one step further by positing the obligation of physicians to view each of their patients as having equal moral worth. Thus physicians are not free to pick and choose among the patients to whom they will give optimal care. All patients are owed the same level of dedication, excellence, loyalty, and fidelity, regardless of their physical or cognitive condition.

These worthy concepts are famously embodied in the Hippocratic tradition. Indeed, medicine may actually have been the first field in which the underlying principles of the equality of life ethic were recognized as applying generally rather than parochially. The Oath, bearing the name of Hippocrates (approximately 470–360 BCE) was created hundreds of years before the advent of Christianity. It required physicians to "apply dietetic measures for the benefit of the sick according to my ability and judgment," to "keep them from harm and injustice," foreswear abortion, and "give no deadly medicine to any one if asked, nor will I make a suggestion to this effect." The Oath taker promised, "Whatever house I may visit, I will come for the benefit of the sick, remaining free of all intentional injustice, of all mischief and in particular of all sexual relations with both female and male persons, be they free or slaves." Physicians further pledged to keep patient confidences, holding what the doctor sees or hears "in the course of treatment" to be "shameful to be spoken about."[66] These life- and dignity-affirming doctrines of the Oath are generally summarized by a familiar summarizing phrase: "do no harm" (the exact phrase is not found in the great document itself, although it is discussed in Hippocratic literature). These principles were and are upheld by physicians in myriad ways: by rendering optimal care to each patient; promoting bodily heal- ing; alleviating pain and suffering; respecting patient dignity; refusing to disclose patient confidences, even in a court of law; and refusing to kill patients.

As we move further into the twenty-first century, the Hippocratic tradition is ailing and in acute danger of collapse. "It was when bioethics came on the scene that the Hippocratic tradition of the physician/patient relationship started to fall apart," philosopher Dianne N. Irving, PhD, a longtime critic of bioethics, told me. "Once it was weakened, bioethics began to replace it with medicine practiced for the greater good of the society rather than the individual patient. That threatens patient welfare and denigrates medicine into a business rather than a profession."[67] Irving's criticisms find support among many mainstream bioethicists who celebrate their calling as "post professional."[68]

A recent study of physician oath taking published in the *Journal of Clinical Ethics*[69] illustrated how far modern medicine has strayed from the traditional values of the Hippocratic Oath. The authors analyzed contemporary medical oaths and compared them to the Hippocratic original. Considering *Roe v. Wade*, it is not surprising that 8 percent of doctors pledged to forswear abortion, but only 14 percent promised not to commit euthanasia (active killing by doctors). In 1977, only 31 percent of oaths required the taker to "respect life," and only 43 percent of present-day oaths require physicians to be "accountable to their profession." There has also been a stunning "nearly complete" disappearance of the proscription against sexual relations between physicians and patients, a key factor in professionalism, since it is a matter "of character and justice ... and not taking advantage of vulnerable patients."[70]

Many of the most prominent doctors and bioethicists could care less. Thus the late author and physician Sherwin Nuland of Yale University School of Medicine wrote in the *New England Journal of Medicine*, "Those who turn to the oath in an effort to shape or legitimize their ethical viewpoints must realize that the statement has been embraced over approximately the past 200 years far more as a symbol of professional cohesion than for its content.... Ultimately, a physician's conduct at the bedside is a matter of individual conscience."[71] Yikes!

When I tell my lecture audiences that most doctors no longer take the Hippocratic Oath upon becoming physicians and that many no longer see it as relevant to their profession, they are shocked and disturbed. They believe, quite correctly, that the Oath exists for *their* protection. They want their doctors to practice a do-no-harm style of medicine. "Why have they abandoned a tradition that has served medicine—and us—so well?" they ask.

The answer to this important question is complex, having much to do with who we are as a culture and a people. According to the late physician and sanctity-of-life bioethicist Edmund D. Pellegrino—who spent a long and productive career as a professor of medical ethics—the Hippocratic system came under attack both from without and within the medical profession: "These constructs first came into question in the mid-1960s as part of the general upheaval of moral values that occurred in the United States. Concomitantly, the character of medicine was being altered by the specialization, fragmentation, institutionalization, and depersonalization of health care. At the same time, the number and complexity of medical ethical issues expanded as the power of medical technology presented new challenges to traditional values."[72]

These challenges could have been met without destroying the "do no harm" tradition. However, medicine, perhaps having lost confidence in its own ethical instincts, "turned to the philosophers"[73] of bioethics. Unfortunately, by this time, the most influential practitioners in the field had enlisted in the relativist branch epitomized by Fletcher rather than the more traditional equality-of-life-affirming approach espoused by Ramsey. In a philosophical milieu in which the most helpless patients were already viewed widely as less than fully human, the Hippocratic tradition didn't stand a chance. This sad fact is illustrated by the treatment given the tradition in *The Principles of Biomedical Ethics*, first published in 1979, in which Beauchamp and Childress blithely dismiss it as "a limited and unreliable basis for medical ethics."[74] As for the do-no-harm ethic the Oath spawned, readers are informed that it is merely a "strained translation of a single Hippocratic passage."[75] So much for more than 2,000 years of applied ethics and medical wisdom.

BIOETHICS AND RELIGION

The antipathy of mainstream bioethics to religion began early. It is not coincidental that Joseph Fletcher, the "patriarch," insisted on forming his views upon the premise that "man is not a worshipper."[76] In recounting the reasons why he believed that bioethics became so influential in such a short time, Daniel Callahan wrote, "The first thing that ... bioethics had to do—though I don't believe anyone set this as a conscious agenda— was to push religion aside."[77] Dan Brock, a prominent philosopher and member of the bioethics elite, was similarly blunt in an article urging the legalization of euthanasia: "In a pluralistic society like our own, with a strong commitment to freedom of religion, public policy should not be grounded in religious beliefs which many in that society reject."[78]

After welcoming theologians in its formative years (ironically, Fletcher was a lapsed Episcopal priest), bioethics now stresses that morality and proper behavior are best determined through "rational analysis" based on secular philosophical precepts. Theology, religious values, spirituality, faith—these are considered "external" and thus "unconvincing" in determining wrong from right.[79] Moreover, unlike most of the general population that bioethics supposedly serves, many (although certainly not all) modern bioethicists are agnostic or atheistic, a personality factor that colors their entire approach to these important issues as much as the Pope's Catholicism does his. Indeed, some bioethicists view religion with utter disdain, as mere "mumbo jumbo," to use Peter Singer's pejorative term.[80] Even those bioethicists who have strong spiritual beliefs—including some Catholic priests—are so worried about imposing their religion upon secular society that they leave their personal faith-inspired values at the door when discussing public health policies.

This near-absolute rejection of religious values as a proper moral underpinning for debating and creating secular public policies is a fatal flaw of modern bioethics. "Ninety percent of the population identifies with the Judeo-Christian tradition," writes the Loma Linda University professor of Ethical Studies James W. Walters. As an obvious consequence, "our society's most fundamental moral views are rooted in religion."[81] If Walters is right, then bioethics isn't merely reflecting a new ethic to meet changing times—it is *imposing* it on and applying it to a population that profoundly disagrees with bioethics' most basic assumptions.

That is not to say that religion in the public square does not have its problems. (Murdering doctors in the name of "life" comes readily to mind.) But it is also true that religion played an indispensable role in creating an ethic of humanity that gentles the savage injustices of life.

Consider the modern hospice movement that owes its origin to the dedication and compassion rooted in the deeply held religious values of its founder, Dame Cicely Saunders. Dame Cicely, as she is known affectionately in England, was a nurse and devout Anglican who was a medical social worker in a London hospital in the years immediately following World War II. She met a Jewish émigré named David Tasma, who had escaped the Warsaw ghetto only to lie dying in a London hospital at the age of forty. Tasma was alone in the world, and Saunders made a special point to visit him every day. Their friendship changed our world.

As Saunders and Tasma spoke of his impending death, she began to comprehend "what he needed—and what all of the other dying patients and their families needed." Saunders had an epiphany. She told me, "I realized that we needed not only better pain control but better overall care. People needed the space to be themselves. I coined the term 'total pain' from my understanding that dying people have physical, spiritual, psychological, and social pain that must be treated. I have been working on that ever since."[82] Tasma left Saunders 500 British pounds to begin her work, telling her, "I will be a window in your home." Saunders told me, her eyes moistening, "It took me nineteen years to build the home around that window."[83]

Saunders epiphany was not "rational" but spiritual, coming from a deep empathy inspired by her religious faith. Her work was a "personal calling, underpinned by a powerful religious commitment,"[84] wrote David Clark, an English medical school professor of palliative care and Saunders's biographer, to whom she has entrusted the organization of her archives. So strong was Saunders's faith in what she perceived as her divine call that she began volunteering as a nurse at homes for the dying after work.[85] Urged on by her deep desire to help dying people, she went to medical school at the age of thirty-three, this at a time when there were few women doctors.

Saunders focused her medical practice on helping dying people and alleviating pain. She obtained a fellowship in palliative research and began work in a hospice run by nuns, where pain control was unevenly applied, a nearly universal problem at the time, causing much unnecessary misery. Saunders conceived of putting patients on a regular pain control schedule, which, in her words, "was like waving a wand over the situation."[86]

Saunders's faith pushed her toward founding a hospice based on her concept of treating the total patient. Believing firmly that "the St. Christopher's project [was] divinely guided and inspired,"[87] she became an activist, energetically raising money for the new project and in the process raising the consciousness of the medical establishment. Based as it was on religious inspiration ("I have thought for a number of years that God was calling me to try to found a home for patients dying of cancer," she wrote to a correspondent[88]), Saunders's initial idea was for St. Christopher's hospice to be a "sequestered religious community solely concerned with caring for the dying." But the idea soon expanded from a strictly religious vision into a broader secular application; in Clark's words, a "full-blown medical project acting in the world."[89]

Saunders succeeded beyond even her own wildest hopes. St. Christopher's opened in a London suburb in 1967 and jump-started the modern hospice movement. "We started in-home care in 1969," Saunders said. "The majority of our work is out in the community." Saunders soon exported hospice to North America. In 1971, she sent one of her team doctors to New Haven, Connecticut, to help found the first modern hospice in the United States, from whence it spread nationwide. Hospice has been a certified medical specialty in Britain since 1987.[90]

There is a direct line of compassion, succor, and love from David Tasma in 1948 to the millions of others who have benefited from hospice care since 1967—including my father, who died under hospice care in 1984, and my aunt in 2013. None of this would have happened without the religious values manifesting in the secular milieu of medicine through Dame Cecily, specifically the belief that no matter what our state of health, no matter our age, no matter how much help we need, no matter how we look or smell, we all have equal moral worth.

To promote such values is not to support theocracy. It does not divide a pluralistic society by imposing religion on an unwilling public. Rather, it is a secular application of the sanctity of life. How sterile and harsh the world would be if the values that inspired Dame Cicely were barred from the public square simply because they were founded in religious faith. How dangerous to exclusively base our approach to issues of public health policy and clinical medical ethics on amoral "moral philosophy." It is true that religion not tempered by secular restraint and rationalism can lead to the tyranny of theocracy. But secularism not enriched by the values inspired by spirituality and religious faith, as this book demonstrates, will lead to the creation of "hierarchies of human worth,"[91] the building blocks for a medical culture of death.

BRAVE NEW BIOETHICS

Having rejected the core values and virtues of Western civilization as bases for determining what is moral and good, bioethics turned to secular moral and analytical philosophy for the answers. This approach accepts no moral standard or ethical rule, no matter how deeply valued, as a self-evident truth. Every moral principle must be reassessed and deemed "rational" if it is to pass bioethical muster. Not surprisingly, the people bioethicists deem best able to perform this task *are themselves*, especially those trained in the arcane schools of secular philosophy. Needless to say, that stacks the deck in favor of those values and approaches to morality that the most influential bioethicists embrace personally. Unfortunately, some critics (me included) find that important human values such as "decency, kindness, empathy, caring, devotion, service, generosity, altruism, sacrifice, and love" are too often omitted from their equations because they are perceived to have little value in determining "what is ethical or moral."[92]

Ironically, mainstream bioethics, which explicitly eschews religious values in public policy and medical ethics discourse as well as proudly proclaims itself the epitome of rationality, has itself become something of a secular faith among its adherents. Renée Fox notes, "Bioethics has always been a societal happening, dealing with issues that have religious import and ramifications. It deals with real dilemmas, issues of how society deals with ultimate beliefs. Bioethics uses medicine as a metaphor for discussing with each other issues of ultimate values and belief, questions that are as religious as they are ethical."[93] Adds Leon Kass: "While bioethics is not formally a religion, it is absolutely faith-based and is as equally indemonstrable. They purport to grapple with First Principles. Yet, they step into the public square with no greater claim to wisdom than does someone who believes in the resurrection or in the revelation of the Law at Sinai."[94]

Bioethicist Daniel Callahan clearly perceives bioethics in quasi-metaphysical terms. "Above all," he wrote in 1994, "bioethics needs to develop the capacity to help individuals make good moral decisions in their own lives and to do so in the context of the most basic moral questions: how ought I to live my life? The health of the soul (as they might have put it in an earlier day) is even more important than the health of the body."[95] In the same article, Callahan advocated a bioethics that helps "people shape their inner, private lives, assisting them in knowing how to make good personal judgments..."[96] Thus it seems that bioethics didn't actually "push religion aside," as Callahan wrote elsewhere, as much as it changed the venue of belief.

We have seen what the new secular faith or ideology of bioethics rejects. But what does it embrace? Again, it is important to concede that the field is not monolithic. Not everyone who claims to be a bioethicist necessarily accepts some or all of the concepts I will discuss below, just like not every Christian adheres to the same tenets of faith. That being duly noted, it is fair to say that predominate bioethics adheres to the following general belief systems with the following dominant features:

Utilitarianism: Whether explicit or implicit—in intent or outcome—bioethics advocacy is predominately utilitarian. "All [leading] bioethicists," claims author Anne Maclean, accept "some version of utilitarianism."[97] Professor Keown told me similarly, "Much of modern bioethics is largely utilitarian. Utilitarianism is fast establishing itself as the new orthodoxy."[98] Fox and Swazey write, "Since the mid-1970s ... moral philosophy has had the greatest molding influence on the field," especially "analytic philosophy—with its emphasis on theory ... and its utilitarian outlook."[99] That theme has continued since this book was first published, with the emergence of younger voices in the field, such as Julian Savulescu, professor of practical ethics at the University of Oxford, and Thaddeus Mason Pope, director of the Health and Law Institute at Hamline University.[100]

Generally stated, utilitarians hold that "what people want, is the ultimate measure of right and wrong."[101] Joseph Fletcher was a wild utilitarian, writing that "a moral agent's business is to maximize good," which he defined as "happiness": "Whatever increases human happiness is good; whatever reduces human happiness is evil."[102] Peter Singer, one of the world's foremost contemporary utilitarians, does not look to happiness so much as whether the "interests" of those affected (which in his view includes animals) are furthered or hindered.[103] Peter Singer himself admits that "ethical ideals, like individual rights, the sanctity of life, justice, purity ... are incompatible with utilitarianism."[104] Thus, to the utilitarian, there is neither objective right nor objective wrong: actions are measured subjectively based on desired or actual outcomes and the ends justify the means. Unfortunately, what the Singers and Fletchers of the world forget is that the means themselves often subsume the ends.

Lacking a firm commitment to the sanctity/equality of human life, utilitarians may justify profoundly dangerous and immoral schemes and not even blush. As described by Anne Maclean in her book *The Elimination of Morality*,[105] bioethicist John Harris—whose views on personhood we have already discussed—proposed a scheme to eliminate the shortage of transplant organs under which the few would be murdered to benefit the many: "[E]veryone [shall] be given a sort of lottery number. Whenever doctors have two or more dying patients who could be saved by transplants, and no suitable organs have come to hand through 'natural deaths,' they can ask a central computer to supply a suitable donor. The computer will then pick the number of a suitable donor at random and he will be killed so that the lives of two or more others may be saved."[106]

To the radical utilitarian Harris, saving two or more lives at the expense of one murder would bring greater overall happiness than would the suffering caused by the killing of one man or woman. And since under utilitarianism no individual possesses human rights per se, at least if the exercise of such rights would impede the highest overall utility, why not perform the human sacrifice?

Obviously, Harris's proposal will never become public policy—although it is worth noting here that Belgium and the Netherlands have joined voluntary euthanasia with organ harvesting. (More about that later.) Nor, I hope, will most bioethicists accept his ideas. Still, that Harris's proposal was presented straight-faced as a respectable point-of-view in an important philosophy primer (*Applied Ethics*, edited by Peter Singer) illustrates the amorality of utilitarian thought and much of what has gone so dreadfully wrong in bioethics discourse.

The Quality of Life Ethic: As skeptical as mainstream bioethicists are about "the sanctity/equality of life," they are equally enthusiastic about the "quality of life" ethic. What do they mean by this phrase as applied to health policy and medical practice? In *Clinical Ethics*, a bioethics book designed for everyday clinical use by working medical professionals, Albert Jonsen and his co-authors write, "In general, the phrase expresses a value judgment: the experience of living, as a whole or in some aspect, is judged to be 'good' or 'bad,' 'better' or 'worse.'"[107]

Such issues are, of course, a proper part of medical decision making. For example, I once snapped a knee ligament while skiing. My orthopedist told me that I could have it repaired surgically, but it would be a delicate and painful process that would take more than a year to heal. My other option was to simply quit skiing and engaging in other sports requiring lateral movements. I decided to give up the slopes because I believed that choice best protected my life's quality—although I might have made another decision if the injury had left me in constant pain. The same kind of cost/benefit analysis goes into more serious medical decisions, such as whether to accept a last-ditch round of chemotherapy or ask for medical technology to extend life.

The problem with the concept of quality of life arises when it ceases to be *a* factor in medical decision making and instead not only becomes *the* factor but is used as a measurement of moral worth. When applied in this manner, it is often called the "quality of life ethic," which Peter Singer describes in his book, *Rethinking Life and Death*:

> We should treat human beings in accordance with their ethically relevant characteristics. Some of these are inherent in the nature of being. They include consciousness, the capacity for physical, social, and mental interaction with other beings, having conscious preferences for continued life, and having enjoyable experiences. Other relevant aspects depend on the relationship of the being to others, having relatives for example who will grieve over your death, or being so situated in a group that if you are killed, others will fear for their own lives. All of these things make a difference to the regard and respect we should have for such a being.[108]

The danger of Singer's approach should be obvious to every reader. The standards Singer uses to measure human worth are *his* standards based on what *he* considers important and "relevant." And therein lies the heart of the problem. Subjective notions of human worth, in the end, are about raw power and who gets to do the judging. In our not-so-distant past, for example, decisions denigrating the moral worth of a subset of people (i.e., blacks) were made to justify their oppression and exploitation based on the allegedly relevant characteristics of skin color and cultural stereotypes. The quality of life ethic is no different—only the "relevant characteristics" have changed, not the wrongness of the approach. Quality of life, as a moral measure, strips worth and dignity from people based on health or disability, just as surely as racism does based on skin pigment, hair texture, or eye shape.

Not surprisingly, disabled people are especially worried about using quality of life as a yardstick of moral worth: they are the target. "Many in society consider disability as worse than death and a drain on our limited resources," says attorney Diane Coleman, a disability rights activist and the founder of Not Dead Yet, a national organization that battles medical discrimination against disabled people and resists the legalization of assisted suicide. "There is a great revulsion against disabled people that is visceral. This disdain is masked as pity but many people believe that in an ideal world, disabled people wouldn't be there."[109]

That being true—and who can deny it—what would happen to the rights of disabled people if the equality of life ethic were supplanted in law and in medical ethics by a quality of life approach? Coleman worries, "Anti-disabled bias would become especially dangerous. If it becomes respectable to label us 'inferior' or even, 'less human' based on perceptions of the quality of our lives, it will become acceptable to oppress, exploit, and even kill disabled people. To some degree, this is already happening. People with disabilities are seriously discriminated against in health care as well as in other areas of life."[110]

Coleman is no alarmist. Bioethicists widely embrace the "quality adjusted life year" (QALY) approach to health care rationing—one of the destinations to which the quality of life ethic would take us. Here's a brief—and very simplified—overview of how the QALY system operates: Let's say I have a serious heart ailment. Medicine A will give me two years of life at my current quality of life as an able-bodied man. That would be worth roughly 2 QALYs (fewer if I am elderly, but let's not get too complicated here).

My friend Mark has MS and is a triplegic. Let's say he contracts the same heart illness I have, and Medicine A would also give him two years of life at his current level as a man with a serious disability. *Because he only has the use of one arm, his two years of actual life might only be deemed a .5 QALY.*

The cost/benefit for providing the medicine is determined by a QALY formula to judge whether the cost of Medicine A is worth the number of QALYs it would provide. Let's say that the total cost of the heart medicine for two years is $100,000 for 2 QALYs. The technocrats in charge of the rationing system might think this price is worth paying for my care.

But even though Mark would receive the *same actual efficacy* from the medicine, his supposed lower quality of life changes the equation dramatically. Mark might be denied coverage for the medicine because the $100,000 would only pay for .5 QALY: pure health care discrimination.

The United Kingdom already imposes the QALY system on the National Health Service. It isn't yet used in the United States. Indeed, the Affordable Care Act prohibits using the QALY system in its eventual goal of establishing cost/benefit guidelines. But note: that prohibition might not stand. Powerful forces wish to repeal that protection in the law and import QALY rationing to America, including the *New England Journal of Medicine*.[111]

As this book will document, the growing acceptance of the quality of life ethic has already led to immoral and life-devaluing public policies and medical practices—with more threatened—undermining the virtue of our public policies and the ethics of health care.

The Georgetown Mantra: Having rejected the sanctity/equality of human life, the Hippocratic tradition, and concepts of objective right and wrong, bioethicists realized they needed to forge new analytical guidelines that would "be respected unless some strong countervailing reason exists to justify overruling them."[112] This need was filled in 1979 by the philosophy professors and bioethics pioneers Tom L. Beauchamp and James F. Childress in their book *Principles of Biomedical Ethics*.

Beauchamp and Childress posited four primary guidelines that have generally directed bioethics analysis ever since. The "four clusters of principles" are:

- Autonomy: "respecting the decision making capacities of autonomous persons";
- Beneficence: "providing benefits and balancing benefits against risks and costs";
- Nonmaleficence: "avoiding the causation of harm"; and
- Justice: "distributing benefits, risks, and costs fairly."[113]

Since bioethics is generally a relativist pursuit, these four principles are not cast in stone but merely "general guides that leave considerable room for judgment in specific cases and that provide substantive guidance for the development of more detailed rules and policies."[114] Still, they are taught in medical schools, nursing schools, medical professional continuing education courses, short bioethics courses given to members of hospital ethics committees, community patient ombudsmen, hospital administrators, health insurance executives, and, indeed, to almost everyone who has taken a course in bioethics in the last twenty years. "The four-principle tradition is now so widely accepted," Dr. Pellegrino wrote, "that some of its more whimsical critics have labeled it a mantra, implying that it is often supplied automatically and without sound moral grounding."[115] The influence of the Georgetown Mantra (so called because of the author's affiliation with Georgetown

University) in the application of bioethics in health policy and clinical decision making is hard to overstate

There is of course nothing inherently wrong with any or all of the guidelines that make up the Georgetown Mantra and very much that is right with them. But in the relativist context in which they exist, unanchored in objective morality (such as equality/sanctity of life), these guidelines are entirely malleable and subject to manipulation in order to justify an answer desired by the ethics analyzer. Thus rather than being proper guides for principled decision making, as was envisioned by their creators, the guidelines are often reduced to mere outcome justifiers: A bioethicist or medical clinician decides what action or inaction to take in a particular situation and then selects the particular Mantra guideline that best justifies the previously made decision. Thus the four guidelines can be manipulated to justify nearly any ends. (The same kind of unprincipled decision making sometimes happens in law. A lawyer may sense that a judge wants to make a favorable ruling, despite it being contrary to the weight of law. The lawyer then looks for any law or previous court ruling for the judge to use as a cover to rationalize the already made decision. Among lawyers, this is known as "providing the judge with a hook upon which to hang his hat.")

The ultimate amorality of the Georgetown Mantra is amply illustrated by an article written by K. K. Fung, PhD, in *the American Journal of Economics and Sociology* entitled "Dying for Money." Fung, a professor of economics at Memphis State University, recommended allowing seriously ill and disabled people to convert their health insurance benefits into a lump-sum cash payment—at less than the market exchange rate—if they agree to commit assisted suicide. How did Fung justify such an odious, exploitative proposal? Why, with the Georgetown Mantra:

> Benefit conversion coupled with dignified death go a long way towards resolving these conflicting principles [of the Mantra]. Because resources released from one patient's refusal of medical treatment (autonomy) can be specifically requested to be used for other patients or beneficiaries with greater need (full beneficence), autonomy and full beneficence need not conflict. Once the patient is allowed to choose death, the caregiver does not have to impose treatment for fear of malpractice liability. Thus, patient-centered beneficence is satisfied. Since benefit

conversion is equally available to all who are insured, and the amount
of converted benefits varies only with the severity of the illness, justice
is also served. All that remains to be done is to educate the terminally
or chronically ill how to allocate their converted benefits once death is
chosen. Because these four ethical principles [of the Mantra] are largely
taken care of, the sense of tragedy connected with the death and denial
of treatment to the hopelessly ill can be mitigated.[116]

As to the abuses that even Fung admits would follow if his proposal were
accepted, they are of little concern. Proving that economists can be as
amoral as bioethicists, Fung shrugs, "the world is full of slippery slopes."[117]

Bioethicists are fond of pointing out that there is no going back to
the era when the West was culturally homogenous and primarily Judeo/
Christian in outlook, or to a time in which health care decisions were
relatively simple. They note correctly, the United States, Canada, and
Western Europe are now fundamentally heterogeneous societies, racially
and culturally mixed, and fundamentally secular in civic and public
policy outlook. Moreover, they argue, the era in which medicine was
primarily concerned with keeping people alive for as long as possible and
public health policy sought essentially to uphold a (misapplied) religious
approach to the sanctity of human life is archaic in a Darwinian world in
which too many people compete for too few resources.

The purposes of modern medicine have indeed expanded beyond
preserving life, treating maladies, and promoting wellness. Healthcare
is now deemed to achieving individual life goals and fulfilling personal
desires. And, yes, we now contend with more complicated ethical issues
than our forbears faced: cloning, genetic medicine, the societal and
individual consequences of increased life expectancies, the impact of
permitting wide latitude in individual medical choices, and the difficulties imposed by limited resources.

But this doesn't mean that ethical analyses need to be as complex as
bioethicists make them, nor that contemporary bioethics ideology has the
best answers to these emerging moral problems. In a question that evokes
the case of the emperor's new clothes, Anne Maclean cogently asks, "Why
should we attach more weight to the pronouncements of philosophers
on moral issues than to those of other people?"[118]

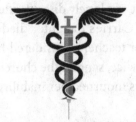

CHAPTER 2

LIFE UNWORTHY OF LIFE

"Three generations of idiots is enough," United States Supreme Court Chief Justice Oliver Wendell Holmes declared in authorizing the involuntary sterilization of Carrie Buck, age twenty-one, in Virginia.[1]

What had Carrie done to deserve this cruel fate? She was born poor and powerless, the daughter of a prostitute. In 1924, at the age of seventeen, she became pregnant out of wedlock, apparently after being raped by a relative of her foster father. To cover up this heinous act, Carrie's foster family had her declared morally and mentally deficient, after which she was institutionalized involuntarily in an asylum.

Adding to Carrie's woes, in 1924, the state of Virginia enacted a law permitting "mental defectives" to be involuntarily sterilized to better the welfare of society. Asylum doctors, believers in the pernicious theories of eugenics, decided that Carrie was a splendid candidate for sterilization. She was, after all, "a human defective." Her mother was institutionalized and Carrie's baby, aged seven months, did not look "quite normal" either.[2] Best for society that Carrie's genes be removed from the human race.

Carrie's guardian tried to stop the involuntary surgery in court— although he may have been in collusion with those who wanted her sterilized. In any event, the trial judge ordered the sterilization to proceed, relying on "experts" who testified that Carrie had unfit genes. The case was eventually accepted for decision by the United States Supreme Court, where Chief Justice Holmes and seven of his colleagues sealed Carrie's reproductive fate with but one lonely dissent, after which she was quickly sterilized and released. (Carrie's daughter died in the second grade of an intestinal ailment. Her teachers considered her very bright.[3] During her life, Carrie married twice, sang in the church choir, and took care of elderly people. She always mourned her inability to have more children. She died in 1983.[4])

Carrie Buck's fate—and that of approximately 60,000 other "defective" people involuntarily but legally sterilized in the United States between 1907 and 1960[5]—was sealed by advocates of a pseudoscience in the scientific, artistic, and progressive political communities known as eugenics. The history of eugenics, its fundamental precepts, the manner in which it was imposed on society and in law, and the horror that flowed from its popular acceptance, are highly relevant to our exploration of modern bioethics. First, its history shows the inhuman consequences that invariably follow when the equality/sanctity of human life is disregarded in science, medicine, law, and greater society. Second, striking and disturbing parallels exist between the manner in which eugenic theories were developed and put into practice and the way in which bioethics ideology is coming to dominate the ethics of medicine and the laws of health. Third, modern bioethics, like eugenics before it, creates hierarchies of human worth intended to justify medical discrimination. Now, after decades of quiescence, eugenics itself is making something of a comeback as a result of the development of new genetic technologies and futuristic ideologies such as "transhumanism."[6] (We will look more closely at this movement later in the book.)

Eugenics originated with the English mathematician and statistician Francis Galton. A cousin of Charles Darwin, Galton believed that heredity "governed talent and character" just as it does eye color and facial features.[7] Profoundly influenced by Darwin's theories of natural selection and Gregor Mendel's pioneering genetic experiments, Galton proposed, in 1865, that humans assume responsibility for their own evolution by using selective breeding techniques to improve society's physical, mental, cultural, and social health. In 1883, Galton coined the term "eugenics" to apply to his theories, a word he derived from the Greek meaning "good in birth."[8]

Eugenics took the same path to acceptability as bioethics would nearly one hundred years later. It first became the rage in the academy and then spread rapidly in the early years of the twentieth century among the cultural elite and the intelligentsia of the United States, Canada, England, and Germany. By 1910, "eugenics was one of the most frequently referenced topics" in the *Reader's Guide to Periodic Literature*.[9] In its boom years of the 1920s, eugenics, like bioethics today, became a serious and influential social and political movement. Courses in eugenics were taught in more than 350 American universities and colleges, leading to the widespread popular acceptance of its tenets.[10] At one time, eugenics was endorsed in more than 90 percent of high school biology textbooks.[11] As would happen later with bioethics, eugenicist societies formed for the promulgation and discussion of theories; academic eugenics journals sprouted; and philanthropic foundations, such as the Rockefeller and Carnegie Foundations, embraced the movement, financing eugenics research and policy initiatives. Many of the political, cultural, and arts notables of the time supported eugenics, including Theodore Roosevelt, Winston Churchill, George Bernard Shaw, and Margaret Sanger, leading to further expansion of the movement's popular support.

The parallels of eugenics with contemporary bioethics extend into the realm of ideology. Both movements reject equal human moral worth. Both are utilitarian based, seeking to improve overall human happiness and reduce human suffering—sometimes at the expense of individual human rights. Like today's bioethics theories, eugenics was taught in some of the world's most prestigious universities, quickly becoming an integral part of professional training. And, again mirroring modern bioethics organizations, most eugenics societies "were dominated by professionals such as professors, social workers, lawyers, doctors, teachers, and ministers."[12]

To be fair, there are important differences between the eugenics of yesterday and bioethics today. Eugenics equated human fitness and morality with overall intelligence,[13] a concept that is not accepted generally in bioethics, although the depersonalization of infants and people disabled by significant cognitive injury or illness seems a disturbing echo of the past. Moreover, absolutely unlike contemporary bioethics, the

eugenics movement was overtly racist, proclaiming the white race superior to blacks and Asians. (One eugenicist pronounced perniciously that
the average black person in the United States had the average mental age
of a ten-year-old.[14]) Eugenicists were profoundly self-satisfied, promoting
the racial and personal characteristics *they possessed* as the highest human
ideal. At the same time, they degraded the characteristics they associated
with the lower economic classes and "inferior" races as those to be "bred"
out of the human condition through eugenic practices. (Among the many
"negative" human characteristics and/or behaviors eugenicists believed
were genetically caused and which they wished to eradicate were feeble-
mindedness, epilepsy, criminality, insanity, alcoholism, and pauperism.[15])

There were two general approaches to effectuating the eugenics theory. Proponents of "positive eugenics" sought to persuade young people
who possessed worthy traits to marry among each other and procreate
liberally toward the end of strengthening these characteristics within the
human gene pool. Worried that the "proper" people were not procreating
in sufficient numbers, eugenicists filled the popular culture with notions
of the ideal family, urging the "betters" among the population to have
many children. (Four per marriage was "was the number thought necessary to maintain a given stock."[16]) There were even prizes given to large
families thought to be promoting the best eugenic human traits.

The real tyranny that eugenics unleashed flowed out of what came
to be known as "negative eugenics," which came to dominate the field.
Negative eugenicists presumed the right to prevent those with undesirable physical and moral characteristics from procreating at all. (That was
a big point of Margaret Sanger's birth control push.) And if the so-called
unfit wouldn't limit their own kind, then eugenics theory held that society
could force these limitations coercively through medical acts and public
policies that exploited and oppressed the weak and medically defenseless.

Although eugenics originated in England, it was soon imported to the
United States. In 1899, the *Journal of the American Medical Association*
published an article that advocated the use of the newly developed vasec-
tomy as a "surgical treatment" to keep undesirables such as "habitual
criminals, chronic inebriates, imbeciles, perverts, and paupers" from
reproducing.[17] In 1902, an Indiana physician named Dr. Harry Sharp
urged passage of mandatory sterilization laws that would require all men
in prisons, reformatories, and paupers' houses to be sterilized. (Before

any law was passed permitting it, he had involuntarily sterilized more than 500 men.[18]) Following Sharp's lead, in 1907, Indiana became the first state to pass a eugenics-based sterilization law. By 1912, eight states had sterilization laws. Eventually nearly thirty states followed suit, including Virginia, leading to the oppression of Carrie Buck.

"USELESS EATERS"

Eugenics helped feed—and was itself nourished by—the particularly harsh ethos of social Darwinism, which applied Darwin's biological theories of natural selection and the struggle for survival to the human realm and relations among people and societies. "To the social Darwinists ... human society had always been a battleground for competing individuals and races in which the fittest survived and the unfit were cruelly eliminated; and, for the sake of human progress, this struggle for existence must be allowed to continue unchecked by governmental intervention or social reform."[19] Believers in social Darwinism, thus, viewed the exploitation of the weak as a natural process. At the same time, social Darwinistic theories worked hand-in-glove with eugenic notions of hierarchies of human worth to classify exploited people as inherently inferior and thus deserving of their fate. This explosive combination never quite reached critical mass in the United States or Canada. In Germany, however, it combusted into the conflagration known as the Holocaust.

In 1806, German physician Christoph Wilhelm Hufeland wrote presciently—and in words that remain relevant today—"It is not up to [the doctor] whether ... life is happy or unhappy, worthwhile or not, and should he incorporate these perspectives into his trade ... the doctor could well become the most dangerous person in the state."[20] Hufeland's point is that the ethics of medicine are a good indicator of the moral health of society and that when medical practice is corrupted, society is soon to follow. "Physicians are central to the quality of life in any society," agrees the American physician and notable Nazi hunter Michael Franzblau. "The minute physicians begin to see some of their patients as having greater worth than others, they will gain power over their patients that is unbelievable. That is what happened in Germany, beginning around 1910."[21]

Most people believe that the medical horrors of the Holocaust were the sole creation of Adolph Hitler. In fact, the path to medical evil was laid long before Hitler was even a storm cloud on the German horizon. "Physicians in the pre-Nazi period began to view their skills as appropriate for killing as well as healing," Franzblau says. Because of eugenic theories, social Darwinistic beliefs, and the deprivations caused by the war, half of Germany's mental patients were starved to death during World War I. "But that was a mere prelude," Franzblau told me. "In 1920, Binding and Hoche published their book, which really set the tone for what was to come."[22]

That book was a tome entitled *Permission to Destroy Life Unworthy of Life* (*Die Freigabe der Vernichtung lebensunwerten Leben*).[23] Its authors were two of the most respected academics in their respective fields: Karl Binding, a nationally renowned law professor, and Alfred Hoche, a physician and noted humanitarian. *Permission to Destroy Life Unworthy of Life*, in reality two extended essays—one by each author—was a full-throated assault on the Hippocratic tradition and the sanctity/equality of human life. The authors accepted wholeheartedly the concept that some humans had greater moral worth than others. The latter were disparaged as "unworthy" of life, a category that, like some contemporary euthanasia advocacy, included the dying, people who were mentally ill or retarded, and badly deformed children. People deemed life unworthy of life, the authors argued, should be allowed to be killed (euthanasia). More than that, the authors *professionalized and medicalized* the entire concept, making it seem compassionate by promoting medicalized killing of those deemed unworthy of life as a "purely a healing treatment" and a "healing work"; they also justified euthanasia as a splendid way to divert money from being spent on caring for unworthy life toward other important societal needs.[24]

Binding and Hoche listed three categories of patients who doctors should be allowed to kill ethically and legally:

1. Terminally ill or mortally wounded individuals, described by the authors as those "who have been irretrievably lost as a result of illness or injury, who fully understand their situation, posses and have somehow expressed and urgent wish for release."[25]

2. "Incurable idiots," whose lives Binding and Hoche viewed as "pointless and valueless," and as emotional and economic burdens "on society and their families." Hoche put it this way: "I have discovered that the average yearly (per head) cost for maintaining

idiots has till now been thirteen hundred marks.... If we assume an average life expectancy of fifty years for individual cases, it is easy to estimate what incredible capital is withdrawn from the nation's wealth for food, clothing, heating—for an unproductive purpose."[26]

3. The "unconscious," if they ever again were roused from their comatose state, would waken to nameless suffering.[27]

Permission to Destroy Life Unworthy of Life was thus a prescription for the medical cleansing of the most weak and vulnerable among Germany's population, a prescription that would be filled with murderous precision by German doctors between 1939 and 1945.

Binding's and Hoche's philosophical approach was eerily similar to that espoused today by many contemporary bioethicists. It was utilitarian. It eschewed the Hippocratic tradition in favor of the quality of life ethic (ditto bioethics). Indeed, the Georgetown Mantra could be used to justify Binding and Hoche arguments (e.g., they described voluntary euthanasia as merely a matter of fulfilling the patient's "urgent wish" [autonomy]; defined killing ill and disabled people as a "healing" act [beneficence]; and promoted euthanasia as necessary to fulfill other urgent societal needs that were going wanting because of the cost of caring for disabled people [distributive justice]).

Although modern bioethicists object to the manner in which Binding and Hoche's proposals were ultimately implemented in Germany, and most would certainly object to the authors' bigoted use of language, it is clear that the anti-sanctity of life values expressed in and the utilitarian philosophical foundation of *Permission to Destroy Life Unworthy of Life* fit snugly within the mainstream of the modern bioethics movement. As just one example, in 2010, Oxford bioethicists Dominick Wilson and Julian Savulescu advocated "organ donation euthanasia," in which the dying unconscious could be killed via *the process* of organ harvesting.[28]

Permission to Destroy Life Unworthy of Life created a sensation among Germany's intelligentsia, whose leadership—in conjunction with the growing acceptance of Social Darwinism, anti-Semitism, racial hygiene, and eugenics—helped the Binding/Hoche view to become soon accepted by much of German society. For example, a 1925 poll of the parents of disabled children reported that 74 percent of them would agree to the painless killing of their own children.[29] Thus, by the time the Nazis came to power in 1933, much of Germany, including its medical establishment, accepted the existence of some human beings as "life unworthy of life."

Upon assuming leadership of Germany, Nazi rulers immediately sought to act against these "useless eaters." In 1933, the German government sought to legalize voluntary euthanasia. (A front-page *New York Times* article described the proposal as making it possible for physicians to end the torture of incurable patients.) Protective guidelines were to be included in the law, many of which were remarkably similar to those espoused by euthanasia advocates today, including voluntary requests "expressly and earnestly" made and, if decided by relatives for incompetent patients, that the motive for killing (ironically) "not contravene morals."[30]

These proposals were eventually withdrawn because of vehement opposition from German churches. However, mandatory sterilization laws were officially enacted within six months of Hitler becoming Germany's chancellor, which made the sterilization statutes in the United States seem pale by comparison. Based on eugenics theories, special "Hereditary Health Courts" were established to judge the "hereditarily sick." Among those targeted were people who were mentally retarded, mentally ill, alcoholics, with epilepsy, and had "grave body malformations." At the law's inception, it was estimated that more than 400,000 people would be sterilized from the hospitals and mental institutions alone. Sterilization was actually imposed on up to 350,000 disabled and other "undesirable" people between 1933 and 1945.[31]

Throughout the 1930s, the idea of actually killing useless eaters gained increased popularity, and not by accident. The Nazi government molded German public opinion. Popular entertainment became an especially effective tool in this unremitting propaganda campaign, particularly motion pictures, an industry that Joseph Goebbels effectively controlled.

The movie *I Accuse* (*Ich klage an*), one of the most notable of these many propaganda films, is particularly relevant to today's medical climate. Wildly popular among German audiences (more than 15 million paid to see it),[32] *I Accuse* was an all-out call for legalizing voluntary euthanasia and an apologia for murdering disabled infants. According to Professor Sobsey, the *I Accuse* filmmaker/propagandists cleverly promoted killing as an acceptable answer to medical difficulties by both intensely personalizing the issue of suffering caused by serious illness while, at the same time, depersonalizing killing as it related to disabled infants to make their murder easier to accept.

The movie was pure melodrama. The primary plot concerned a woman pianist who grows progressively disabled because of multiple sclerosis. Unable to play her beloved piano and deeply worried about becoming a burden to her physician husband, she begs for euthanasia. "The audience was supposed to relate to her deeply and accept as correct and compassionate her desire to die," Sobsey says. Thus, *I Accuse* promotes euthanasia as beneficial, compassionate, and supportive of autonomous decision making in the same manner as do contemporary euthanasia activists.

As the wife and husband struggle with her MS, a subplot develops that is deeply utilitarian and dismissive of the moral worth of disabled people. The third main character, a university professor, lectures students on how in nature, only the "fit" survive. He illustrates his teaching with graphic documentary scenes of asylums from Nazi film archives, which depict the patients as grotesque and inhuman. It is in this context that the parents of a disabled infant beg the doctor to kill their child as an act of mercy. "The movie never shows the baby," Sobsey says. "This is as a way of depersonalizing the infant and make its ultimate killing less shocking."[33]

At the same time, as the husband desperately searches for a cure for MS, he cripples a mouse in his research laboratory and then thoughtlessly abandons it to suffer. A woman lab worker promises the mouse she will take care of him and later surreptitiously gives the animal a lethal injection as an act of compassion. The message is blunt and unremitting: the unfit should die, both as a matter of mercy and to keep the society healthy.

The parents of the disabled child continue to beg for the same consideration for their baby, and finally have their way. The baby is killed off camera, and depicted as a difficult but eugenically correct act that protects the overall health of the *Volk*. The wife commits suicide with her husband's help, a scene played, to the sound of a mournful piano, for all the pathos it is worth. He is arrested. The movie ends with the husband's impassioned accusation to the judges against the law for preventing euthanasia (the real accusation in *I Accuse*):

No! Now, I accuse! I accuse the law which hinders doctors and judges in their task of helping people. I confess . . . I have delivered my wife from her sufferings, following her wishes. My life and the lives of all people who will suffer the same fate as my wife, depends on your verdict. Now, pass your verdict.[34]

These words could have been taken from a transcript from one of the trials of Jack Kevorkian, many of whose victims were non-terminally ill women disabled by multiple sclerosis. Moreover, the word "deliverance" was once the favorite euphemism used by the Hemlock Society (now compassion and choices) to describe killing by euthanasia or assisted suicide. And that isn't all. As we shall see, the moral values, philosophy, and even the words expressed through and in *I Accuse* are alive, well, and in practice in the United States, Canada, and much of the West more than seventy years after its release.

Indeed, in addition to the Kevorkian trials, the Debbie Purdy case in the United Kingdom tracks almost exactly with the view of the featured couple in *I Accuse*: Like the wife in the movie, Purdy was growing progressively disabled from MS and wanted her husband to be free from prosecution if he took her to a Swiss suicide clinic. In 2009, she won a case in the British Supreme Court requiring the public prosecutor to clarify prosecution standards.[35] The clarification determined that family members would generally not be so prosecuted so long as their assistance in suicide was not done with improper motives. (Purdy died in hospice on December 23, 2014 after refusing to eat.[36])

Back in 1930s Germany, the eugenicists and government propaganda continued to soften the ground for the eventual killing of "useless eaters." One task remained before implementation could commence: that the medical profession had to reject the Hippocratic requirement that its sole loyalty is to be to each and every individual patient. "Between 1933 and 1945, German physicians did not take the Hippocratic Oath," Dr. Franzblau told me. "Instead, they took an oath to the health of the state, known as the *Gezuntheit*. Thus doctors had a dual loyalty, to their patients yes, but their first loyalty was to Germany."[37]

German doctors, to recall Dr. Hufeland's warning, were now among society's most dangerous members. Many physicians accepted wholeheartedly the eugenics-based theories, reinforced by Nazi racial ideology, that disabled people, mentally retarded people, and, of course, Jews, Gypsies, and others were life unworthy of life. At the same time, their first loyalty shifted to the state, away from their individual patients. Forced sterilization of the "unfit" had become commonplace and popularly accepted. Physicians and midwives voluntarily reported every child born with disabilities to authorities. Binding and Hoche's notions of killing as a "healing" practice were accepted widely as ethical and moral. Dr. Karl Brandt, who Hitler had placed in charge of promulgating euthanasia bureaucratic procedures, had a plan of implementation firmly in place. The table was now set for the mass murder of hundreds of thousands of disabled people—the opening overture of the Holocaust.

Disabled infants became the first to suffer medical cleansing when Hitler signed a secret executive order in early 1939 permitting infanticide based on disability. No doctor was forced to kill patients. However, illustrating how effectively the Hippocratic tradition and the belief in the equality of all human life had been undermined over several decades in Germany, many physicians (as well as nurses and midwives) enthusiastically supported the policy, either directly by killing patients or indirectly by referring disabled babies to "health centers." "The tragedy is that these doctors were not ogres," Dr. Franzblau told me. "They were mainstream physicians who were exquisitely trained in German medical schools, which at the time were the best in the world. They went utterly wrong, in my judgment, because they no longer perceived these [disabled] patients as fully human."[38] Thus the German medical establishment participated in the euthanasia Holocaust, not because they were Nazis—although many had joined the Party—but because they had convinced themselves that they were performing, in Binding and Hoche's words, a "healing" service for the child, the family, and the Reich.

Hitler and Brandt were so pleased with the success of their infanticide program that Hitler next issued an executive order expanding the categories of those to be medically cleansed to include disabled and mentally retarded adults. The order stated simply: "Reich Leader Bouhler and Dr. Brandt are charged with the responsibility for expanding the authority of physicians, to be designated by name, to the end that patients considered incurable according to the best available human judgment of their state of health, can be granted a mercy death [Signed,] Adolph Hitler."[39] This was the infamous "T-4 Program," named after the address of the German Chancellery, Tiergarten 4. "Killables" included people with epilepsy, polio, schizophrenia, senile diseases, paralysis, and Huntington's disease. As with the infanticide program, T-4 was officially a secret; death certificates listed phony causes of death.

Adult euthanasia victims were sent to specially designated hospitals that had been converted into centers of mass murder. Like the later Jewish genocide, T-4 was highly bureaucratized. Government workers "coldly and calculatingly organized the murder of thousands of people" and kept meticulous records of what they were doing. Secretaries, for example, "shared their offices with jars of foul-smelling gold-filled teeth, listening to dictation which enumerated 'bridge with three teeth,' 'a single tooth,' and so on."[40] With so many people involved in the killing, it wasn't long before much of Germany became aware of what was going on. There were some public protests. Catholic Archbishop Clems August Graf von Galen even preached openly against the euthanasia policy,[41] and dared the Gestapo to arrest him, stating that he would meet them in full regalia. Even some Party members objected, assuring themselves that the *Führer* must not know.[42] Himmler soon recognized that the jig was up and pronounced euthanasia "a secret that is no longer a secret."[43]

Because of public pressure, Hitler rescinded the T-4 program, although not the infanticide directive. Nevertheless, German doctors continued to murder disabled and ill infants and adults in a process known as "wild euthanasia" until stopped by the Allies at the end of World War II. The death toll is estimated to have been about 250,000 people. Every one of these deaths "required a physician's review and order to determine that the individual's life was not worth living."[44] Among those who participated in the killing programs were Dr. Ernst Wetzler, ironically the inventor of an incubator for prematurely born children, and Dr. Hans Joachim Sewerling, who was elected in the 1980s to the presidency of the World Medical Association but forced to resign due to the efforts of Dr. Franzblau and the American Medical Association. Neither German doctor ever expressed remorse. Indeed, Dr. Wetzler called his participation in the murder of disabled infants as "a small contribution to human progress."[45] Dr. Sewerling sought refuge in anti-Semitism, claiming his political troubles were the result of a "Jewish conspiracy."[46] Rather than receiving the calumny of his peers, after being forced to resign as president of the WMO Dr. Sewerling was named an honorary member of the German Medical Association's board of trustees.[47]

IMMORAL MEDICAL EXPERIMENTS

Adding to the infamy of German medicine were the SS physicians who engaged actively in genocide and human medical experimentation. For example, at Auschwitz, doctors helped create "the murderous ecology" of the camp. They performed selections and supervised the killing in the gas chambers. They determined when all of the gassed victims were dead. Doctors lethally injected debilitated inmates and helped work out details of body disposal.[48]

A few SS doctors also carried out inhumane "medical" experiments on people in concentration and death camps, during which inmates, almost all of them Jewish, were subjected to horrible crimes of bodily violation. The horror of this is impossible to overstate: women had their cervixes injected with caustic substances in an attempt to invent sterilization-by-injection; men were subjected to intense X-ray exposures of their genitals to induce sterilization, with later castration to study the damage radiation caused to the testes; inmates were intentionally exposed to typhus contagion to determine the efficacy of various sera. At Auschwitz, Joseph Mengele engaged in a sadistic study of identical twins, including children who he physically examined over several months, measuring every part of their body and taking their blood, and then lethally injected them prior to dissection.[49] "German physicians in the name of science," Dr. Franzblau has stated, "froze people to death, asphyxiated them by denying them oxygen at high altitudes, forced them to drink seawater to the point of serious illness, injected them with tubercle bacilli, cut off arms and legs of war prisoners and attempted [tissue] grafting, and perfected the use of Zyklon B gas, the preferred method of death in the concentration camps."[50]

CRUCIAL LESSONS LEARNED

The depth of depravity to which some German physicians sank seems unthinkable to us today. But it was unthinkable when it happened, too. How could German doctors, of all people, have gone so far astray? To exclusively blame the Nazis is to miss the mark and give us false comfort about our own flirtation with unethical health policies. Adolph Hitler did not blaze the road to medical depravity. He just goose-stepped with full fascist regalia down the boulevard already paved by Binding and Hoche with their advocacy that there is such a thing as a human life unworthy of life. *Permission to Destroy Life Unworthy of Life* gave the imprimatur of the academy to a subjective measurement of human life—the intellectual essence of the modern-day quality of life ethic. Indeed, Binding and Hoche's book is so important to our understanding of the evil that followed that Lifton calls it the "crucial work."[51] For, as Dr. Franzblau noted sagely, "Once you breach the firewall of Hippocratic morality, only bad things can happen."[52]

A second fundamental lesson of the euthanasia Holocaust is that doctors must never allow themselves to be seduced into accepting dual loyalties. Subject to the rules required in protecting public health, the welfare of each individual patient—not that of society, the patient's family, the finances of health insurance companies, government mandate, or the doctor's individual pocketbook—must be each physician's unequivocal concern. For doctors to place other agendas before the welfare of their patients is to expose those in their care to significant danger of exploitation and oppression.

Finally, let us heed the words of Dr. Leo Alexander, who served as an investigator in the Nuremberg trials and became one of the world's foremost experts on the medical aspects of the Holocaust. In 1949, Dr. Alexander attempted to summarize what he had so painfully learned through years of investigation. In the *New England Journal of Medicine*, he wrote:

> Whatever proportions these crimes finally assumed, it became evident
> to all who investigated them that they started from small beginnings.
> The beginnings at first were merely a subtle shift in emphasis in the
> basic attitudes of physicians. It started with the acceptance of the atti-
> tude, basic to the euthanasia movement, that there is such a thing as a
> life not worthy to be lived. This attitude in its early stages concerned
> itself merely with the severely and chronically sick. Gradually the sphere
> of those to be included in this category was enlarged to encompass
> the socially unproductive, the ideologically unwanted, the racially
> unwanted and finally all non-Germans.[53]

Dr. Alexander then issued a prophetic warning:

> In an increasingly utilitarian society these patients [with chronic diseases] are being looked down upon with increasing definiteness as unwanted ballast. A certain amount of rather open contempt for the people who cannot be rehabilitated ... has developed. This is probably due to a good deal of unconscious hostility, because these people for whom there seem to be no effective remedies have become a threat to newly acquired delusions of omnipotence.... At this point, Americans should remember that the enormity of the euthanasia movement is present in their own midst.[54]

In today's enlightened world, we soothingly tell ourselves that the spirit of Binding and Hoche has been exorcised. But that is self-deception. In fact, it still lurks in hospital corridors, university seminars, medical school classrooms, legislative cloakrooms, and most particularly in the depth and breadth of bioethics advocacy. This is not to say, of course, that today's bioethicists are similar to Nazi doctors. (But then, Binding and Hoche weren't Nazis either.) Nor is it to say that Western health policies are the same as those of fascist Germany. But we are heading in a very wrong and dangerous direction. There are, after all, many ways to fall off an ethical cliff.

Neglecting Disabled Infants to Death: In 1972, *Life* magazine reported that Mrs. Phyllis Obernauer gave birth to a daughter with Down syndrome. The girl's condition was complicated by heart problems and an intestinal blockage, the latter a common occurrence with Down's babies. The Obernauers decided they didn't want a disabled baby and ordered their doctors not to perform surgery to clear up the intestinal blockage. Their intent was that their baby would die by starvation. The doctors refused to deprive the child of life's basic necessities, and the baby lived.[55]

Beginning at about the time of the Obernauer case—a mere fifty years after the publication of *Permission to Destroy Life Unworthy of Life*—some of the world's most respected doctors and philosophers began to again suggest openly that it should be ethical to kill or neglect disabled babies to death. Many of these death advocates were among the cream of the scientific community. For example, Harvard professor and Nobel laureate

James D. Watson, the co-discoverer of the genetic makeup of DNA, reacting to the emergence of new reproductive technologies argued, "we have to reevaluate our basic assumptions about the meaning of life." Analogizing to the ancient practice of exposing disabled infants on hills, Watson further declared, "No one should be thought of as alive until about three days after birth," adding that parents would then "be allowed the choice" to keep their baby or "allow" their child to die.[56] Similarly, another Nobel laureate involved in the discovery of DNA, Francis Crick, declared in 1978 that "no newborn should be declared human until it has passed certain tests regarding its genetic endowment and that if it fails these tests it forfeits the right to life."[57]

Demonstrating the prescience of Dr. Alexander's 1949 worries about American medical ethics, such advocacy took root. In 1982, Baby Jane Doe's doctors engaged willingly in the very medical neglect that Baby Obernauer's doctors refused to countenance only ten years before. Like the Obernauer infant, Baby Doe was born with Down syndrome and an intestinal blockage. Routine surgery to clear the blockage could have saved the baby's life. But the mother's ob-gyn told Jane's parents that they could refuse surgery. Deciding that she—and they—would be better off if she died, Jane's parents refused consent to surgery and ordered the doctors to withhold food and fluids for their child, dooming her to death by dehydration.

When the news broke that Baby Jane was being neglected to death because she was disabled, several couples came forward asking, even begging, for the opportunity to adopt her. But Jane's parents wanted their baby dead, not adopted. They refused to allow others to intervene. The matter was brought to court, where a judge sided with Jane's parents and against Jane's equal moral status as a human being. She died six days after her birth. If a "normal" child were neglected to death in this way, the parents and doctors would be brought to the docket for child abuse. But because Jane was disabled, she was made to die and no legal sanctions were applied against either the parents or the participating doctors, this despite that on her way to death, she became parched, dried out, and spit blood.[58]

Similar cases have occurred elsewhere in the United States, England, Canada, and the Netherlands. In England, a woman gave birth to a

Down's baby who did not have an intestinal blockage. Upon learning that her baby was disabled, she said, "I don't want it, Ducks." Despite the fact that the child had no physical abnormalities other than the genetic condition that causes Down's, she ordered the doctors not to feed the baby. Dr. Leonard Arthur ordered the baby to be given morphine but not fed. The baby died at the age of four days. Dr. Arthur wasn't tried for homicide but paradoxically for "attempted murder." Several of Dr. Arthur's medical colleagues testified that such medical neglect directed at babies born with significant abnormalities is "normal medical practice." Sir Douglas Black, president of the Royal College of Physicians, told the jury that he thought it ethical for a "rejected child" to be put "upon a course of management that would end in its death," declaring "it is ethical that a child suffering from Down syndrome ... should not survive." After only two hours, the jury decided the doctor was not guilty to sounds of rejoicing in the courtroom.[59]

Babies with spina bifida have suffered similar fates. Spina bifida is a condition in which the spine is exposed at birth, with hydrocephalus (water on the brain) a frequent accompanying malady. The proper treatment for the condition is to close the wound in the back and drain the fluid from the brain with a shunt. Babies with spina bifida generally are disabled by paralyzed legs and are sometimes incontinent.

Dr. John Lorber was once a leading proponent of treating babies with spina bifida. At some point, he had a change of heart and became a leading advocate for nontreatment, developing protocols for deciding which spina bifida babies to care for and which to abandon to death by neglect. He subsequently traveled to the United States and Canada, urging pediatricians not to operate on these helpless infants. His justification?

> Humanity demands that such badly affected infants should not be put through such constant and severe punishment. Criteria had to be found, preferably on the first day of life which could reliably separate those infants who may die early but even more importantly those who would live but would suffer from severe multi-system handicaps and would be unable to live an independent and dignified existence in spite of the best possible treatment.... [In such cases,] nothing should be done to prolong life.[60]

What does this mean in actual practice? According to the approving Peter Singer, who interviewed Dr. Lorber, "The wound should be left open. If an infection develops, no antibiotics should be given. If excess fluid accumulated in the head, this should not be drained. If the babies did not eat and lost weight, they should not be tube-fed.... Few if any would live longer than six months."[61]

How does this practice differ from those of German doctors circa 1939–1945? Then, countless disabled babies were similarly neglected to death or killed based on doctors' decisions as to which children had livable lives. Now, as then, a decision is made to take action, or rather, not to act, thus ensuring that the babies die. As before, the physicians believe they are providing a service to their soon-to-be-made-dead patients, the babies' families, and society. (And this doesn't include prenatal eugenic cleansing in which approximately 90 percent of fetuses testing positive for Down's are aborted.[62]) Binding and Hoche would approve.

In response to the Baby Doe tragedy, the federal government passed regulations to prevent medical discrimination based on disabilities, which, unfortunately, were invalidated by courts. Congress then passed amendments to federal child abuse statutes as they affect the laws of the states to prevent medically beneficial treatments from being withheld due to quality of life criteria. The law permits the withholding of treatment for babies in irreversible comas if treatment would only prolong dying, if it would be virtually futile, and if it would be inhumane. Do these laws actually protect disabled infants? That is unclear. Former Surgeon General C. Everett Koop, who was instrumental in getting the Baby Doe laws enacted, has opined that they "are probably not legally effective" and that the "greatest protection that handicapped newborns have in the [United] States today is the concern on the part of physicians and sur-geons who care for newborns that someone is watching."[63] Considering the increasingly utilitarian state of medical ethics and the pressures placed on doctors by managed care health insurance companies to cut the costs of health care, that protection may be scant indeed.

Active Infanticide: Most people know that it is wrong to kill babies. They view the intentional killing of medically incompetent people as murder. At least, they used to. As modern bioethics looms, that certainty comes under increasing attack.

In the 1970s, Joseph Fletcher, the patriarch of bioethics, advocated killing disabled children, an act he euphemistically called "post birth abortion,"[64] dismissing the ethical and moral constraints against infanticide as a mere "taboo." For Fletcher, the rightness of killing disabled babies could be determined through a simple utilitarian equation: If killing a baby increased happiness or reduced overall human suffering, than the baby should be made dead. If not, the baby should live. He wrote, "This view assigns value to human *life* rather than merely being *alive* and holds that it is better to be dead than to suffer too much or to endure too many deficits of human function."[65] (Emphasis in original.)

What was shocking in the 1970s is shocking no longer. Arguing in favor of infanticide is now respectable and mainstream. The Australian moral philosopher and Princeton bioethicist Peter Singer began arguing decades ago that infants have no moral right to live because, as discussed in the previous chapter, they are not "persons." He views infanticide at the request of parents as an ethical act so long as it will promote the overall interests of family or society.

Singer originally suggested that parents have twenty-eight days within which to keep or kill their newborn child. He then broadened this putative license, telling an interviewer, "I no longer think that will work. It's too arbitrary. I don't think you would get people to recognize that there's a big difference in the wrongfulness of killing a being at twenty-seven or twenty-nine days. So, what do you do? I think you need to look at it on a case-by-case basis given the seriousness of the problems and balance that against the age of the child."[66] Earlier in the interview, Singer supposed that a child became a person "sometime during the first year of life," and thus his "case-by-case" approach could apply to murdering a baby for many months after the child is born.

When Singer's views are discussed in the media, he is often portrayed as "only" calling for the infanticide of "severely disabled" babies. In and of itself, that would be terribly wrong, but this alleged mitigation simply isn't true. Singer views *all* infants, not only disabled babies, as nonpersons who are "replaceable ... in much the same way as ... non-self conscious animals [e.g., bird and fish]."[67] Since nonpersons have no right to life, so long as utilitarian principles are applied properly, there is nothing in his philosophy that explicitly limits infanticide to the killing of babies born with disabilities.

That being duly noted, Singer knows that it would not pay for him to discuss the killing of healthy babies, and so he almost always addresses the issue in connection with disabled infants. But even here the examples he gives of babies whom it should be ethically and legally permissible to murder are not "severely disabled." In *Practical Ethics*, for example, Singer supported infanticide of newborns with hemophilia, writing: "When the death of a disabled infant will lead to the birth of another infant with better prospects of a happy life, the total amount of happiness will be greater if the disabled infant is killed. The loss of the happy life for the first infant is outweighed by the gain of a happier life for the second. Therefore, if the killing of the hemophiliac infant has no adverse effect on others it would … be right to kill him."[68]

Thus, to Singer, it is okay to kill a child for the benefit of hypothetical future siblings who have not yet been conceived!

Singer reiterated his anti-disability bias using a different type of disability as an illustration in *Rethinking Life and Death: The Collapse of Our Traditional Ethics* (1994, St. Martin's Press, New York, NY), in which he wrote:

> To have a child with Down syndrome is to have a very different experience from having a normal child. … (W)e may not want a child to start on life's uncertain voyage if the prospects are clouded. When this can be known at a very early stage of the voyage we may be able to make a fresh start. … Instead of going forward and putting all our efforts into making the best of the situation, we can still say no, and start again from the beginning.[69]

Singer's advocacy of infanticide (and for the morality of euthanizing profoundly cognitively disabled people as an ethical act) caused a tremendous uproar in Europe, particularly in Germany and Austria, countries with an acute memory of the euthanasia Holocaust. Indeed, so many Germans and Austrians despise Singer's views that he is unable to lecture in those countries because of angry demonstrations that erupt against him whenever he appears to speak. These protests deeply disturb Singer. As a child of German/Austrian Jews who lost family members in the Holocaust, he resents his philosophy being linked in any way to the Nazis.

Singer defends himself by claiming that the acts he espouses are nothing like those of the German doctors who participated in infanticide, claiming that his proposals are merely predicated upon "avoiding pointless suffering." But that was precisely what Binding and Hoche claimed when they labeled their proposal to kill disabled people a "healing process." Singer also says that the German doctors' *motives* in killing babies were different from the ones he espouses. That is not entirely true. As we saw, most German doctors who participated in killing believed fervently that they were benefiting all concerned: baby, family, and society. Singer attempts to distinguish himself further by claiming that he does not agree with racial hygiene theory. That much is true, but so what? A murdered baby is a murdered baby is a murdered baby, regardless of why the baby is killed. That Singer does not grasp that basic moral concept speaks volumes about his philosophy.

Another tack Singer takes to distance himself from the German experience is by claiming that "Nazi euthanasia was never voluntary."[70] Here, Singer is simply wrong.

The first known German government-approved infanticide, the killing of Baby Knauer, occurred in early 1939. The baby was blind and had a leg and an arm missing. Baby Knauer's father was distraught at having a disabled child. So he wrote to Chancellor Hitler, requesting permission to have the infant "put to sleep." Hitler had been receiving many such requests from German parents of disabled babies over several years and had been waiting for just the right opportunity to launch his euthanasia plans. The Knauer case seemed the perfect test case. He sent one of his personal physicians, Karl Rudolph Brandt, to investigate. Brandt's instructions were to verify the facts, and if the child was disabled as described in the father's letter, he was to assure the infant's doctors that they could kill the child without legal consequence. With the Führer's assurance, Baby Knauer's doctors willingly murdered their patient at the request of his father. Brandt witnessed the baby's killing and reported back to Hitler, who was pleased all went as planned. Based on this case of requested infanticide, Hitler signed the order permitting doctors to kill disabled infants.[71]

The murder of Baby Knauer is *precisely* the scenario Singer espouses when he argues that parents should be allowed to have their unwanted babies killed. Indeed, Baby Knauer's father was quoted by Lifton in *The*

Nazi Doctors, stating in 1973 that Brandt assured them "we wouldn't have to suffer from this terrible misfortune because the *Führer* had granted us the mercy killing of our son. Later, we could have other children, handsome and healthy, of whom the Reich could be proud."[72] Note the *exact juxtaposition* of Brandt's justification for murder with Singer's philosophy.

It appears that the protesters in Germany and Austria who see a moral equivalence between Singer and the German euthanasia Holocaust don't have it so wrong after all. While there is not an exact match at every level of substantive ideas—Singer does not support the involuntary killing of physically disabled people, and most babies were killed without their parents' consent—the similarities between Singer's beliefs and those of the German doctors who willingly slaughtered tens of thousands of disabled babies are too striking to be ignored.

In addition to being a utilitarian philosopher, Singer is also a very political animal. Having received much grief for infanticide promotion, a few years ago he (sort of) walked back his advocacy, stating at a bioethics conference held at Princeton: "Maybe the law has to have clear bright lines and has to take birth as the right time, although maybe it should make some exceptions in the cases of severe disability where parents think that it is better for the child and better for the family that the child does not live."[73] In other words, "maybe"—Singer always advocates odious acts with such equivocal language—we should be able to kill babies, but only if they would have very difficult lives, and then, only because we care.

Singer and Fletcher are far from the only bioethicists to seriously advocate permitting infanticide in some situations. An icon of bioethics in Britain, Jonathan Glover, wrote quite bluntly that infanticide is not morally wrong because babies are "replaceable."[74] Glover's reasoning, like Singer's, doesn't require that the killed baby be disabled: "It is wrong to kill a baby who has a good change of having a worth-while life [a life worthy of life], but ... it would not be wrong to kill him if the alternative to his existence was the existence of someone else with an equally good chance of a life at least as worth-while."[75]

As to those who oppose infanticide because babies cannot "choose" to be killed—autonomy, after all, being an overarching value in bioethics—Glover casually dismissed the objection: "Killing someone overrides his autonomy where it goes against his own preference for staying alive. This objection to killing provides no argument against infanticide, for newborn babies have no conception of death and so cannot have any preference for life over death.... The objection to infanticide is at most no stronger than the objection to frustrating a baby's current set of desires, say by leaving him to cry unattended for a longish period."[76]

Since the first edition of this book, other bioethicists have jumped enthusiastically onto the infanticide bandwagon. In 2014, for example, the prominent Canadian bioethicist Udo Schuklenk—an enthusiastic adherence to the quality of life ethic—wrote, in essence, that infants judged to have a life unworthy of life should be euthanized: "A quality-of-life ethic requires us to focus on a neonate's current and future quality of life as relevant decision making criteria. We would ask questions such as: Does this baby have the capacity for development to an extent that will allow him or her to have a life and not merely be alive? If we reach the conclusion that it would not, we would have reason to conclude that his life is not worth living."[77] What makes a life worth living? Well, that would be in *the eye of the utilitarian beholder, wouldn't it?*

As Binding and Hoche did in *Permission to Destroy Life Unworthy of Life*, Schuklenk cited strained resources as a rationale for committing medical infanticide: "The question of whether it would be a wise allocation of scarce health care resources to undertake the proposed surgical procedures invariably arises in circumstances such as this. Continuing life-prolonging care for the infant would be futile, it would constitute a waste of scarce health care resources. Health care resources ought to be deployed where they can actually benefit patients by improving their quality of life."[78] And he expressed zero qualms about violating the sanctity and equal dignity of all human life:

> A quality-of-life proponent could just as well argue that respect for human dignity demands that the infant's life be terminated on compassionate grounds. Human dignity is mostly a rhetorical cloak for other—more controversial—ideologic convictions. Incidentally, this applies to other types of nonarguments, too. For instance, opponents of infanticide frequently ask whether we would want to live in a society that permitted such a course of action. Proponents could simply reply

affirmatively. We would be better served to avoid this kind of rhetoric in public and professional discourse altogether.[79]

How does that old song go? "Everything old is new again."

Usually, arguments in bioethics for infanticide escape public notice because they take place in professional journals or at symposia where academics read their papers to each other. For example, Schuklenk wrote in the *Journal of Thoracic and Cardiovascular Surgery,* hardly a publication on most people's "must read" list.

But once in a while, people get a glimpse of what utilitarian bioethicists have planned for them, leading often to angry controversy. That is what happened in 2012 after the *Journal of Medical Ethics* published "After Birth Abortion: Why Should the Baby Live?" by Alberto Giubilini and Francesca Minerva. The article argues, á la Singer, that infants are not "persons," and hence—harking back to Fletcher—"after-birth abortion" is morally permissible.[80] But unlike many infanticide-promoting articles, Giubilini and Minerva confront head-on the question of whether healthy and able-bodied babies can be killed, arguing that whatever justifies abortion—and in the USA, that means anything and everything—also supports a right for parents to have unwanted born babies painlessly killed.

Such logic flows easily from the rejection of the idea that human life matters morally simply because it is human. Moreover, that premise allows rank bootstrapping to justify expanding the killing license. Never mind that abortion wasn't legalized to grant a woman the "right" to a dead fetus but to ensure a woman's right to control her own body. Thus once the baby is born, the entire issue of protecting "choice" should be factually irrelevant.

But having blithely dismissed intrinsic human value, the authors easily inflate autonomy to include a *putative right not to be personally inconvenienced or burdened by the infant or the child she would later become.* And since an infant isn't a "person"—having yet to develop desires or goals—the baby's life is of secondary concern to the desires of her mother.

The article is too lengthy to completely recount, but here are a few representative excerpts:

- "In spite of the oxymoron in the expression, we propose to call this practice 'after-birth abortion,' rather than 'infanticide,' to emphasize that the moral status of the individual killed is comparable with that of a fetus ... rather than that of a child."

- "Therefore we claim that killing a newborn could be ethically permissible in all circumstances where abortion would be."
- "If the death of a newborn is not wrongful to her on the grounds that she cannot have formed any aim that she is prevented from accomplishing, then it should also be permissible to practice after-birth abortion on a healthy newborn too."
- "Merely being human is not in itself a reason for ascribing someone a right to life."
- "Why should we kill a healthy newborn when giving it up for adoption would not breach anyone's right but possibly increase the happiness of the people involved? ... On this perspective ... we also need to consider the interests of the mother who might suffer psychological distress from giving up her child for adoption."[81]

Unlike most pro-infanticide journal articles, this one was published online and noticed by the popular media—leading to the rare case when a major bioethics article received widespread public scrutiny, sparking a firestorm of popular outrage. Indeed, the criticism became so intense that the *Journal of Medical Ethics* took it offline and the authors wrote a public non-apology apology—not recanting anything they wrote, mind you, but claiming to be harmless philosophers merely chewing intellectual cud: *"When we decided to write this article about after-birth abortion we had no idea that our paper would raise such a heated debate. 'Why not? You should have known!' people keep on repeating everywhere on the web. The answer is very simple: the article was supposed to be read by other fellow bioethicists who were already familiar with this topic and our arguments [as] ... this debate has been going on for 40 years."*[82]

But that is precisely why it was important that the public reacted so viscerally. As I described in the last chapter, bioethics is not a mere debating society. Rather, the field is—and has been since its inception—*about changing societal values and public policies.* Moreover, bioethicists haven't discoursed about infanticide for forty years because they enjoy exploring novel concepts, but rather because it isn't easy to convince people—not even bioethicists—that killing babies is acceptable. Should infanticide ever become "unexceptional," in Richard John Neuhaus's formula, killing babies would become the launching pad for the next radical proposal.

Giubilini and Minerva disingenuously pretend they are not part of that process of persuasion: "We never meant to suggest that after-birth abortion should become legal. This was not made clear enough in the paper. Laws are not just about rational ethical arguments, because there are many practical, emotional, social aspects that are relevant in policy making (such as respecting the plurality of ethical views, people's emotional reactions etc.). But we are not policy makers, we are philosophers, and we deal with concepts, not with legal policy."[83]

Whatever. That which we don't condemn we may ultimately allow. Thus the strong public pushback against Giubilini and Minerva's philosophical apology for infanticide was not only justifiable but absolutely necessary. Indeed, the fact that bioethicists deem promotion of infanticide debatable—even those who "respectfully disagree" with permitting it—speaks volumes about the danger posed by the contemporary bioethics movement.

Killing Babies in Holland: Peter Singer and Udo Schuklenk's infanticide-friendly philosophy has been turned into lethal practice in the Netherlands, where seriously disabled and terminally ill babies are killed in their cribs by pediatricians and neonatologists. According to a 1997 study published in the British medical journal *The Lancet*, approximately 8 percent of Dutch infants who died in 1995 were killed by doctors who administered drugs "with the explicit aim of hastening death."[84] If the study, which looked into the deaths of 338 infants between August and November 1995 is accurate, and with approximately 1,000 infants dying in the Netherlands each year (1,041 in 1995), approximately 80 babies are murdered each year by their doctors without legal consequence. A follow-up investigation in the same journal in 2005 came to a nearly identical conclusion.[85] According to the 1995 study, 45 percent of surveyed neonatologists and 31 percent of surveyed pediatricians had "given drugs explicitly to end life."[86]

Most of the babies were killed because the doctors believed they would not survive, but 18 percent of the killings were due to "a poor prognosis,"[87] meaning disabilities. Life was shortened by *more than five years* in 16 percent of the cases. Some of the killed babies didn't even need life support to survive: "… a drug was given to hasten death to neonates not dependent on life-sustaining treatment in 1 percent of all death cases," which "represents 10–15 deaths of this type per year in the Netherlands."[88] Most—but not all—of the killings were at the request of parents, as per the Peter Singer and Udo Schuklenk formulas.[89] Despite legal requirements that euthanasia deaths be disclosed to the coroner's office for review, "physician-assisted deaths for neonates is ... virtually never reported."[90]

Few cases of infanticide have been prosecuted in the Netherlands; those that have been have not been attempts to punish doctors but rather to establish a "precedent." (Dutch prosecutions are not necessarily adversarial in nature, particularly as they involve physicians involved in euthanasia. As Dutch lawyer and euthanasia proponent Eugene Sutorius told me, "The public prosecution, as a body, sees that this is not criminality in the normal sense.... So, even the prosecutor, while bringing the case, he's more interested in making sure that we have strict definitions and order than he is in punishing the professional. He's trying to create a precedent."[91])

The first Dutch infanticide precedent that essentially decriminalized infant euthanasia involved a Dutch gynecologist named Henk Prins who killed a three-day-old infant who was born with spina bifida, hydrocephalus, and leg deformities. When prosecuted (in order to create a precedent), Dr. Prins testified that he killed the child with her parents' permission because of the infant's poor prognosis and because the baby screamed in pain when touched. Yet the child was in agony because she was neglected medically. The open wound in her back, the primary characteristic of spina bifida, had not been closed; the fluid had not been drained from her head either, even though these treatments are standard in spina bifida cases and would have substantially reduced the infant's pain.

The trial court refused to punish the doctor for killing the baby. Indeed, the judge praised Dr. Prins for "his integrity and courage" and wished him well in any further legal proceedings he might face.[92]

The Royal Dutch Medical Association (KNMG) published a report in 1990 that set forth guidelines for killing incompetent patients, including infants. The standard for pediatric euthanasia is what is called "a livable life,"[93] a more tactful way of expressing the Binding and Hoche idea of a life unworthy of life. According to Dutch medical ethics, and echoing Fletcher's "humanhood" concept described in the last chapter, the "livableness" of an infant's life depends on a combination of factors, including the following:

- The expected measure of suffering (not only physical but emotional);
- The expected potential for communication and human relations, independence (ability to move, to care for oneself, to live independently);
- The child's life expectancy.[94]

If the infant's prospects don't measure up to what the doctor and parents believe is a life worth living, the child can be medically neglected to death, or if that doesn't work, killed by the doctor via lethal injection.

Dutch infanticide came completely out of the shadows—albeit remaining technically illegal, for what that might be worth—in 2004 with the publication of the "Groningen Protocol for Euthanasia in Newborns" by the Groningen University. The protocol was drawn up by doctors at the Groningen Academic Hospital, led by Dr. Eduard Verhagen, head of the hospital's pediatric department. Infanticide is a clear violation of the existing euthanasia law, which requires competent patients to voluntarily request death.

No matter. Verhagen explained, "It's time to be honest about the unbearable suffering endured by newborns with no hope of a future," adding that he hoped the Groningen protocol would serve as a nationwide guide to the killing of seriously ill or disabled infants.[95]

Even more alarmingly, some of the world's most respected bioethical and medical journals embraced the Groningen protocol as a respectable approach. It was published, for example, with all due respect in the *New England Journal of Medicine*.[96] The bureaucratic infanticide checklist was even applauded in the *Hastings Center Report*—in which, reminiscent of Binding and Hoche—bioethicists Hilde Lindermann and Marian Verkerk lauded the protocol because it allows the infanticide of babies who aren't dying: "Critics charge that the protocol does not successfully identify which babies will die. But it is precisely those babies who could continue to live, but whose lives would be wretched in the extreme, who stand in most need of the interventions for which the protocol offers guidance."[97]

Bioethicists and euthanasia advocates claim that modern infanticide differs from wartime German euthanasia because most cases in the Netherlands involve parental consent, while most German cases involved physician decision making without parental involvement. But this is a distinction without a significant moral difference. Infants are people, not chattel. Parents have no more right to decide to have them killed than do doctors, or, for that matter, government bureaucrats.

The first sentence of the Universal Declaration of Human Rights states, "Whereas recognition of the inherent dignity and of the equal and inalienable rights of all members of the human family is the foundation of freedom, justice and peace in the world."[98] If that is true, it must apply to all of us, not just the healthy and able-bodied. Unless we want to devolve to the ancient morality that allowed disabled and unwanted infants to be abandoned on hills, we must condemn infanticide unequivocally, whether in actual practice, as in the Netherlands, or as a matter of "respectful intellectual debate," as occurs within bioethics and among some euthanasia advocates.

DEHYDRATING COGNITIVELY DISABLED PEOPLE

Disabled infants are not the only ones at risk of medical cleansing. Today, in the United States, as a matter of almost medical routine, cognitively disabled people who receive their food and fluids medically through a "feeding tube" are intentionally dehydrated and starved to death, and it is deemed ethical and moral.

In few areas of modern medicine have bioethicists been so influential and destructive to the tenets of the equality of human life than in the care of brain-damaged, cognitively disabled people. First, they dehumanized them. Next, they gave moral permission to families and physicians to withdraw basic sustenance. Then, waving the medical consensus they forged like a bloody flag, they urged legal authorities in court cases and in statute writing to make dehydration a matter of the legal "right to die." Due largely to the energetic efforts of bioethicists, causing death by dehydration to cognitively disabled people who receive their sustenance medically is legal in all fifty states.

The first individuals to be targeted for dehydration were people diagnosed as persistently unconscious. The medical term for this condition (coined in 1972) is "persistent vegetative state" (PVS), perhaps the only medical diagnosis that contains a pejorative—from which comes the dehumanizing term "vegetable," as if any human being can be a carrot or a turnip. PVS is "a form of eyes-open permanent unconsciousness in which the patient has periods of wakefulness and physiological sleep/wake cycles, but at no time is the patient aware of him or herself or the environment."[99] People in PVS "are not terminally ill." What they need to survive is simply what every other human being does: food, water, warmth, shelter, cleanliness, and movement (in their cases, by way of turning). With one crucial exception, these services are considered humane care, which can never be withdrawn ethically (although even *that* patient protection is now under attack in bioethics, as we shall discuss below).

That exception is food and water when it is delivered via a feeding tube, which is considered a medical *treatment*, not a basic human requirement. Defining artificial nutrition and hydration (ANH) as a treatment was a crucial step in crafting the medical culture of death. As will be described in more detail later on, medical treatment, unlike humane care, can be withdrawn or withheld from patients legally and ethically as a matter of respecting the patient's personal autonomy—even if the decision is expected to lead to death.

Not too many years ago, it was considered unethical—indeed, potentially a criminal act—to stop feeding and hydrating an incompetent patient. Then, beginning roughly in the early 1980s, some bioethicists began to grapple with their belief that profoundly disabled and frail elderly people were living too long. At that time society would not have accepted euthanasia—and to be fair, some prominent bioethicists opposed mercy killing. (A few still do.) A consensus solution was required to solve this newly conjured "ethical problem." Bioethicists found it in intentional dehydration. Thus, in 1983, Callahan wrote, "A denial of nutrition may in the long run become the only effective way to make certain that a large number of biologically tenacious patients actually die. Given the increasingly large pool of superannuated, chronically ill, physically marginalized elderly, it could well become the non treatment of choice."[100]

For several years the debate raged among bioethicists as to the appropriateness of pulling feeding tubes from people diagnosed as persistently unconscious, who, after all, are not terminally ill. A few resisted the rising tide. Paul Ramsey, for instance, argued that only the "objective medical condition of the patient" should be considered when determining whether to cut off treatment, "not the subjective, capricious, and often selfish evaluations of the quality of future life that are often to the detriment of the most vulnerable and voiceless."[101] Ramsey's point—a good one—was that when someone is *actively dying* and can no longer assimilate food and water, they will often stop eating. At such times, it is humane to allow nature to take its course by not forcing food and water on an unwilling patient; indeed, the practice is a proper and compassionate component of good end-of-life care in particular circumstances. But withholding sustenance from an aged or disabled person to *cause* death is simply wrong, as such decisions are not based on the patient's actual medical needs but rather on the perceived moral worth of a human life.

Dr. Fred Rosner, director of medicine at Queens Hospital Center, also agued strenuously, if in vain, against countenancing intentional dehydration as an ethical medical act. Denial of food and fluids is different than other forms of care, he wrote in the *New York State Journal of Medicine*, because it is "biologically final"; that is, it can have only one result: death. Second, unlike surgery or other forms of treatment, "food and fluids are universal human needs." Rosner worried that for physicians to remove food and fluids "attacks the very foundation of medicine as a profession." He further suggested that just because nutrition is delivered through a tube, it "does not change into an exotic medical substance"; food and fluids do not become medical therapy simply because another person is needed to provide them.[102]

Ramsey, Rosner, and the relatively few others who fought against transforming ANH from humane care to medical treatment were unable to stanch the fast-running tide. And although Ramsey had been one of the first bioethics luminaries to promote the appropriateness of ceasing life-supporting medical treatment at the patient's request, few of his colleagues were swayed by his doubts.

The advocacy of bioethics profoundly influenced court decisions and legislation on the issue of removing food and fluids from people diagnosed as persistently unconscious. In a 1983 California case, for example, an appeals court refused to sustain an indictment of doctors who had withdrawn food and fluids from a patient in PVS, citing bioethics literature as assisting the court in its reasoning.[103] That case was soon followed up by another appeals court decision overturning a trial judge's refusal to permit the dehydration of another man in PVS at the family's request. Indeed, the court ruled, families can order doctors to pull feeding tubes from people in PVS without asking a supervising court's permission.[104]

At about the same time, in 1986, the American Medical Association (AMA) issued a momentous ethical opinion. While asserting that doctors should never "intentionally cause death," the AMA opined that it was ethical to terminate life support, even if "death is not imminent but a patient's coma is beyond doubt irreversible." In and of itself, that wasn't big news. What was significant is that, for the first time, the AMA listed "artificially supplied ... nutrition and hydration" as a form of medical treatment.[105] Needless to say, despite the AMA's declaration that doctors should never "intentionally cause death," removing all sustenance necessarily causes that very result.

The ultimate legal blow came in the landmark United States Supreme Court case of Nancy Beth Cruzan, who, on January 11, 1983, lost control of her car on an icy road in Missouri and crashed. She was thrown from her car and landed facedown in a water-filled ditch. Nancy's heart stopped, but paramedics revived her. Nancy's injuries included profound cognitive disability: a diagnosis of PVS. While that diagnosis is disputed in some circles, there is no contradicting the fact that her care did not require "high tech" medicine. She was not on a respirator. She did not need kidney dialysis. She was not terminally ill.

In May 1987, the Cruzans filed suit in Missouri seeking to force hospital employees where Nancy resided to remove their daughter's food and fluids. Hospital administrators and especially nurses who treated her daily and who saw her as a living, breathing human being who was deserving of respect and proper care resisted the request. The trial judge disagreed. Nancy was ordered dehydrated.

The state of Missouri appealed, basing its disagreement on a state law requiring clear and convincing evidence that a patient would want life support removed before allowing it to be done. On this basis, the Missouri Supreme Court reversed the trial judge, ruling, "This is not a case in which we are asked to let someone die.... This is a case in which we are asked to allow the medical professional to make Nancy die by starvation and dehydration."[106]

The Cruzans appealed to the United States Supreme Court. But the Supreme Court affirmed the lower ruling, finding the evidentiary standard constitutional, ruling that such a strict standard was properly in keeping with the state's obligation to protect the lives of its citizens. Since no clear and convincing evidence had been offered at trial that removing food and fluids was what Nancy would have wanted—as opposed to what her parents wanted for her—Missouri could properly require her life support to continue.

What at first appeared a resounding victory for those who opposed Nancy's dehydration soon turned to ashes. First, it became clear that the Supreme Court, by implication, had agreed that tube-supplied food and water was a medical treatment that could be withdrawn. The Cruzans went back to court in front of the same trial judge who had originally ordered Nancy dehydrated. This time there was testimony from two of Nancy's former coworkers of a few vague conversations with Nancy that she would not want to live in a coma. Nancy's exact words could not be described, and whether she made the statement or simply agreed with someone else's opinion could not be proven. But that sparse testimony was all the judge needed to rationalize doing what he had wanted to do all along. Once again, he ordered Nancy dehydrated. This time Missouri did not appeal the decision and none of the many opponents of Nancy's killing had legal standing to enter the case. Nancy Cruzan died on December 26, 1990, twelve days after the removal of her feeding tube.

The death of Nancy Cruzan was a true watershed moment in bioethics, demonstrating the power of philosophers and activist physicians to recreate medical ethics, public policy, and influence popular opinion. With the Cruzan case, virtually all institutional and legal opposition to dehydrating people in PVS at the request of caregivers collapsed. Such people are now dehydrated routinely in all fifty states. If other family members dispute the decision—as happened most famously in the Terri Schiavo case described below—it will rarely be to any avail. Indeed, they will often be accused of bad-faith meddling and roundly castigated in the media. And it only took about ten years from the beginning of the bioethics debate about dehydration for people in PVS to be viewed in medicine, law, theology, and among the general public, as the patriarch Fletcher hoped they would eventually be, as "objects," "vegetables," "mere biological life," a disposable caste whose intentional killing by dehydration is proper and compassionate.

The attitude that it is better to die than live cognitively disabled has so pervaded the culture of medicine that some doctors report that there is a rush to judgment to write off newly unconscious patients and consign them to death by cutting off life support before they have had a chance to recover.

There is no question that in 2005, the rush to dehydrate almost took the life of eleven-year-old Haleigh Poutre, beaten nearly to death by her adoptive mother and stepfather. The beating left her unconscious and barely clinging to life.

Within a week or so of the beating, her doctors had written her off, telling Haleigh's court-appointed guardian, Harry Spence, that she was "virtually brain-dead." Even though he had never visited her, Spence quickly went to court seeking permission to remove her respirator and feeding tube.[107] The court agreed, a decision affirmed recently by the Supreme Court of Massachusetts. And so, no doubt with the best of intentions, a little girl who had already suffered so much was stripped by the Commonwealth of Massachusetts of even the chance to fight to stay alive. If she didn't stop breathing when the respirator was removed, which doctors expected, she would slowly dehydrate to death.

Then came the unexpected: Before "pulling the plug" on Haleigh, Spence finally decided to visit her. He was stunned. Rather than finding a little girl with "not a chance" of recovery, as doctors had described Haleigh's condition to him (as reported by the Boston Globe), Haleigh was conscious. She was able to give Spence a yellow block when asked to by a social worker and respond to other simple requests.[108]

Laudably, Spence immediately called off the dehydration. In the following months, Haleigh steadily improved to the point that the supposedly "nearly brain-dead" little girl was able to eat by mouth and receive education. The story had a happy ending: Haleigh was adopted by a loving family, and today, while disabled, at age twenty-two she loves going to church, listening to music, and interacting with her family.[109]

Think about this. Think about it hard. None of this good news would have happened had the quality of life ethic, pushed vociferously in mainstream bioethics, been implemented against Haleigh by state bureaucrats. Indeed, *she would have died by dehydration* had it not taken months to complete the bureaucratic procedures.

It is a very dangerous thing to create invidious categories of people denigrated by medical technocrats as having lives not worth living—or paying for. So the next time a bioethicist argues that we must dehydrate a child or other cognitively disabled person to death in "their best interests," remember Haleigh Poutre. Sometimes doctors are wrong. Sometimes "miracles" do, indeed, happen. If we are to err, it should be on giving life a chance. At the very least, we should not be in a rush to dehydrate the newly brain injured. We can never know when the unexpected will happen.

The Terri Schiavo Case: When Terri Schiavo collapsed on the evening of February 25, 1990—cause unknown—she could have had no idea that twenty-five years later people the world over would know her name and care very much about the manner in which she died. What began as a private tragedy—a vivacious young woman stricken in the very prime of her life with a brain injury that left her profoundly disabled—ultimately became a multiyear international cultural conflagration that sowed widespread popular distrust for the courts and political branches of government; forced a state legislature, a popular governor, both houses of Congress, and the president of the United States into tight political corners; and even attracted the concerned attention of a dying Pope John Paul II. Now, more than ten years after her death, "the Terri Schiavo Case" is still bitterly debated all around the world.

Terri's cardiac arrest left her profoundly cognitively impaired—diagnosed as persistently unconscious, although that is disputed by Terri's defenders who insist she had some interactive capacities. (From my perspective, it shouldn't matter.) At first, husband Michael and parents Bob and Mary Schindler worked together, seeking treatment and rehabilitation, including an experimental intervention in which electrodes were placed in Terri's brain. Eventually, Michael—as Terri's guardian—sued for medical malpractice, obtaining a seven-figure award, from which some $300,000 was paid to Michael for his loss of companionship and consortium, and $750,000 to Terri—put in a trust account—to care for her throughout what one of Michael's expert witnesses testified should be a normal life span.

Michael and the Schindlers' previous good relationship soured shortly after the lawsuit money was banked. Michael told CNN interviewer
Larry King that Bob Schindler wanted a cut of the settlement,[110] which
seems highly unlikely since the Schindlers would eventually spend most
of their assets trying desperately to keep their daughter alive. (Full dis-
closure: I wrote repeatedly in defense of Terri's life during the controversy
and became an informal adviser to the family.) For his part, Bob claimed
that Michael reneged on his promise to pursue further rehabilitation,
sparking a heated argument between the two in her room.[111] In any event,
Terri never received any rehab from that day on, and the breach between
Michael and Terri's blood family became permanent and increasingly
bitter.

In late spring 1993, Terri developed an infection. Michael ordered that
she receive no antibiotics, later testifying in a deposition that he didn't
think she would want to live in such an impaired condition—a matter
he neglected to tell the malpractice jury. The Schindlers didn't want their
daughter to die and sued for guardianship. Eventually, the dispute was
settled, with Michael authorizing continuing medical support for Terri
while remaining Terri's personal guardian.

In the intervening years, Michael went on with his life. He fell in love
and moved in with another woman, eventually siring two children by her
even though still legally married to Terri. Then, in 1998, he petitioned a
Florida court for permission to remove Terri's feeding tube. The proverbial sewage was about to hit the metaphorical fan.

Such intra-family legal disputes over medical care are relatively rare
but not unheard of. Usually they garner some local publicity and are soon
forgotten after they reach their conclusion.

Not this time. It wasn't planned. Events spontaneously developed, one
after the other, eventually achieving critical cultural mass. The intense
personal, cultural, legal, and political struggle over Terri Schiavo's life
and death deserves far more attention than I can possibly devote to it
here. Nor, in the limited space available—books have been written about
the case—can I possibly unpack the many factual and legal disputes that
developed over more than a decade of intra-family acrimony and years
of bitter litigation. But here is a general overview of what happened.[112]

The original case. The question of whether Terri Schiavo would be
dehydrated to death was heard in the courtroom of Judge George Greer.

At first, it seemed that the dehydration might not happen. Terri's guardian *ad litem*, Richard L. Pearse, Jr., worried that since Terri's trust fund held $713,828.85, "Mr. Schiavo will realize a substantial and fairly immediate financial gain if his application for withdrawal of life support [tube-supplied food and water] is granted."[113] Of perhaps even greater concern was the acute personal conflict of interest between Michael's duty as a guardian for Terri and the new life he had created for himself in the years after her collapse. Pearse described this matter tersely as Michael "getting on with his life."[114] Pearse perceived these conflicts of interest as crucial evidence in determining how to properly decide Terri's fate, writing in his report to the court in December 1998, "Given the inherent problems already mentioned, together with the fact that the ward has been maintained on the life support measures sought to be withdrawn for the past 8 years, it is the recommendation of the guardian *ad litem* that the petition for [tube] removal be denied."[115]

Pearse was soon dismissed as Terri's guardian *ad litem* based on allegations of bias asserted by Michael Schiavo's lawyers, and no new *ad litem* was ever appointed in the state guardianship case to represent Terri's interests (even though Florida statutory law required *ad litem* guardians in cases such as Terri's.) Once Pearse was out of the picture, the conflicts-of-interest issue lost all traction.

At trial, Michael testified that Terri told him on a few occasions during their marriage that if she were ever in a situation of being artificially maintained, she would want life support removed.[116] His assertion that Terri wouldn't want to live in her impaired condition was supported by Michael's brother Scott, who testified that she told him she wouldn't "want to be kept alive on a machine." (Terri wasn't on a "machine." But Judge Greer interpreted this statement to also mean a feeding tube.) Michael's sister-in-law, Joan Schiavo, testified that after watching a movie, Terri stated she would not want "tubes" and approved of pulling the life support from the dying baby of a mutual friend and said that if she ever wrote a "will" she would say that she didn't want "tubes."

Others told a different story. For example, one of Terri's friends testified that Terri opposed removing life support from Karen Ann Quinlan, but this was disregarded by Judge Greer when issuing his first death order because the witness had used present tense verbs when describing the purported conversation instead of past tense verbs.[117]

In any event, Judge Greer found "clear and convincing evidence"—the highest legal standard in non-criminal cases—that Terri wouldn't want to live in her impaired state and ordered Terri's feeding tube removed. The Schindlers appealed. Soon afterward, the "Terri Schiavo Case" became one of the most disputed and heated public bioethics controversies in history.

In the court of public opinion. Terri's plight only became known widely because of the Internet. Knowing the importance of public relations in the modern age, Terri's parents created a website, www.terrisfight.org, dedicated to uniting public opinion around saving Terri's life. The site issued press releases, carried news of the case, linked copies of court documents, and provided a personal story of Terri's history. Most importantly, understanding that pictures speak louder than written words—and, more particularly, that videos are far more convincing than pictures—the Schindlers uploaded powerful videos of Terri apparently reacting to the world around her.

In one scene, Terri is asked by a doctor to open her eyes. For a moment, nothing. Then, Terri's eyes flutter and she opens them. She is apparently so eager to please—and this really touched my heart when I first saw it—that she opens her eyes so wide her forehead wrinkles.

In another scene, Terri's mother comes into the room. She talks happily to her daughter, "Hi! Hi, it's Mommy. How are you?" As Mary Schindler adjusts Terri on the bed, it sure appears like she understands that it is her mother, and she smiles happily. In a third scene, Terri appears to respond happily when music is turned on.

These videos humanized Terri in a way that mere word descriptions never could. Her case burst into the highest levels of public awareness, aided in particular by radio talk show hosts Glenn Beck and Sean Hannity (among other media personalities on the starboard side of the political spectrum) and the kind of visibility that social media sharing can engender. Michael's supporters and proponents of Terri's dehydration within the bioethics community insisted that the appearance of interactivity in the videos were actually mirages and reflexes, that Terri was PVS.

Whatever the truth of her condition, Terri's case became the talk of the country, dividing society—or perhaps, better stated, exposing already existing bitter discords—about whether human life has intrinsic value or, as many in bioethics contend, it is relative depending on the quality of the life lived. Indeed, on the public airways, particularly on talk radio programs, in newspaper opinion columns, Internet chat rooms, and in private conversations, people argued about whether Terri should live or die.

Terri's Law. As the Schindlers lost every legal appeal and the time of Terri's death quickly approached, tens of thousands of people from all around the country began to pressure Florida Governor Jeb Bush in letters, emails, telephone calls, and petitions to intervene in the case. Bush sent Judge Greer a letter asking that he appoint a guardian *ad litem*; otherwise, Bush kept a prudent silence.

The Schiavo case did not allow fence sitting, but rather, it compelled people at all levels of society to decide whether it is right or wrong to dehydrate a young woman to death when her blood family wanted to care for her the rest of her life, as her husband declared he was faithfully following her wishes. Moreover, this was high-risk politics of the most intense kind. Bush was the younger brother of the president of the United States—adding to the political import of what he did or did not do. Soon, Terri Schiavo's fate had become a new and volatile front in America's decades-long "culture war."

Then her feeding tube was removed and she began to dehydrate. On October 21, 2003—when Terri had been without any sustenance for six days—the Florida Senate debated "Terri's Bill," passed the previous evening in the Florida House of Representatives. If the bill became law, it would allow Bush to immediately restore Terri's feeding tube, pending further investigation of Terri's case.

Pushing politicians to let Terri's dehydration reach completion were bioethicists; members of the medical intelligentsia; "right to die" advocates; and Terri's husband, Michael Schiavo, and his attorney, George Felos. On the other side were disability rights advocates, right-to-lifers, Governor Jeb Bush, Terri's parents and their stalwart lawyer, Patricia Anderson, and the tens of thousands of people from all over the country and the world whose months of insistent emails and telephone calls had resulted in such overwhelming political pressure that Florida's government felt compelled to act.

Finally, Terri's Bill passed by a huge margin in the Senate, and after a brief reconciliation with the House version, the bill became Terri's Law.[118] But if the supporters of Terri's life thought she was *ipso facto* saved, they were naïve; the struggle was just beginning.

Terri's Law required the courts to appoint a guardian *ad litem* to write a report to the governor about Terri and the case. Attorney Jay Wolfson received the appointment, and he quickly set to work, delivering his thirty-eight-page, closely detailed report on the controversy and its history on December 1. Curiously—some would say inexplicably—he never once mentioned Michael Schiavo's new family.

Wolfson also seemed to buy into "personhood theory," the predominate view in bioethics that people with severe cognitive impairments are less than fully equal persons and hence have fewer rights. Expressing his belief that Terri was in a persistent vegetative state and that her behavior recorded on videos was "reflexive, rather than cognitive," and thus she was "neither conscious nor aware," Wolfson referenced Descartes's proposition, "*Cognito, [sic] ergo sum*" (I think, therefore, I am). "This logic would imply," he wrote, "that unless we are aware and conscious, we cease to be."[119]

Still, Wolfson took his responsibilities to Terri very seriously and performed his work in good faith. Unlike Judge Greer, who never laid eyes on Terri—one would think that sentencing someone to a slow death would compel at least *one visit*—Wolfson attended to her bedside frequently and, to his credit, admitted that Terri "has a distinct presence about her."

Most importantly, Wolfson recommended that Terri be allowed a swallow test, writing that if she "has a reasonable hope of regaining any swallowing function" that her feeding tube should not be removed. Terri shouldn't have been forced to justify her existence by passing any tests, of course. But if the several medical and rehabilitation experts who opined in affidavits that Terri was a good candidate for relearning how to swallow were correct, Wolfson's recommendation could have been the crucial turning point that ultimately saved Terri's life.

But the judge in charge of the Terri's Law case proceedings, David A. Demers, chief judge of the Sixth Judicial Circuit and who had appointed Wolfson, rejected the request and refused to renew Wolfson's authority[120]; this despite Governor Jeb Bush specifically informing Demers that he needed further information from the guardian *ad litem* to properly carry out the governor's responsibilities under Terri's Law.

In the end, none of that mattered. Terri's Law was subsequently declared unconstitutional by the Florida Supreme Court as a violation of the separation of powers doctrine.[121] The continuation of Terri's life was once again in the hands of Judge Greer. He again ordered her sustenance withdrawn.

The federal Terri's Law. As Terri was again in the throes of dehydration, her parents turned to the federal government for help. Senate Majority Leader Bill Frist (R-TN) sponsored a bill that would grant the federal courts jurisdiction to review the state proceedings in Terri's case: "In such a suit, the District Court shall determine de novo any claim of a violation of any right of Theresa Marie Schiavo within the scope of this Act, notwithstanding any prior State court determination and regardless of whether such a claim has previously been raised, considered, or decided in State court proceedings."[122]

Time was of the essence, as Terri would soon be dead. But getting the bill to the floor of the Senate for a quick vote required "unanimous consent." In other words, if just *one* senator refused to allow a vote, it would not be able to pass in time to save her life.

Contrary to revisionist accounts that have depicted the effort to pass the federal bill as an exclusively Republican effort, the federal law was one of the most bipartisan passed during the George W. Bush presidency. Not only did liberal Democrats such as Tom Harkin of Iowa cooperate in pushing the bill through the Senate, but *not one Democrat senator objected*—not Hillary Clinton, Barack Obama, Joe Biden, or Ted Kennedy.

With unanimous consent given, the bill passed the Senate without objection in an unrecorded voice vote. It was quickly brought to the House of Representatives—then in an Easter recess—which soon followed suit by a 203-58 vote, including 47 Democrats (with 178 representatives not voting). President Bush quickly signed the bill, and Terri's parents sued to have Terri's case reviewed in federal court.[123]

The "Act for the Relief of the Parents of Terri Schiavo" granted standing to Bob and Mary to ask the federal court to undertake a de novo review of the case, i.e., to have a federal judge hold a new trial, complete with testimony and other evidentiary fact finding. But United States District Court Judge James D. Whittemore refused to engage in an independent review of the case or enjoin Terri's dehydration, ruling: "Terri Schiavo's life and liberty interests were adequately protected by the extensive process provided in the state courts."[124] In other words, Whittemore concluded that Terri's constitutional rights had been protected because Florida courts had issued rulings so stating after extensive litigation. That was not a de novo review: it was a rubber stamp.

It was also the last nail in Terri Schiavo's coffin. As people protested outside her hospice—including civil rights leader Jesse Jackson—Michael and the Schindlers continued to argue, including over the conditions under which her family could visit. Then, the end: Terri Schiavo dehydrated to death on March 31, 2005.

Her death was not easy. Brother Bobby Schindler, who was with her near the end, told me, "Terri's skin had turned patchy, bluish in one place and jaundiced in another. Her skin became so dry from the dehydration it reminded me of aged leather. Her face became very drawn and her mouth fell open, so that her upper teeth seemed to protrude forward, giving the false appearance of buck teeth. Her breathing became very labored, and her eyes darted back and forth in a frantic manner. Perhaps the worst thing was seeing blood pooling her eyes. It was what nightmares are made of."[125]

The aftermath. Before the Terri Schiavo case, people could say, "I didn't know" that helpless people are dehydrated to death because they are cognitively devastated. Afterward, people had to choose whether they supported such actions. Polls showed that, apparently, majorities do.

Part of the reason for the public's attitude may have been reporting around the autopsy report claiming the findings supported Michael's assertions. Many commenters asserted (and still assert) that the autopsy proved she was in a vegetative state. But that's flatly not true. Indeed, to the contrary, the report noted, "Neuropathic examination alone of decedent's brain—or any brain, for that matter—cannot prove or disprove a diagnosis of persistent vegetative state or minimally conscious state."[126]

Much was also made in the media that the autopsy found her brain to be half the weight of a normal organ. Indeed, the autopsy report found that Terri's brain weighed just 615 grams compared to Karen Ann Quinlan's brain, which weighed 835 grams "after ten years in a similar persistent vegetative state." But there is a crucial difference between the two cases: Unlike Terri, Karen was not dehydrated to death. Indeed, *dehydration causes brain shrinkage*, as a story in the *Washington Post* about children in Africa dying of thirst clearly demonstrated:

I asked Jeffrey Berns, president-elect of the National Kidney Foundation and a nephrologist at the University of Pennsylvania, what these children may be going through.... "People are going to be miserable." The body is about 60 percent water, and under normal conditions, he said … If it's not replaced over time and dehydration becomes severe, cells throughout the body will begin to shrink as water moves out of them and into the blood stream, part of the body's efforts to keep the organs in fluid. "All the cells will shrink," he said, "but the ones that count are the brain cells. They don't operate normally when they're shrinking." Changes in mental status will follow, including confusion and ultimately coma, he said. As the brain becomes smaller, it takes up less room in the skull and blood vessels connecting it to the inside of the cranium can pull away and rupture. Without water, blood volume will decline and all the organs will start to fail, he said. Kidney failure will soon lead to disastrous consequences and ultimately death as blood volume continues to fall and waste products that should be eliminated from the body remain.[127]

This is precisely the process that took the life of Terri Schiavo.

The media also reported, almost breathlessly, that the autopsy found that "no amount of therapy would reverse her condition." But nobody ever said Terri would one day get out of bed and tap dance. Rather, the core question was whether it was right and proper to dehydrate her to death—regardless of whether she was unconscious or minimally conscious—and second, who should decide on her care: a husband who had moved on with his life by starting a family with another woman, or her parents and siblings who wanted to care for Terri for whatever time she had left.

Terri is long in her grave. But she is not forgotten. Her life and death changed the culture and stimulated a much-needed discussion of the importance of advance directives and good family communication about medical care in the event of incapacity. Her name continues to be a cultural flashpoint. My deeply held views are clearly discerned in these pages, and no doubt my readers have their own strongly held opinions. This much is sure: No one is neutral about Terri Schiavo.[128]

Targeting the Conscious: The medical death culture is never static, never satisfied. It aspires to expand steadily until it fills all available space.

Even before Terri Schiavo's dehydration, bioethicists were advocating to expand the dehydratable to include severely brain-damaged—but clearly conscious—patients.

One of the most disturbing examples of which I am aware was the case of Marjorie Nighbert, a successful Ohio businesswoman felled by a stroke while visiting her family. Marjorie was quickly stabilized. She was not terminally ill. She was somewhat disabled by the stroke but was expected to benefit from rehabilitation. Accordingly, she was moved to the Crestview Nursing and Convalescent Home in Florida, where everyone hoped that Marjorie could relearn how to chew and swallow without danger of aspiration. To ensure she was nourished, Marjorie was provided a feeding tube.

This presented an excruciating quandary for Marjorie's brother Maynard, who was made her medical decision maker in his sister's power of attorney. Marjorie had once told him she didn't want a feeding tube if she were terminally ill. He interpreted that statement as indicating that if she were unable to be weaned off the tube, she would have wanted doctors to remove it. Finally, when she did not improve, he ordered the tube removed. Marjorie was expected to die within three weeks.

Then, the unthinkable: As she was slowly dehydrating, Marjorie began to *ask the staff for food*. "She was saying things like, 'Please feed me, I'm hungry, I'm thirsty, and I want food,'" attorney William F. Stone told me, who briefly represented Marjorie as a court-appointed guardian.[129] In response to her pleas, members of the nursing staff surreptitiously gave her small amounts of food and water. One eventually blew the whistle, leading to a state investigation and a restraining order directing the nursing home to continue Marjorie's nourishment pending a quick investigation.

Stone was appointed Marjorie's temporary guardian by Circuit Court Judge Jere Tolton, who instructed Stone to conduct a twenty-four-hour inquiry, the sole issue being whether Marjorie was competent to rescind her power of attorney and make her own decisions. After the rushed investigation, Stone was forced to report to the judge that she was not competent *at that time*. She had, after all, been intentionally malnourished for several weeks. Stone particularly noted that he had been unable to determine whether she was competent when the dehydration commenced.

With Stone's report in hand—and even though she had asked for food—the judge allowed the dehydration to be completed, apparently on the theory that Marjorie did not have the competence to request the medical treatment of food and water. Nighbert died on April 6, 1995. Stone told me he would have appealed but he—and his client—ran out of time.

The dehydration bandwagon has hit a few snags. A recent Wisconsin Supreme Court decision refused to allow a cognitively disabled, conscious Alzheimer's patient to be dehydrated at the request of her sister/caregiver, ruling that they had established a "bright-line rule" limiting dehydration to people who are PVS in part because conscious people might feel the agony of dehydration and to prevent Wisconsin from falling down a "slippery slope for the consequences may be great."[130] Unfortunately, Wisconsin is the exception, not the rule.

This isn't to say that every legal case over the last twenty years has allowed helpless cognitively disabled patients to be dehydrated. Two notable victories against removing food and fluids—Michael Martin in Michigan and Robert Wendland in California—illustrated that the advance of the quality of life death agenda has not been static nor a straight road.

The cases of Michael Martin in Michigan and Robert Wendland in California were remarkably similar to the later-occurring Terri Schiavo brouhaha, although they received far less public notice. Both involved wives of disabled middle-aged men—brain-damaged in auto accidents—who decided to dehydrate their husbands based on their belief that their husbands would prefer to die than live in a profoundly disabled condition. In both cases, the mother and sister of the disabled patient opposed dehydration. Both Michael Martin and Robert Wendland had relatively high levels of functioning, particularly as compared to Terri. Both cases were extended, bitter, and emotionally traumatic for all concerned.

Michael Martin was interactive with caregivers. He enjoyed watching television and listening to country and western music. He was also able to nod his head yes and no and respond to simple requests. In April 1992, he learned how to use a communication augmentation system in which he pointed to letters to express himself. Through the system, he was able to communicate, "My name is Mike."[131] According to the therapist's report, when asked to spell a word, "Mike spelled out the word [water]. When asked to find the character to clear this page, Mike was able to do it independently. Mike also indicated to us in response to a yes/no question, that the scanning device was too slow for him and he wanted it a little faster. When directed to the feelings page, Mike responded to the question of how he was feeling by indicating happy."[132]

In October 1992, as part of the ongoing court case, Dr. Robert K. Kreitsch, a board-certified physician specializing in physical medicine and rehabilitation, evaluated Michael and reported:

> When I first entered the room his radio was on and he agreed to allow it to be turned off. When asked if he is able to see television and follow some shows, he indicates with an affirmative and also again, with a "yes" head nod when asked if he likes certain shows. He brightened up with a large grin when asked if he liked cartoons.... When shown his poster with country western music stars, he again became quite animated with his expression, using a large grin, and was very cooperative in identifying by head nod and attempted to point with his right hand on questioning who were the different stars that I pointed to.... He was 100% accurate on identifying all of these.[133]

Dr. Kreitsch also reported that when asked if he felt at any time it was not worth going on, Michael indicated, "No."[134]

The principal medical expert testifying in favor of dehydration was Ron Cranford, the same doctor who had previously testified in the Cruzan case, and would later in Schiavo. Cranford reported that Michael's left side was completely paralyzed and his right side had limited movement. He was unable to speak or swallow. His ability to answer yes and no questions was "consistently inconsistent." He got some answers wrong, such as whether he wears diapers or whether he is disabled. Moreover, of key concern to Cranford were Michael's pre-injury statements, indicating that he would not want to live with a profound cognitive disability. According to Cranford, Michael smiled when told his daughter had been killed in the accident that caused his own injuries, indicating he didn't understand what he was hearing. Cranford opined, "The horror in this case is that you don't know what he is thinking for sure, you don't know what he's feeling."[135] Michael's wife, Mary, joined Cranford in believing fervently that it was in his best interest to be dehydrated.

Michael's mother and sister stood up for the right of Michael to live. While his life was certainly not what he would have chosen for himself before he was injured, that does not mean that his pre-injury statements reflected his current wishes or that it justified his life being ended by slow dehydration.

The trial court and the court of appeals sided with Mary. But the Michigan Supreme Court ruled 6-1 that conscious, cognitively disabled people can only be dehydrated if it can be demonstrated by clear and convincing evidence—the most stringent standard in civil court—that they would not want to live with their disability and (unlike the standard applied in the Terri Schiavo case) that they *would want to die in the manner that removing food and fluids would cause.* The court ruled wisely, "If we are to err ... we must err in preserving life."[136]

It wasn't long before a similar intra-family struggle broke out in Stockton, California. Like Michael Martin, Robert Wendland was in an automobile accident that left him physically and cognitively disabled and dependent on others for his care. Like Martin and Schiavo, he was not terminally ill. He was not hooked up to machines. All he required to continue on was a feeding tube because he couldn't swallow well enough to eat.

Robert's wife, Rose, decided to dehydrate her husband based primarily on a statement he made in the aftermath of her father's death—three months before the accident—that he would not want to live if he could not "be a husband, father, and provider." [137] It is pertinent that the last time Robert made such a statement—one week before his accident—he and Rose were arguing over his heavy alcoholism and repeated drunk driving. Indeed, Robert's mood was so sour, according to Rose, that he claimed his death or incapacitation would have no impact on the family[138]—as much an indication of depression as a clear and reasoned statement about life.

Robert's mother, Florence Wendland, and half-sister, Rebekah Vinson, were warned of Rose's plan by an anonymous call from a hospital nurse whistleblower. Stunned, they immediately sued to save Robert's life.

Robert was indisputably not PVS, and his ability to perform some activities could not be denied. Thus, Rose's attorney, Steven Scott, and Doran Berg, a San Joaquin deputy public defender appointed to represent Robert in the trial (who decided that her own client should die), tried to convince Judge Bob McNatt to permit Robert's dehydration. Dr. Cranford (yes, again) and other bioethicists and physicians testified in favor of dehydrating Robert, opining that his abilities meant little, amounting to mere "training" rather than truly human behavior. Some of the witnesses even likened his activities to that of trained animals. One went so far as to claim that Robert "is unable to think at all in the manner we conceive humans do."[139] Similarly, the appellate attorney retained by the County of San Joaquin to represent Robert after the trial followed in Berg's footsteps, arguing that his own client should be dehydrated, maintaining that Robert "can respond to simple stimuli somewhat in the manner that an animal might."[140]

What these so-called experts and advocates saw as demeaning, meaningless, and akin to animal behavior could also be described as wonderful victories for someone who progressed from a total sixteen-month unconsciousness to the point where he could:

- Maneuver a manual wheelchair down a corridor;
- Drive an electronic wheelchair down a hospital corridor;
- Retrieve and return colored pegs into a peg-board when asked;
- Take and return a ball when asked;
- Write the letter "R" of his first name when asked as well as some other letters of his name; and
- Use buttons to accurately answer yes and no questions some of the time (e.g., is your name Robert? Yes. Is your name Michael? No.).[141]

Robert could also feel pain. This was significant, considering the agony that dehydration can cause to conscious people.

What kind of pain and suffering accompany dehydration when the patient is not otherwise in the stage of active dying? The same as would be experienced by any of us in such a circumstance. In 1999, a journal article on palliative medicine reported that conscious patients undergoing dehydration suffer "Confusion and restlessness; dry mouth, impaired speech, thirst, increased risk of bedsores, circulatory failure, renal failure … cardiac arrest … confusion, constipation, nausea, myoclonus [rapid, uncontrollable muscle spasms], seizures."[142]

Dr. William Burke, a professor of neurology at St. Louis University Medical Center, summarized for me the suffering caused by dehydration in conscious, non-dying people even more bluntly: "A conscious person would feel it [dehydration] just as you or I would. They will go into seizures. Their skin cracks, their tongue cracks, their lips crack. They may have nosebleeds because of the dryness of the mucus membranes and heaving and vomiting might ensue because of the drying out of the stomach lining. They feel the pangs of hunger and thirst. Imagine going one day without a glass of water! Death by dehydration takes ten to fourteen days. It is an extremely agonizing death."[143]

Even Dr. Cranford, who testified in the Wendland case that he participated in withholding food and fluids from his PVS and conscious, cognitively disabled patients, admitted during the trial that the lips, eyes, and tongue of a person being dehydrated "get extremely dry," although he claimed it is rare for them to crack and bleed, while acknowledging that "anything that is dry for a long period of time may crack. And anything that may crack may bleed...." He also testified that patients undergoing dehydration can experience seizures, although that is rare. That being duly noted, even Dr. Cranford's description of the dehydration process demonstrates the awfulness of the procedure, a process he testified usually takes between ten and fourteen days but in some cases up to twenty-one days:

> After seven to nine days [from commencing dehydration] they begin to lose all fluids in the body, a lot of fluids in the body. And their blood pressure starts to go down. When their blood pressure goes down, their heart rate up.... Their respiration may increase and then the patient experiences what's called a mammalian's diver's reflex where the blood is shunted to the central part of the body from the periphery of the body. So, that usually two to three days prior to death, sometimes four days, the hands and the feet become extremely cold. They become mottled. That is you look at the hands and they have a bluish appearance. And the mouth dries a great deal, and the eyes dry a great deal and other parts of the body become mottled. And that is because the blood is now so low in the system it's shunted to the heart and other visceral organs and away from the periphery of the body....[144]

Proponents of dehydration claim that these symptoms can be palliated by the proper use of eye drops and ice chips for dryness, and morphine for pain. Dr. Cranford also testified that he sometimes puts his dehydrating patients into a coma. But this is a circular—not to mention deeply ironic—argument. The patient wouldn't require strong drugs to palliate suffering except for being denied the basic humane provision of food and water.

But do attempts at palliation really control the suffering? In Robert's case, Dr. Cranford testified that the amount of morphine he would be given would be "arbitrary" because it would "be hard to tell whether he's suffering or not" due to Robert's inability to communicate effectively. If that is true for Robert Wendland, it is also true of other conscious, cognitively disabled people who are dehydrated in nursing homes and hospitals throughout this country.

When dealing with these food and fluids cases, bioethicists often describe dehydration as being "in the best interests of the patient." But that is questionable. What is actually behind many of these decisions is a utilitarian view that some lives are simply not worth living. Read the testimony of Dr. Cranford, in this regard, in the Wendland case and judge for yourself who was really intended to benefit from his death:

> MS. SIESS [Florence and Rebekah's lawyer, Janie Siess]: Why in your opinion as a clinical ethicist should ... the error not be on the side of caution ... and just let Robert live?
>
> (Objection and the Court's overrule omitted.)
>
> THE WITNESS [Dr. Cranford]: The harm to continuing treatment ... is, first of all, there wouldn't be a lot of harm to per se as he is now because he has a minimal level of cognition. It's hard to talk about harm although he has some suffering. It's harmful *to the family* because ... they know his wishes are not being observed. They know he is in limbo or living death if you want to call it that. That's not what *they* want for Robert. I think it's very harmful *for a family* to again feel like they're prisoners of medical technology about his treatment. So—you can go on and on about the psychological harm *to the family. I think the family should be able to go through the grieving process. Four years is enough.* And so I think for people to start functioning again—because it is *really harmful to families* when you get into a situation like this— that *the family should be allowed to live their lives.* They can still love

Robert and remember Robert, *but Robert should be allowed to die so the family can grieve* and go through the normal grieving and knowing that Robert's wishes were respected.... I think it is counterproductive to what medicine should be doing in an era *where we have to look at resources*. Not just money and everything, but to give futile treatment like we do in the United States in situations like this which doesn't benefit the patient and doesn't benefit the family is one major problem for health care costs. So, *I think it is harmful to society to do it.* I think there's a lot of harm that's done by erring on the side of caution. I think it's ridiculous to err on the side of caution when there's [no] doubt in my mind and any reputable person will say he's never going to recover. He's beyond that point.[145] (Emphasis added.)

So, the primary issue for Dr. Cranford and many other bioethicists isn't really the individual patient but rather the impact of profound impairment on family and society. And that presents a cogent ethical challenge to us all.

Judge McNatt refused to permit Rose to dehydrate Robert. Following the clear and convincing evidence standard set forth in *Martin*, and stating that he believed Rose only had Robert's best interests at heart in her decision, McNatt ruled: "In our society, the rules under which Rose must make surrogate decisions are the same ones that someone less compassionate, less ethical would also operate.... To allow termination of Robert's life over the objections of other family members and on the legal basis of the evidence presented would allow the opening of a door that other families with less noble motives might follow through.... To allow it would be to start down a treacherous road."[146]

The California Supreme Court ultimately decided the case. (I filed an amicus brief in the case on the side of Florence and Rebecca.) Even though Robert died of pneumonia after the oral arguments, the high court issued an important unanimous ruling granting important protections to *some* cognitively disabled people (e.g., the conscious) that as a matter of protecting the right to life of conscious, cognitively disabled patients, a court-appointed conservator must prove by "clear and convincing evidence" that withholding tube-supplied food and fluids is in the patient's "best interests" or would have been what the patient wanted.[147]

That much was fine. But, frighteningly, the court also ruled that such basic constitutional protections do not extend to people who are diagnosed as permanently unconscious. In other words, according to the California Supreme Court, Robert Wendland enjoyed full constitutional rights when he was an auto parts salesman. But he lost at least some of these protections during sixteen months of unconsciousness, only to regain them when he awakened. Or, to put it another way, the court declared that unconscious people have lesser rights and their lives are entitled to fewer legal protections than those of conscious people, a radical decision that may mark the beginning of a personhood theory of constitutional jurisprudence in the United States.

Forcing Nursing Homes to Withhold Spoon-Feeding: In 2014, bioethicists and right-to-die advocates opened a new front in the food and fluids cases. Previously—as discussed above—the fight over removing or refusing sustenance involved *medical treatment* (e.g., ANH) from incompetent patients based on what they would have wanted or what was deemed in their best interests. But what about incompetent people who did not require medically provided sustenance but had previously indicated they would not want to live under the now-existing circumstances? Since they can't be legally euthanized in most jurisdictions—Netherlands and Belgium permit such medicalized killings of the incompetent—the portentous question has been raised whether under these circumstances nursing homes and other care facilities should be *required to withhold spoon-feeding*—even if the patient willingly eats, and, one presumes, even like Marjorie Nighbert, the patient asks for food.

This is not an alarmist fantasy but already the subject of multiple articles in bioethics journals and, as of this writing, at least one lawsuit. Indeed, as has occurred with the question of tube-supplied sustenance in the 1980s, the intellectual groundwork is now being laid for legislation or court orders requiring nursing homes, hospitals, and other facilities to withhold spoon-feeding from incompetent dementia patients if they requested to be starved and dehydrated to death in an advance medical directive.

Consider the Bentley case in Canada: The family of an Alzheimer's patient named Margot Bentley filed a lawsuit in 2013 in British Columbia. Bentley had signed an advance directive instructing that she be refused life-sustaining treatment—or be euthanized—if she became unable to recognize her children. She eventually was diagnosed with Alzheimer's disease. But she did not require life-extending medical treatment that could be withdrawn, such as ANH or a respirator. Moreover, she willingly accepted food and water by mouth. Thus, there was no legal way of making sure she died immediately.

Bentley's family thought her continued existence unjust and asked a court to order her nursing home to starve her to death. The trial court refused, in part because Bentley's advance directive did not specifically reject spoon-feeding. Thankfully, that determination was upheld on appeal.

The Canadian court's ruling should not make us sanguine. The Bentley case was merely the first skirmish in what promises to be a longer conflict. Already, bioethicists are publishing articles in prominent medical and bioethics journals arguing that nursing homes and hospitals should be required to starve dementia patients who directed their lives be so ended in an advance directive. For example, Hamline University law professor and bioethicist Thaddeus Mason Pope argued in the Spring 2014 *Journal of Clinical Ethics* that Margot Bentley should be starved because she is now incompetent and thus is legally unqualified to change her mind about dying, writing in part:

> It seems remarkable to hold that, when a spoon or glass is pressed to the lips of someone with severe dementia, the mere opening of her or his mouth evidences decisional capacity to continue eating and drinking. Mrs. Bentley may have the capacity to "communicate a choice." But this is just one component of capacity. She does not understand the relevant information, does not appreciate the situation and its consequences, and cannot reason about treatment or care options."[148]

In other words, Pope asserts that patients in Bentley's condition should *not be allowed* to thwart a previously stated desire to die by the act of willingly taking nourishment.

Similarly, an article published in the prestigious *Hastings Center Report* also supported forced starvation of dementia patients who requested to be so killed in an advance medical directive. Writing in the May/June 2014 edition, Paul T. Menzel and M. Colette Chandler-Cramer argue:

Such directives are ... arguably already legal. They follow logically from the intersection of two existing legal rights: directives for refusing life support and VSED ["voluntary stop eating and drinking," discussed later]. The principle behind [advance medical directives] is that people do not lose their rights when they become incompetent; someone else just has to exercise those rights for them. The driving element behind VSED is that forcing people to ingest food is as objectionable an intrusion on bodily integrity, privacy, and liberty as imposing unwanted medical treatment. Thus, if incompetent people do not lose their rights to refuse life-saving treatment, then people do not lose their right to VSED when incompetent either.[149]

This is rank sophistry. No court has ever deemed that spoon-feeding is a medical treatment. To the contrary, it is basic, *humane care*—no different ethically from turning a patient to prevent bedsores or providing hygiene. Patients have the right to refuse medical treatment in a written directive, but not humane care. Thus just as written instructions that a patient not be kept clean should be disregarded, so too should an order from the patient that she be starved if she becomes incompetent.

If this early advocacy for forced starvation prevails, the pretext that removing feeding tubes is merely the withdrawal of unwanted medical treatment will be exposed as a mere pretext applied to justify killing patients with profound cognitive impairments. But rather than retreating from such slow-motion imposed deaths and allowing these patients to live, the cruelty of starvation would instead become the justification for lethally injecting these helpless patients as the "compassionate" and "gentle" method of putting these unwanted lives into their graves.

CHAPTER 3

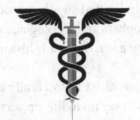

THE PRICE OF AUTONOMY

"I don't want to be hooked up to medical machines when I am dying."

How often I have heard those words during question-and-answer sessions after speeches and on talk radio. People's fear of being tethered to high-tech medical machines against their will is persistent and consistent across the entire political, religious, and moral spectrums of American life: Pro-lifers are as concerned as pro-choicers; conservatives as liberals; the young as the elderly. Indeed, if I were asked to choose the most common worry people have about their own deaths, it is this nightmare scenario.

Fears about being forced to stay alive beyond reason are often based on real-life experiences of loved ones and friends who had "bad" and elongated death experiences in hospital ICU wards, the last place people want to die. But the worry about being "forced" to remain alive is growing outdated. Today, with the changing economics of medicine, getting the machines when you *want* them is fast becoming the more pressing problem.

It is true that doctors once believed they had a duty to use every weapon in medicine's armamentarium to prevent death. But those days

are long gone—thanks in large part to bioethics. In the 1960s, the medical community began quiet professional discussions about how to move
end-of-life care toward a better balance. Other issues were also joined in
this professional soul searching, such as how to justly distribute medical treatments that were in limited supply, particularly access to kidney
dialysis machines. Philosophers and theologians were invited to enter the
fray, and, as the old saying goes, the rest is history: Bioethics, as it came
to be known, was born.

Ironically, the first bioethicist to forcefully approach the subject of
respecting people's rights to say no to life-preserving treatment was Paul
Ramsey, a devout believer in the sanctity of human life. In the late 1960s,
Ramsey gave a series of lectures on the topic, which he later expanded
into *The Patient as a Person*,[1] a book that bioethics historian Albert R.
Jonsen describes as the "first truly modern study of the new ethics of
science and medicine."[2] Here, Ramsey argued forcefully against keeping
dying patients alive against their will with what were then called "heroic"
measures. (At the time, physicians and ethicists made a distinction
between "extraordinary care" and "ordinary care," a concept that is still
accepted by many among the public but that has been rejected in bioethics, in medical ethics, and in law.)

Ramsey argued that there came a time when it was morally acceptable to "only" give palliative care for people who were actively dying
while ceasing curative or life-prolonging treatment that was "no longer
merciful or reasonable."[3] Using language that presaged the approach of
the modern hospice movement that was even then aborning, Ramsey
advocated "systemic change" in the medical approach to dying:

> If the sting of death is sin, the sting of dying is solitude. What doctors
> should do in the presence of the process of dying is only a special case
> of what should be done to make a human presence felt to the dying.
> Desertion is more choking than death and more feared. The chief prob-
> lem of the dying is how not to die alone. To care, if only to care, for the
> dying is, therefore, a medical-moral imperative; it is a requirement of us
> all in exhibiting faithfulness to all who bear a human countenance....
> "The process of dying" needs to be got out of the hospitals and back
> into the home and in the midst of family, neighborhood, and friends.[4]

The difference between Ramsey's advocacy and the "quality of life" approach that permeates contemporary bioethical discourse cannot be overstated. To Ramsey, that each individual life is precious in and of itself has incalculable value—regardless of physical condition. To care without trying to cure is not to reject the human value of dying people or denigrate their moral worth; it is not to label them pejoratively as "non-persons," mere organisms, or human objects. To the contrary, Ramsey advocated *increasing* our human commitment to dying people. Don't hide them in hospital ICUs tethered to machines, he said. Embrace them, value them, be present for them by ensuring that at their time of dying they receive the most personal and beneficent gifts we are capable of giving: unconditional love, true compassion (which means to suffer with), and unequivocal commitment to their overall medical well-being.

Ramsey—along with Dame Cecily Saunders's forceful contemporaneous promotion of modern hospice care—lit a fuse. Soon, others within bioethics, both the "sanctity of life" and "quality of life" perspectives, took up the cause. Within a few years, the often-contentious branches of bioethics of that era reached rare agreement that when it came to accepting or rejecting rigorous medical interventions, patients, not doctors, should be in ultimate control of what happened with their own bodies.

These bioethics debates did not arise in a vacuum, of course. Other societal factors energized the emergence of patient autonomy as a central tenet of modern medicine. For example, the consumer movement taught that people could exert power in their professional relations. The furious cultural debate over abortion in the wake of *Roe v. Wade* made autonomy a primary issue in medicine. In the wake of Viet Nam, the idea of "questioning authority" resonated with much of the public. Many people no longer wanted doctors to be altruistic dictators, and doctors no longer wanted that responsibility. For both better and worse, the traditional physician/patient relationship in which patients put their health care completely in the hands of their doctors became obsolete.

This confluence of powerful cultural shifts within a few short years sparked legal and ethical reform, leading to a new culture of medicine that stressed the inviolability of patient autonomy in health care decision-making. The doctor's duty was to sufficiently inform the patient about the intended benefits, potential risks, and alternatives of treatment or testing, and to give recommendations. But now, it was up to patients to decide for themselves in which direction they wanted to go.

The new approach, it is important to note, evolved when health care was not in a financial crisis. Indeed, the cultural, medical, and financial incentives in these years were heavily weighted toward providing rather than restricting care. Thus the primary focus of "informed consent" was to guarantee the patient's right to say no to medical care that was still readily accessible and where the prospect of "death panels" was not even a dark cloud on the horizon.

The triumph of autonomy was soon complete. Today, it is profoundly unethical to force competent people to receive unwanted treatment, and, indeed, doctors can be sued if they do. Except in a few extraordinary situations, patients must give their explicit permission before being medically treated, including those times when refusing treatment will likely to lead to death. Thus mentally competent patients who don't want to be hooked up to medical machines don't have to be hooked up to medical machines. If they don't want to be hospitalized, they can refuse to be admitted. If they want to leave the hospital, even when their doctors disagree, they can be discharged against medical advice. If they wish to refuse chemotherapy or any other urgent treatment needed to stay alive, then so be it. This patient-empowering reform in health care was a profound victory for patients that improved the practice of modern medicine and helped move the health care system toward a more patient-centered medical ethic. For this, it must be said, bioethics deserves much of the credit.

AUTONOMY OR ABANDONMENT?

And yet, patient choice does not occur in a social vacuum. Indeed, the preexisting cultural biases of medicine have been turned inside out. Whereas providing intensive treatment used to be the standard of care, today's biases push forcefully against providing expensive care, particularly when the patient is elderly, dying, or significantly disabled. In fact, as we saw in the first pages of this book, patients or families who request "disfavored" treatments often find themselves pushed, pressured, and cajoled by doctors, nurses, social workers, hospital chaplains, and bioethics committees to change their minds. Moreover, the intense emphasis placed on autonomy by bioethics training has made it far easier for health care professionals to accede to requests to terminate life-saving care made by vulnerable and depressed people in their darkest hours. Indeed, bio-ethics' campaign against medical paternalism may have succeeded too well, allowing "respect for persons" to sometimes mask acts of discrimi-nation against people with significant health problems or disabilities.

An early "right to die" case that occurred in California in the 1980s illustrates the point. Elizabeth Bouvia decided she wanted medical help in starving herself to death. Bouvia was suicidal after undergoing one devastating emotional crisis after another: her brother died, she was in deep financial distress, she had a miscarriage, she was forced out of graduate school, and she divorced—all within approximately two years. She decided to commit suicide by self-starvation and checked into a hos-pital where she hoped to be given palliative measures to ease the agony of dehydration. Instead, the hospital inserted a feeding tube to keep her from dying.

If the stated reasons for wanting to self-destruct had been the emo-tional blows listed above, it is doubtful that she would have received significant support in her quest to die. But Bouvia was quadriplegic, disabled from birth by cerebral palsy. In many minds, the mere fact of her significant disability made her request for help in dying rational and reasonable.

When the feeding tube issue arose, so did the controversy over patient autonomy.

The American Civil Liberties Union leaped to her aid, as did mem-bers of the growing "right to die" movement. Her attorney, Richard Scott, had been the first legal counsel for the assisted suicide advocacy organization the Hemlock Society. One of the psychological experts who testified that she should be allowed medical help in starvation was Faye Girsh, who later became the executive director of the National Hemlock Society and today remains active in assisted suicide advocacy as a senior adviser to the Final Exit Network.

After two trial judges ruled against Bouvia, the case ended up in a California Court of Appeals. In language dripping with the pervasive societal prejudice against disabled people, Judge Lynn Compton wrote, "In Elizabeth Bouvia's view, the quality of her life has been diminished to the point of hopelessness, uselessness, unenjoyability, and frustra-tion. She, as the patient lying helplessly in bed, unable to care for her-self, may consider existence meaningless. She is not to be faulted for so concluding.... We cannot conceive it to be the policy of this State to inflict such an ordeal on anybody."[5]

The Bouvia case became a landmark in establishing the right of people to refuse unwanted medical treatment and in defining tube-feeding as medical treatment rather than humane care. But did the court's order forcing Bouvia's doctors to cease suicide prevention and tube-feeding really serve to overcome, in bioethicist heavyweight Robert M. Veatch's words, "the oppression of the physician's paternalism"?[6] Most bioethicists and civil libertarians say yes unequivocally, viewing the case as an important blow for patient autonomy. But many among the disability rights community were appalled at the decision. The late Paul Longmore, a national disability rights leader and professor of history at California State University San Francisco, followed the case closely. He told me, "Throughout the litigation and in the court's ruling, there was a pervasive prejudicial assumption that she wanted to die because of her disability. The fact that she had suffered tremendous and severe emotional blows that could seriously undermine anyone's desire to go on living was virtually ignored in the courts and the media. Such thinking represents oppression and a profound disrespect for the value of her life."[7]

Which was it: respect for autonomy or abandonment of someone deemed by able-bodied observers and judges to have a life not worth living? The ironic denouement of the Bouvia case provides us with some important clues. Despite winning the right to refuse tube-feeding as she starved herself to death, Bouvia soon resumed eating and left the hospital. To the best of my knowledge, as of this writing in March 2015, she lives independently, if not altogether happily, with the help of a personal assistant. Her attorney is the one who ultimately committed suicide.

Perhaps what Bouvia really needed most at that time of profound emotional crisis was not cold "autonomy" but intervention and sufficient time to recover her equilibrium. Perhaps her most urgent need wasn't "choice" but for others to value her life more than she then did. Whatever can be said about her doctors' "paternalism," it saved her life. Had she been given her way immediately upon request, she would probably be dead today.

Bioethicist Art Caplan gives a clearer example of the principle of autonomy gone wrong. One day, Thomas W. Passmore, a man with a history of mental illness, looked at his hand and was horrified to see the numbers 666—the sign of the devil. Completely lost in his hallucination, intent on saving his soul, Passmore cut off the offending hand with a circular saw. He was taken quickly to a hospital, where, according to Caplan, things took a "crazy turn." Passmore, still believing that his hand carried the symbol of evil, refused to permit surgeons to reattach his hand. A psychiatrist was called in; lawyers were consulted; a judge refused to intervene. In the end, no one would act to save the hallucinating man from himself.

This was a profound and unsettling abandonment of a mentally ill, self-destructive man in desperate need of help from the medical professionals whose responsibility it was to care for him. Instead, because of the increasingly extreme view of self-determination that permeates modern medicine, those who should have helped Passmore became morally paralyzed. As Caplan so aptly put it, "A nation that has created a health-care system in which doctors, nurses, and administrators are not sure whether it the right thing to do to sew a mentally ill man's severed hand back onto his arm is a society gone over the edge regarding autonomy."[8]

A more recent case illustrates how respecting individuals' autonomy more than their life has the potential to harm people with disabilities. Georgette Smith, age forty-two, was shot in the spine by her mother in a dispute about the older woman being placed in a nursing home. The wound literally broke Smith's neck, leaving her unable to move and completely dependent on a ventilator to breathe, much like the physical circumstances faced by the late actor Christopher Reeve after his horseback riding accident.

Smith was understandably distraught over her quadriplegia. Not only that, but she also had been shot by *her own mother*, which surely added to her despair. Only three months after her injury, she decided that she had nothing left to live for and instructed her doctors to remove her ventilator. Her children supported her decision and a court quickly confirmed Smith's autonomous right to refuse unwanted medical treatment. Within a few days, she was dead.

Smith's death caused only mild controversy and then primarily over whether or not Smith's mother should be charged with murder. Perhaps the system's rush to honor her desire to die by ending treatment should have caused more reflection. Read the words of the chief of staff at the hospital where Smith died, Dr. Juan P. Suarez, about the case:

Georgette Smith did not commit suicide. *A person can only commit suicide if he or she is alive.* Smith was kept alive artificially.... By keeping Smith alive against her wishes, we would have hurt her.... Life as a [high] quadriplegic is not easy. These patients can't walk away from their ventilators; their mobility is gone. Yes, [Christopher] Reeve looks good and appears cheerful. But the only images we see of him are the ones that television grants us. We don't see the special hospital bed he lives on, or the catheter he carries for urination or the ventilator that is hidden away from the cameras. The reality is that he can't breathe on his own, and if his ventilator would stop, he would die quickly.[9] (Emphasis added.)

These are cold words. Smith was not really "alive" because she needed medical intervention to sustain her life. Well, so do diabetics and people who require kidney dialysis. Are we really at the point where we want to distinguish between truly "alive" people and "artificially alive" people? Dr. Suarez also seems to be saying that her life would probably never be worth living because of the many physical difficulties caused by paralysis. Isn't that just another way of saying that we value the lives of healthy, able-bodied people more than we do disabled or sick people who may require intensive medical treatment to keep on living? Besides, it is a false premise. Many people who become quadriplegic from illness or injury, given time, go on to lead rich and satisfying lives.

It is certainly true that Smith did not commit suicide but not because she wasn't really alive. Her death resulted from her injury, not from an outside cause such as poison. But that does not mean that her death was unavoidable or should not have been delayed. The thought lingers like a sour stomach: What if Georgette Smith would have later changed her mind and decided to get on with her life like Elizabeth Bouvia did? Seen in this light, by removing her ventilator only three months after her injury, did we simply respect patient autonomy or actually abandon her at the moment of her darkest despair?

After a terrible tragedy, people sometimes need to be carried. That isn't condescension; it is love. Perhaps a mild dose of potentially life-saving paternalism, including psychiatric intervention and counseling by members of the disabled community, would have been the right prescription for Smith; not forever certainly, and not in the pejorative sense of the term as meant by bioethicists but as an expression of society's unequivocal commitment to her equal moral worth. Indeed, in cases like Smith's, shouldn't every reasonable effort have been made to give the patient sufficient time and information to permit her to change her mind?

As part of her rehabilitation process, Smith could have been urged to visit at length with disabled people who would have come to her bedside with a different perspective than she might have been receiving from her family and doctors. Disabled people could have been living demonstrations to Smith that there were valid reasons to go on, that there is indeed life—often good life—after quadriplegia. For as disability rights activist Diane Coleman told me, "The disability culture is rich and diverse and welcoming. We have a lot to offer and people who are newly disabled, who often come to see that we have a lot to live for." Unfortunately, many newly disabled people, their family members, and the medical professionals who care for them do not only "not know" that but they can't even imagine it—often with lethal results. "Our priorities are all mixed up," Coleman says. "When we demand services that would help us to live in liberty we are resisted at almost every turn. But if we ask to die, lawyers, doctors, bioethicists, and everyone else comes out of the woodwork and are more than happy to help."[10]

The case of Larry McAfee proves that such interventions work. McAfee, who was disabled with quadriplegia in a motorcycle accident, asked to have his feeding tube removed because, "every day when I wake up, there is nothing to look forward to."[11] McAfee convinced a judge to permit his feeding tube to be withdrawn. But then something wonderful happened. Because his story made headlines, people rushed to the young man's assistance. Disabled people with rich and fulfilling lives visited him and assured him his life could change. He was given a computer, which he was able to operate because of a software program that allowed him to control the machine by using his head, thereby allowing McAfee to pursue his interest in architecture and engineering. Then he left the nursing home in which he had been warehoused and lived with other disabled men with the aid of personal assistants who helped him with tasks of daily living—people he could hire and fire—meaning that he was again in control of his own life. McAfee changed his mind and decided he wanted to continue. He lived for several more personally rewarding years—he died in 1996—that he would have been denied had he carried out his "autonomous" desire to die. Perhaps the same happy result awaited Smith had she been given sufficient time and access to similar "paternalistic" outreach and love.

The Bouvia approach has grown stronger in the intervening years. As noted in the last chapter—and will be later in this discussion—many in bioethics support doctors helping elderly and disabled people to commit suicide through self-starvation, supported and promoted by the euthanasia movement.

Reflecting the general attitude within bioethics on these issues, Robert Veatch (who was the director of medical ethics at the Kennedy Institute of Ethics, Georgetown University) believes, "No matter how tragic, autonomy should always win if its only competitor is the paternalistic form of beneficence,"[12] an interestingly absolutist statement for a bioethicist to make, considering the relativism that generally permeates the movement. But such a rigid approach as surely dooms some people to deaths that they might not want in the future as never permitting people to refuse care dooms them to lives they don't want to live. Death will wait. In appropriate cases, why not give life every reasonable chance to be embraced before acquiescing to action that can never be rescinded?

PULLING SOMEONE ELSE'S PLUG

The exercise of autonomy, by definition, requires mental competence. But all are not capable of making their own medical decisions. Infants and children are too young. People with serious mental conditions, such as Alzheimer's disease, psychosis, or diagnosed persistent unconsciousness, may not have the mental capacity to make informed and reasoned choices. Whatever the reason, when a patient is incapable of giving informed consent or refusal, a health care "proxy" must step in, be it a spouse, sibling, adult child, court-appointed conservator, public guardian, or recipient of decision-making powers in the patient's advance medical directive.

In the past, when most physicians felt duty-bound to keep their patients alive for as long as possible, surrogate decision making wasn't a significant issue. When it came to deciding whether or not to prolong life medically, there was usually only one answer: yes. However, when patients won the right to refuse unwanted life-prolonging medical treatment, a new complication entered the picture. It is one thing to pull your own plug, but pulling someone else's is something else again.

Paul Ramsey, the Christian bioethicist who first advocated granting patients the right to refuse unwanted medical treatment, presciently worried that surrogate decision making could endanger the lives of devalued people. Accordingly, he tried to rally the bioethics movement behind protocols that would ensure that proxy decisions would be strictly based on the *medical needs* of the incompetent patients—as distinguished from basing non-treatment decisions on the biases and prejudices of the decision makers toward the disabled, elderly, and seriously ill. Straying from such an objective approach, he warned, could shift "the focus from whether *treatments* are beneficial to patients to whether patients' *lives* are beneficial to them."[13]

The right of patient proxies to refuse life-prolonging medical treatment reached critical mass in New Jersey when the parents of Karen Ann Quinlan, a young woman who had been unconscious for several years, sued her hospital to compel them to remove her respirator. The case went all the way to the New Jersey Supreme Court, which in 1976 ruled (properly, in my view) that Karen's parents, not her doctors or hospital administrators, had the right to decide about her care. Further, this right included the power to refuse treatment even if it meant the patient would likely die. (Karen's respirator was removed, but unexpectedly she breathed on her own and lived for approximately ten more years before succumbing to pneumonia. Her parents never considered removing her food and water.) Most other states quickly followed New Jersey's lead, as did the federal government.

That still left a huge problem: *How* were these decisions to be made for people unable to decide for themselves? Upon whose values should the decisions be based? What standards of decision making should apply? How could the lives of the most vulnerable among us be protected from wrongful ending on one hand while still permitting autonomy on the other? And how might doctors be compelled to accede to surrogate decision making if they are not willing to do so?

Advance Medical Directives: The answer to many of these questions was the advance medical directive, a legal document that instructs caregivers and/or physicians about the signers' desires for future medical care—whether they want treatment or not and under what circumstances. The directives are used if and when the patient becomes so incapacitated that they are unable to give informed consent.

Advance medical directives have the potential to be a positive anti-
dote to overzealous doctors keeping patients alive through unwanted
medical treatment or to prevent care wanted from being cut off. Too
often, advocacy and education about advance directives when they first
appeared on the scene seemed aimed at persuading people to refuse
treatment. But in recent years, improvements have been made allowing
people to more easily determine both the kinds of care they want and the
interventions they choose to reject.

There are two primary forms of advance directives. The first is generically known as a "living will," which provides instructions to physicians about the provision or withholding of treatment. There are several
problems with living wills, the worst one perhaps being that none of us
can anticipate the exact medical circumstances under which we may be
unable to make medical decisions.

The better approach is to appoint a trusted family member, friend,
or clergy member to become your surrogate decision maker, who can be
trusted to follow instructions on the advance directive and make person-
alized decisions consistent with your values. This document is usually
called the "durable power of attorney for healthcare." As Rita Marker,
executive director of the Patients Rights Council, has written, "The most
protective and the most flexible type of advance directive is the durable
power of attorney for health care. With this type of document you des-
ignate someone else to make healthcare decisions on your behalf if you
are ever temporarily or permanently unable to make those decisions for
yourself. The person you name is usually called an 'agent,' although some
states refer to this individual as an 'attorney-in-fact,' a 'healthcare proxy,'
a 'healthcare representative,' or a 'healthcare surrogate.'"[14]

If everyone prepared an advance directive, many of the headaches
associated with end-of-life surrogate medical decision making would
disappear. Unfortunately, most people do not have advance directives,
forcing proxies to try and figure the decisions out for themselves. (This
question became acutely visible during the Terri Schiavo debacle.)

But what about patients who do not prepare advance directives?
After all, in such cases, decisions will still have to be made for patients
unable to decide.

There are two general approaches in medicine and law that are used
in such circumstances. The *substituted judgment* standard has the proxy

figuratively "stand in the shoes" of the person for whom the medical decision is being made. The proxy then accepts or rejects treatment based on what the incompetent person would have probably chosen under the same circumstances. This may be easy or difficult, depending on how well the proxy knew the patient and how precise the patient was about his or her desires. When families are in dispute over supplying or withholding life support, for example, in the interests of protecting vulnerable people, strong evidence of the patient wanting to refuse care may be required, as occurred in the Michael Martin and Terri Schiavo cases discussed in the last chapter.

The other primary approach to proxy decision making is known as the *best interests* standard. When deciding whether to accept or reject treatment, the proxy weighs the burdens and benefits of care, the risks and the costs, the potential for pain, and other factors, such as whether the treatment will restore health or functioning. The best interest standard is usually the one utilized by parents on behalf of infants, for example, since parents are expected to have their baby's best welfare at heart. However, there is a pronounced danger here. In an increasingly utilitarian health care system, disfavored people such as premature infants, demented elderly people, or others with marginal physical or mental abilities can fall victim to decision making based on the notion that their lives are unworthy of being lived.

Most of us want to avoid our loved ones fighting over end-of-life or continued care disputes. Happily, these goals are readily attainable by signing an advance medical directive, preferably the durable power of attorney—although, as we will see later, many bioethicists now urge that doctors and hospital ethics committees be enabled to essentially veto advance directives that request all efforts be engaged to keep the patient alive.

POLST: In recent years, a new medical instruction document has come into widespread use that provides doctors, nurses, and other caregivers readily accessible instructions on the kind of treatment to provide to—or withhold from—a hospitalized patient or resident of an assisted living or extended care facility. POLST ("physician's order for life-sustaining treatment") or MOLST ("medical orders for life-sustaining treatment") forms are signed by the patient or duly appointed surrogate when entering a medical or caregiving facility. Once completed and signed, it is countersigned by the doctor, or perhaps a physician's assistant or certified nurse practitioner, and then filed in the patient's chart. (They are readily recognized by title and being printed on brightly colored paper.)

POLSTs allow the patient or duly appointed surrogate to quickly—in a checklist format—give instructions regarding common questions such as whether to provide CPR in the event of a cardiac arrest, whether a nursing home patient should be sent to the hospital if she experiences a life-threatening medical event, whether treatments such as antibiotics or blood transfusions are desired, whether to provide ANH in the event the patient is unable to swallow, and the like. Many forms permit temporary treatment to be ordered pending further instructions—which is the approach I ordered on the POLST form I signed as the surrogate medical decision maker for my late aunt.

A POLST is supposed to be wholly voluntary—although what constitutes "voluntary" may depend on the interpreter. Special care is required when signing a POLST, as the instructions provided can mean the difference between living and dying. In this regard, it is worth noting that there are fewer protections creating a POLST than an advance medical directive. For example, the person who signs an advance directive (AD) must be competent, and it usually has to be witnessed or notarized. Not so the POLST, which can be signed by a surrogate—and that, at least in theory, could be contrary to the terms of an AD.

Perhaps most important, a POLST *follows the patient* from facility to facility. This can be a problem. For example, assume eighty-eight-year-old Margaret enters a hospital with serious pneumonia and refuses CPR by agreeing to a do-not-resuscitate order (DNR) on the POLST. She later recovers and is restored to full vitality. She may forget the DNR exists, but unless she invalidates or changes the instructions, the DNR remains in full force and effect—and indeed will control her care in a later facility admission—even if under the then-existing circumstances the DNR no longer reflects her desires.

The laws surrounding POLSTs are quickly evolving, and I cannot do the issue justice in a general discussion nor guarantee that the text has kept up with the times. For a more detailed discussion and up-to-date information on POLSTs, I strongly suggest researching the material offered by the Patients Rights Council at www.patientsrightscouncil.org.

The Liverpool Care Pathway: ADs and POLST forms can be an important element of ensuring quality care for patients unable to make their own decisions. But despite the protections these documents provide, pulling the plug of those unable to decide for themselves will always remain a delicate and sometimes hazardous enterprise. This is particularly true in hospitals straining under the burden of limited resources and where busy nursing homes may be tempted to practice medicine by-the-numbers and/or make treatment withdrawal decisions by rote.

The Liverpool Care Pathway is a terrible case in point. Conceived in the UK to remedy the National Health Service's abysmal record of treating pain in dying patients, well-meaning pain-control experts created a protocol—known as the Liverpool Care Pathway (LCP)—which, among other provisions, informed doctors when to apply a legitimate medical palliative intervention known as palliative sedation. The protocol was recommended for adoption by the National Institute on Clinical Excellence (NICE)—the NHS's rationing and quality oversight board—and there you go: problem solved.[15]

Except it wasn't. Indeed, as so often happens in centralized systems, the bureaucratic remedy for one problem led to even worse trouble—a form of backdoor euthanasia—down the line.

To understand what went so badly wrong in the implementation of the LCP—and why it is important to understand in a time of increasing centralization of health care—we must first detail the crucial moral and factual distinctions between the legitimate pain-controlling medical treatment known as palliative sedation (PS) and a slow-motion method of euthanasia sometimes called terminal sedation (TS). The two are too often conflated, particularly by euthanasia advocates seeking to blur important moral distinctions and definitions.

A very good article published in the *Journal of Pain & Palliative Care Pharmacotherapy* clearly distinguishes between sedation applied to control pain and sedation used as a method of killing.[16] First, author Michael P. Hahn, a respiratory therapist with Loma Linda University, notes that palliative sedation applies the least amount of sedative to obtain the needed relief: "Ideally, the level of palliative sedation is provided in a fashion that is titrated to a minimal level that permits the patient to tolerate unbearable symptoms, yet the patient can continue to periodically communicate."[17]

PS is tailored to the needs of the individual patient. For example, the level of sedation may be varied to the extent that it "may ... be provided intermittently or continuously."[18] In other words, palliative sedation is a *medical treatment* applied *when necessary* to relieve intense suffering; it offers *individualized* relief from pain and suffering (caused by conditions such as severe agitation) *as the situation may warrant*. It is *not directed at causing death or ending the patient's life*. If the patient dies, it is usually from the underlying condition or as an unwanted side effect, which can happen with any medical treatment.

In contrast, terminal sedation *intends to kill* by putting the person into a permanent artificial coma conjoined with depriving the patient of food and fluids. TS-induced deaths usually are caused by dehydration over a period of about two weeks. In this sense, Hahn notes, PS and TS, while both using consciousness-altering drugs, are mirror opposites.

With the above in mind, we now return to the Liverpool Care Pathway and what went wrong. It is clear that the LCP's authors never intended it to become a form of TS. For example, an educational document prepared for health care professionals by the Marie Curie Palliative Care Institute (Liverpool)—under which auspices the Pathway was created—notes that the specific "aim" of the Pathway was to "improve care of the dying in the last hours or days of life," stating specifically that a "blanket policy" of withdrawing ANH "is ethically indefensible."[19]

Alas, many NHS hospitals and nursing homes instituted just such an indefensible "blanket" approach to the LCP. The serious problems with the Pathway first came to light in 2009 when the *Telegraph* published an open letter signed by palliative physicians and other pain-control experts complaining that hospital personnel were applying the LCP in a "tick-box" manner that threatened the lives of patients who did not need sedation based on their medical conditions.

> Just as in the financial world, where so-called algorithmic banking has caused problems by blindly following a computer model, so a similar tick-box approach to the management of death is causing a national crisis in care. The government is rolling out a new treatment pattern of palliative care into hospitals, nursing homes, and residential homes. It is based on experience in a Liverpool hospice. If you tick all the right boxes in the LCP, the inevitable outcome of the consequent treatment is death.

This, the letter writers warned, had resulted in some patients who were not actively dying—a core requirement for application of the LCP—being sedated: "As a result, a nationwide wave of discontent is building up, as family and friends witness the denial of fluids and food to patients. Syringe drivers are being used to give continuous terminal sedation, without regard to the fact that the diagnosis could be wrong.... Experienced doctors know that sometimes, when all but essential drugs are stopped, 'dying' patients get better."[20]

A concurrent *Telegraph* story reported that an alarming *16.5 percent* of patients who died in 2007–2008 expired while under "continuous deep sedation."[21] Soon, disturbing stories in the press added credence to the open letter writers' fears. Again, the *Telegraph* led the way, reporting Rosemary Munkenbeck's claim that her father, hospitalized with a stroke, was quickly deprived of fluids and medications. She further claimed that doctors wanted to sedate him under the Pathway protocols until he died. The family refused, but not before Munkenbeck's father went five days without sustenance.[22]

The *Sunday Times* of London soon reported another case, headlined "Daughter Saves Mother, 80, Left by Doctors to Starve":

An 80-year-old grandmother who doctors identified as terminally ill and left to starve to death has recovered after her outraged daughter intervened. Hazel Fenton, from East Sussex, is alive nine months after medics ruled she had only days to live, withdrew her antibiotics and denied her artificial feeding. The former school matron had been placed on a controversial care plan intended to ease the last days of dying patients. Doctors say Fenton is an example of patients who have been condemned to death on the Liverpool Care Pathway plan. They argue that while it is suitable for patients who do have only days to live, it is being used more widely in the NHS, denying treatment to elderly patients who are not dying.[23]

Fenton lived to tell the tale. Not so for seventy-six-year-old Jack Jones. As reported by the *Daily Mail*, Jones was hospitalized in the belief that his previous cancer had recurred and was now terminal. The family claimed he was soon denied food and water and put into deep sedation. But his autopsy showed that *he did not have cancer at all* but actually a treatable infection. The hospice denied wrongdoing but paid £18,000 to Jones's widow.[24]

As time progressed, it became abundantly clear that despite the LCP's good intentions, as applied in clinical settings, the protocol often became a form of backdoor euthanasia. "At many hospitals more than 50 per cent of all patients who died had been placed on the pathway and in one case the proportion of foreseeable deaths on the pathway was almost nine out of ten."[25]

Space does not permit a full description of the history of, and argumentation about, the LCP. In the end, everyone came to understand that a well-intended policy had gone badly off the rails, causing the needless deaths of multiple patients and eroding faith in the British health care system. The NHS phased out the LCP in 2013.[26]

The LCP debacle carries a strong warning for the United States, particularly given the passage in 2010 of the Affordable Care Act. The ACA did not establish socialized medicine of the kind operating in the UK. But it did centralize federal bureaucratic control over much of the American health care system and authorized the government to offer incentives to doctors and medical institutions to follow predefined approaches of providing "excellence." Indeed, many of the architects and implementers of the ACA have stated that they hope to emulate NICE-style cost containment/quality care methods—the very approach that subverted proper application of the LCP. As the country searches for ways to curb health care spending, consideration of the cost-effectiveness of health interventions will unavoidably be part of the health care debate, alongside considerations of possible payment- and delivery-system reforms. As these debates go forward, the lessons to be learned from the LCP failures should remain foremost in our minds.

SUICIDE NATION

In July 1999, Surgeon General of the United States David Satcher warned that suicide had become one of our most pressing public health concerns. Matters have not materially improved in the intervening years. According to the Foundation for Suicide Prevention, suicide is the tenth leading cause of death in the United States, with more than 41,000 reported in 2013. From 1986 to 2000, rates in the US dropped from 12.5 to 10.4 suicide deaths per 100,000 people in the population. But over the next twelve years, however, the rate generally increased, and by 2013 stood at 12.6 deaths per 100,000.[27]

Perhaps it isn't totally coincidental that the latter time period also encompassed the years of intensified assisted suicide advocacy. The United States is growing progressively pro-suicide. Where once suicide was culturally disfavored and the humane and compassionate response was deemed to be prevention, today suicide is promoted widely as an acceptable answer to life's most pressing difficulties. Indeed, there are reportedly more than 100,000 suicide sites on the Internet. Many are "highly graphic, with copies of suicide notes, death certificates, and color photographs," designed to encourage self-destruction.[28]

Meanwhile, the book *Final Exit*, written by Derek Humphry, cofounder of the Hemlock Society (now called Compassion and Choices under different management), was a best seller when it was first published in 1991 and still sells briskly. When I checked Amazon.com in March 2015, it was ranked the number-one selling book in "self-help, death, grief." The fact that some dead teenagers used the book when committing suicide has not, apparently, reduced sales or caused Mr. Humphry any pause in his suicide advocacy.

Some groups even sell plastic suicide bags with Velcro sewn around the opening so it fits snugly around the neck. I bought a suicide bag from an assisted suicide organization for $32, plus $10 for the suicide instructions as a visual aid in my lectures. The cheery promotional material that attracted me to the macabre product assured in bold letters that it is "Proven effective!" and that "the customized EXIT BAG is made of clear strong industrial plastic. It has an adjustable collar (with elastic sewn in back and a six-inch Velcro strip in front) for a snug but *comfortable* fit.... It comes with flannelette lining inside the collar so that the plastic won't irritate sensitive skin. AND it comes with an optional separate *terry-cloth-neckband* to create a 'turtleneck' for added comfort and snugness of fit."[29] (Emphasis within the text.)

Then, there is the pro-suicide Final Exit Network that "counsels" suicidal people on how to kill themselves with helium and a plastic bag. They also "attend" the suicides and apparently "clean up" afterward so that investigators are unaware of the helium element in the deaths. There have been a few felony convictions for these activities among FEN's suicide "counselors," but the group continues its dark work generally unimpeded.

If suicide isn't popular, what are we to think of the popularity of the murderer Jack Kevorkian? If public opinion polls are to be believed, Kevorkian is popular despite—or, better stated, *because*—he helped kill about 130 suicidal people. Many among the media and cultural elite certainly approved of him. Mike Wallace and Larry King were fans and *Time* magazine feted him at its seventy-fifth anniversary party where actor Tom Cruise rushed up to shake his hand. Kevorkian was even positively portrayed by A-list movie star Al Pacino in an award-winning HBO motion picture.[30]

When it comes to suicide, America is Dr. Jekyll and Mr. Hyde. Oregon voters legalized assisted suicide for people diagnosed with a terminal illness in 1994 and the law went into effect in 1997. Yet when local newspapers ran headlines about the state's soaring suicide rate among adolescents, nobody connected the dots. Such willful "compartmentalization" isn't restricted to Oregonians. Some newspapers that editorialized in favor of implementing Satcher's fifteen-point suicide prevention program had also editorialized in favor of legalizing assisted suicide.

"Rational Suicide"*: The popular culture is beginning to view suicide as "just another option" among many that should be available to suffering people. Bioethics has had a major hand in this; its radical notion of autonomy has helped fuel this cultural transformation. For example, many university and medical bioethics classes, professional articles, and symposia claim that there are two kinds of suicide: those that should be prevented and those that should be respected and perhaps facilitated, both as a matter of respecting personal autonomy and not engaging in non-maleficence by forcing people to stay alive. For example, the bioethics primer *Principles of Bioethics*, one of the most influential textbooks in the field, asserts that respecting suicide desires may be required in some cases to prevent "paternalism." "Often," Beauchamp and Childress write, "the burden of proof is more appropriately placed on those who claim the [suicidal] patient's judgment is not autonomous.... [T]hose who propose suicide intervention require a solid moral justification that fits the context. There are occasions in health care (and elsewhere) when it is appropriate to step aside and allow a suicide, and even assist in a person's suicide, just as there are occasions under which it is appropriate to intervene."[31]

This pro-suicide agenda has been given a name: "rational suicide." Alarmingly, "rational suicide" is promoted widely not only in mainstream bioethics but also among allied psychiatrists, psychologists, and social workers, the very people who serve as the last line of defense to protect the lives of suicidal people. Indeed, many within these related professions are working actively to dismantle society's cultural revulsion against suicide and transform our attitudes toward self-killing into yet another issue of "choice." All suicides are not wrong, these "experts" opine, just those that are irrational.

Under the theory of "rational suicide," mental health professionals have a duty to stop suicides only if they are impulsive or deemed frivolous. If mental health professionals judge the death desire to have rational bases, their duty to the patient is to nonjudgmentally help sort out the pros and cons of self-destruction and assist the patient in the use of proper decision-making techniques. Indeed, some advocates believe that the proper response of professionals in such cases is to help facilitate the suicide if that is what the patient chooses.

A rough consensus has been crafted about the circumstances that can make suicide a rational action. James L. Werth, PhD, one of the nation's foremost proponents of the concept, has written that a decision to kill oneself, or in his parlance, "to suicide" (he uses the term as a verb), should be viewed as "rational" if the patient has a "hopeless condition." Werth's definition of hopeless condition "includes but is not limited to terminal illnesses, severe physical *or psychological pain*, or *mentally debilitating or deteriorating conditions*, or a *quality of life that is no longer acceptable to the individual*."[32] (Emphasis added.)

Consider this definition closely: Don't all suicidal people *by definition* believe that their quality of life is unacceptable? Otherwise, they wouldn't want to end their lives. And if that is true, how are irrational and "rational" suicides to be differentiated? Most likely based on the biases and opinions of the therapist whose beliefs and values will powerfully influence whether the patient's condition is diagnosed "hopeless" and is thus a proper basis for self-destruction. Another option is for therapists to be lethally nonjudgmental: their only job being to facilitate the decision-making process. In either case, we will be well on the road to a system of near death-on-demand in which the very professionals whose job it is to save their lives abandon people to their deepest despair.

It is important to note that proponents of "rational suicide," while still in the minority among mental health professionals, are respected mainstream bioethicists, academics, and clinical mental health practitioners, professionals who treat suicidal people or teach those who do. More worrisome still, "rational suicide" appears to be catching on. Werth reported that 80 percent of respondents from a survey he sent to the American Psychological Association's Division of Psychology and other prestigious mental health associations supported his definition of rational suicide and the five-step process he created for determining whether a patient's suicide decision-making processes are "sound." An appalling 85 percent of survey respondents believed that a mental health professional who follows Werth's published guidelines would be acting ethically.[33]

Sometimes rational suicide is even promoted as a means of putting ourselves out of our family's misery. Take a 2014 column, published by *Psychology Today*, applauding the courage of an eighty-nine-year-old member of the Society for Old Age Rational Suicide, who had killed herself:

> I would like to think I could mount enough courage to bow out before things got too terrible for me or for my husband and daughters, who would have to watch me suffer and gradually disappear, possibly taking care of me in my dotage in ways that would diminish their joy in their own lives, and would color their feelings about me. Anne had never married and had only her niece to hold her hand, so maybe that's part of why she felt so ready to go. But in a way, maybe those of us with families are the ones whose old-age suicides might be truly "rational," leading us to bow out for the peace of mind of the people we leave behind.[34]

Imagine being told by your doctor that self-killing is a rational course. In this sense, the "rational suicide" movement sends despairing people and society a terribly mixed message. On one hand, surgeons general and mental health advocates worry about suicide rates. On the other, we are told repeatedly in academic forums, professional journals, public policy debates, news stories, and television shows and movies that while suicide may be wrong for some people, for others it is a proper and respectable choice. In a sense, that is like telling people not to smoke—but if you do, use a filtered cigarette.

Assisted Suicide: The assisted suicide movement has been the leading edge for promoting suicide for the last twenty years. If "rational suicide" incubates outside much of the public's field of vision, assisted suicide is at the center of public controversy and political agitation.

Modern assisted suicide advocacy arose out of the struggle to permit people to refuse unwanted life-extending medical treatment. Rather than being about refusing unwanted bodily intrusions—the legal basis for the right to refuse treatment—assisted suicide advocates assert that the issue is about the right to become dead.

Bioethicists are generally advocates for legalizing assisted suicide in medical journals and at symposia, often aiding in the drafting of proposed legislation. A few, such as Daniel Callahan, oppose legalization. Many others, such as Peter Singer, Thaddeus Mason Pope, Margaret P. Battin, Childress, and Beauchamp, vocally support legalization. Most recently, former opponent bioethicist luminary Arthur Caplan changed to the pro side "as a last resort," believing that strict guidelines can prevent abuse.[35]

Assisted suicide is promoted far more publicly than "rational suicide." Public advocacy generally focuses on hastened death as a proper answer to the difficulties associated with significant health problems and disability. And with bioethicists increasingly boarding the euthanasia train, the issue has been gaining respectability and support.

Indeed, assisted suicide advocates have had astonishing success in persuading almost every organ of popular cultural communication to pick up and run with that meme. Most of the women's magazines, at one time or another, have run assisted suicide-friendly articles, such as the "special report" in the January 1997 issue of the *Ladies' Home Journal* on assisted suicide consisting of a "roundtable" discussion with experts and family members of people who had committed assisted suicide. Some roundtable—not one assisted suicide opponent appeared in the piece. Most of the daytime talk shows have featured family members of assisted suicide victims, playing the subject for all the emotion it is worth.

Many popular movies have had pro-suicide/mercy killing themes. Meryl Streep's character commits suicide rather than living out her life with cancer in *One True Thing*, from the popular novel of the same name by Anna Quindlen. Similarly, the title character of *The English Patient* is given enough morphine with which to kill himself at the end of the movie. And who can forget *Million Dollar Baby*, the 2005 Clint Eastwood-directed and Academy Award-winning motion picture that climaxes with Eastwood's boxing trainer character mercy killing his female boxer protégé because she has lost the will to live after becoming quadriplegic in a bout?

Prime-time television has been an especially fertile field for suicide-positive themes. Almost every medical, legal, or police drama—*ER*, *Chicago Hope, Prescription: Murder, Homicide,* and *Law and Order,* to name a few—have aired assisted suicide episodes with almost every one casting a favorable light on mercy killing. Suicide and assisted suicide have even been depicted as the wave of a more humane future: *Star Trek: Voyager* aired an episode in which an immortal alien known as "Q" receives permission from Captain Janeway for an assisted suicide because he was despondent about his life's unending ennui.

You Don't Know Jack is a particularly egregious example of pro-suicide advocacy masquerading as popular entertainment. Advertised as a biopic of Jack Kevorkian, the 2010 HBO-produced movie actually crosses the line into hagiography, with A-list megastar Al Pacino playing the lead role.

The film presents Kevorkian as primarily motivated with the relief of human suffering. The promotional material claimed that Kevorkian launched his "crusade" to give the terminally ill "a humane and dignified option." In real life, Kevorkian's fundamental motive—actually, his obsession—was ghoulish. He wrote in his 1991 book, *Prescription Medicide*: "I feel it is only decent and fair to explain my ultimate aim.... It is not simply to help suffering people or doomed persons kill themselves—that is merely the first step, an early distasteful professional obligation.... What I find most satisfying is the prospect of making possible the performance of invaluable experiments or other beneficial medical acts under conditions that this first unpleasant step can help establish."[36] Bluntly stated, Kevorkian wanted to engage in human vivisection, in the pursuit of naked quackery:

> If we are ever to penetrate the mystery of death—even superficially—it will have to be obitiatry [Kevorkian's term for experimenting on those being euthanized].... [K]nowledge about the essence of human death will of necessity require insight into the nature of the unique awareness of consciousness that characterizes cognitive human life. That is possible only through obitiatric research on living human bodies, and most likely by concentrating on the central nervous system.[37]

Before pursuing his assisted suicide campaign, Kevorkian went from prison to prison asking for permission to experiment on condemned prisoners. Indeed, he only turned his focus to the sick and disabled after being denied access to executions. Jack Kevorkian was a very disturbed man, not the heroic, if eccentric, visionary depicted by Pacino in *You Don't Know Jack.* But depicting him as he really was would not have promoted our popular culture's assisted-suicide-is-compassion reigning narrative.

In the last decade, the news media has almost become a partner with ideological advocates in promoting assisted suicide into law. Perhaps the most notable example is the international media feeding frenzy over the assisted suicide of brain cancer patient Brittany Maynard in November 2014. Even though there had been more than 700 legal assisted suicides in Oregon by the time of Maynard's death at her own hand, she was made into an international media celebrity—before and after committing suicide—prominently featured in *Time*, the *New York Times*, the *Los Angeles Times*, *USA Today*, BBC, PBS, ABC, CBS, CNN—just to name a few—because she announced plans to kill herself. She was even the subject of a cover story in *People*, which lauded her for being fearless because she planned on committing assisted suicide.[38] CNN listed her among 2014's most "Extraordinary People."[39]

Maynard was made the public face of assisted suicide because she was young, pretty, newly wed, tragically dying, and transgressive for killing herself rather than face the rigors of late-stage brain cancer—the perfect icon for our sentimental age. But that alone doesn't explain why she received the kind of conspicuous adulation usually reserved for movie and rock stars, presidential candidates, and Kim Kardashian. If she had chosen to die naturally, cared for humanely by hospice instead of taking a lethal overdose, nobody outside of her friends and family would ever have heard of her.

So what was going on? When we look more deeply at arguments in favor of legalizing assisted suicide, we see that the assisted suicide discussion is really more about what I will call the *aesthetics of dying* than it is about potential pain and symptoms. This is no small matter, nor is it in the least a frivolous concern. Worries about lost looks, dependency, or perhaps how the sick room might smell can be devastating. Indeed, our self-esteem—and perhaps, more important, how we perceive that others view us—can materially impact our mental and emotional states as we approach the end of life. (For example, when I was a hospice volunteer, one of my patients became so distraught by his changed appearance that he covered all the mirrors in his home.)

Maynard's evocative explanation for eschewing hospice out of hand in favor of suicide illustrates how potent aesthetic fears can be: "I considered passing away in hospice care at my San Francisco Bay-area home. But even with palliative medication, I could develop potentially morphine-resistant pain and suffer personality changes and verbal, cognitive and motor loss of virtually any kind. Because the rest of my body is young and healthy, I am likely to physically hang on for a long time even though cancer is eating my mind. I would probably have suffered in hospice care for weeks or even months. And my family would have had to watch that."[40]

The above quote tells us that Maynard apparently fixated on a worst-case scenario for herself. But when others tried to tell the world her dying did not have to be that way, she (and others) bitterly criticized hospice doctors, such as Ira Byock, for daring to point out publicly that many with terminal brain cancer die peacefully at home, their symptoms well managed and their pain controlled.[41] Along the same lines, Maynard told *Elite Daily*, "Not only do I want to save myself from that fate [of suffering and decline], but I love my family too much to make them carry the memories of my deterioration for the rest of their lives."[42]

Yes, Maynard worried about suffering. Who wouldn't? But she seemed even more intent on not forcing her family to suffer by witnessing her loss of beauty, vitality, and capacity—an effort her husband and mother fully supported, marking an alarming trend in suicide advocacy.

The sensationalism around Maynard's death was just one of the more prominent examples of how the media frequently promotes self or mercy killing as an acceptable answer to the serious problems of grave illness and disability, at best portraying assisted suicides as the "most acceptable of unacceptable options"[43] and at worst gullibly publishing false assertions of euthanasia advocates without checking the facts.

A classic case of this misfeasance occurred on the popular CBS news magazine television program *60 Minutes*, a program that led ironically to Kevorkian's undoing. Kevorkian videoed himself as he murdered Thomas Youk, a man with ALS. He then took the tape to *60 Minutes* correspondent the late Mike Wallace, a vocal pro-euthanasia advocate. In the *60 Minutes* presentation, Kevorkian takes Wallace step by step through Youk's murder and tells the newsman that he killed Youk, with permission, to keep him from choking to death on his own saliva.[44] Wallace accepted the excuse without blinking an eye, thereby cruelly allowing people with ALS and their families who were watching the program to believe Kevorkian's lie.

The truth is far more hopeful. Proper medical care prevents people with ALS from choking or suffocating. Dame Cicely Saunders, the creator of the modern hospice movement who personally treated hundreds of ALS patients, told me in no uncertain terms, "We have kept careful notes [about how patients die] for all these years. Patients with ALS do not choke. They are all frightened of it, but they do not choke!"[45] Hospice physician Dr. Walter R. Hunter, chairman of the ethics committee of the National Hospice Organization, confirmed Saunders's report, telling me, "We have very effective medications that control the problem of choking. In addition to medicine, there is an easy treatment, similar to the device used in a dentist's office, that family members can use to keep patients from choking."[46] Accurate information was just a phone call away. Yet Wallace, a legendary newsman who became famous for his hard-hitting, acerbic interviews, apparently didn't bother to verify Kevorkian's assertions before airing the program.

The BBC was similarly egregious in 2011 when it broadcast the death of a famous euthanasia advocate's death at a Swiss suicide clinic. It is worth noting that such stories—particularly the glamorizing coverage of Brittany Maynard's suicide—violate the World Health Organization's published media guidelines for covering stories involving suicide. To keep suicide stories from sparking copycat deaths, the WHO urges, "Sensational coverage of suicides should be assiduously avoided, particularly when a celebrity is involved. The coverage should be minimized to the extent possible. Any mental health problem the celebrity may have had should also be acknowledged. Every effort should be made to avoid overstatement." And get this:

"Glorifying suicide victims as martyrs and objects of public adulation may suggest to susceptible persons that their society honours suicidal behaviour. Instead, the emphasis should be on mourning the person's death."

The WHO guidelines are very specific:

WHAT NOT TO DO

- Don't publish photographs or suicide notes.
- Don't report specific details of the method used.

- Don't give simplistic reasons.
- Don't glorify or sensationalize suicide.[47]

Alas, rather than follow the WHO's advice in "death with dignity" cases, the media permit that people planning to commit suicide are not only presented in a positive light but permitted to advocate for their plan as a positive good for individuals and society.

Such assisted suicide propaganda can cover egregious abuses and justify crimes. When the news broke in July 1995 that Manhattanite George Delury "assisted the suicide" of his wife, Myrna Lebov, because she was disabled by multiple sclerosis, the media immediately swallowed Delury's self-serving story and duly painted the killing as a compassionate, loving, and courageous act. Delury became an instant hero among the true believers of the assisted suicide movement. The Hemlock Society created a defense fund, and William Batt, chairman of the New York chapter, proclaimed his confidence that Myrna had chosen to die because of the extent of her disability. Delury made numerous television appearances, a speech in front of the American Psychiatric Association, and signed a book deal to write his story. Far and wide, he was acclaimed as a dedicated husband willing to risk jail to help his wife achieve her deeply desired end to suffering. He was allowed to quickly plead guilty to a minor crime and served only four months in jail.

The truth about the case, eventually uncovered by the *Forward*, a Jewish weekly; *Newsday*; and *NBC Dateline* demonstrated that Delury was anything but loving and compassionate. It turned out that the person most committed to Lebov's suicide in the Delury-Lebov family wasn't Myrna—it was George. And he wasn't quiet about it, either. For months he coerced, cajoled, and pressured Myrna into killing herself. For example, according to his own diary, at one point Delury told Myrna cruelly, "I have work to do, people to see, places to travel. But no one asks about my needs. I have fallen prey to the tyranny of a victim. You are sucking my life out of my [sic] like a vampire and nobody cares. In fact, it would appear that I am about to be cast in the role of a villain because I no longer believe in you."[48]

That Delury wanted Lebov to kill herself cannot be disputed. On May 1, 1995, he wrote in his diary: "Sheer hell! Myrna is more or less euphoric. She spoke of writing a book today. [Myrna was a published author.] She's interested in everything, wants everything explained, and believes that every bit of bad news has some way out.... It's all too much. I'm not going to come out of this in one piece with my honor. I'm so tired of it all, maybe I should kill *myself*."[49] (Emphasis in the text.)

Delury claimed that on the night she died, Myrna voluntarily swallowed a poisonous pudding he made for her. But Delury's own diary reveals that his wife was not consistently suicidal. Indeed, according to Myrna's sister, Beverly Sloane, "Myrna told me, she told my daughter, she told her swimming therapist, that she did not want to die and that she would not change her mind. This was in May. Myrna died on July 4."

Sloane was particularly galled by the glowing review of Delury's book, *But What If She Wants to Die?*, that appeared in the *New York Times Book Review*, in which Delury is described as having "unquestioning love for his wife,"[50] despite the admissions in his book that Myrna "chose death for my sake," that he withheld her full dosage of antidepressant medication from her so that he could stockpile the drugs for a lethal overdose, and that when the poison didn't kill her, he finished her off by smothering her with a plastic bag.[51]

"People were quick to accept George's excuse for ending Myrna's life," Sloane told me. "But in my opinion he used the assisted suicide controversy as an alibi for intentional homicide. Her disease did not change the essence of Myrna. She was a loving, intelligent, warm, compassionate, sensitive, giving human being. She was a joy to talk to and be with. She was making plans for the future. She was not in pain. She was not terminally ill. She should still be alive enjoying the love of her family and he should still be in jail."[52] (Delury never found the fame he seemed to crave. He committed suicide in 2007, a copy of Derek Humphry's *Final Exit* on his nightstand.)

Then there was the case of Susan Randall, the distraught daughter of Judith Bement, who asked her stepfather, John Bement, an excruciating question: "When you put the [plastic] bag on Mom's head, was she awake? I mean, did she know you were doing that? I just need peace of mind."

Bement did not realize that Susan was cooperating with a police investigation into her mother's death or that she was taping their conversation and conversations with her sister, Cynthia, who had been present for part of the assisted killing. Bement replied, "I don't know. I don't know. She was not totally out but she wasn't conscious."

Bement told Susan that years before, when Judith was first diagnosed with ALS, he promised to assist in his wife's suicide. He claimed that placing a plastic bag over Judith's head after she took twenty Seconals was simply the keeping of that promise.

But Susan didn't see it that way. She had been with her mother on the night of her death, and Judith was happy. She said, "But when I left, we were joking around and everything was fine and it was a split second and everything just went to hell. Do you know what happened?"

"Well, what she wanted was the pills.... I read that book and ..."

"What book?"

"*Final Exit*."

"I never saw it."

"It's a book this guy wrote. So he says whenever you take these drugs that after the person is unconscious, you slip the bag over their head—kind of like insurance because, you know, somebody could survive."

Bement then rationalized his actions: "She wasn't going to get any better. If it wasn't, then it would be a month later, two months later."[53]

Susan is convinced that her mother was not suicidal on the night she died and that she had not given up on life. "My mother had made plans for the future," she told me. "Her moods fluctuated, sure, but they were dictated by the quality of care she was receiving. When she felt valued and loved, she wanted to live. When she was made to feel like she was a burden, she grew despondent. She was not going to die soon. She had not qualified for hospice care because they said she would not die within six months. What Mom needed was quality care and to know that she was loved, not a plastic bag over her head to suffocate the life out of her."

What shocked Susan was not only the manner of her mother's death but her stepfather's actions in its aftermath. "John began to date immediately after Mom's death. His entire lifestyle changed. When Mom was alive and needed him, he would often not come home at night, he said, because of his job as a local truck driver. I know because I stayed with her. As soon as she died, suddenly he started coming home every single night. I would drive by her house and his vehicle was always there."

Even worse for Susan, the townsfolk of Springville, New York, in her words "were conned into believing his sad story of acting out of love for his wife. Before and during John's trial, all their sympathy went to him, even though he never took the stand in his own defense. I was ostracized for a while and only because I tried to stand up for my mom."

Had Judith ever expressed a desire to die? "Yes," Susan said. "When she was first diagnosed, a neurologist in Buffalo told her, 'You are a lost cause. You might as well go home, sit in a chair, and wait to die.' She became despondent after that. Who wouldn't? For two years, she gave up on life. But then my daughter was born, and she started seeing things differently. She had an active life again. Sure, she sometimes got depressed, but she would bounce out of it and get on with life."

Despite Bement's conviction of second-degree manslaughter, the local media and public opinion generally supported the killer, as did the judge, apparently. But despite Bement never having testified at either his trial or sentencing hearing, which would have allowed the district attorney to challenge his motives on cross-examination, he was sentenced to only two nonconsecutive weeks in jail.

Susan is bitter. "With that sentence, the law confirmed what that awful doctor told my mother. Her life had no value. Her death wasn't worth worrying too much about. That was an insult to my mother and to all sick people. I hope that if I ever get into a position where I am vulnerable like Mother was that there is a law that protects my life and prevents others from getting rid of me and then saying it was okay because it was all about compassion."[54]

A lot of people don't see it that way. After years of pro-suicide advocacy in the popular media and medical and psychiatric journals, in legislative halls, and as entertainment, some now differentiate between suicide (bad) and assisted suicide "aid in dying" (compassion), the latter being reserved for cases in which the desire to die arises out of serious illnesses or disabilities.

Such a dichotomy threatens to construct a two-tiered system for measuring the worth of human life. The young and vital who become suicidal would receive suicide prevention—and the concomitant message that their lives are worth living. At the same time, the suicides of the debilitated, sick, and disabled, and people with extended mental anguish—the "hopelessly ill"—would be shrugged off as merely a matter of choice. Such a value system would not only reflect a distorted value about the worth of human life but also send a lethal message to the weak and infirm that their lives are not worth living.

As the culture of death rushes to embrace the false compassion of assisted suicide, critical distinctions are lost:

Assisted suicide is not the same as refusing medical treatment. Too many people have painful memories or have heard stories of loved ones hooked up to medical machines beyond reason when all they wanted to do was die quietly in their own beds. Similarly, people have watched in anguish as their loved ones writhed in agony because they received inadequate medical care for pain. Advocates of legalizing assisted suicide know this and exploit people's deep psychic wounds to convince them to accept killing as the alternative. The good news is that once people learn that they don't have to fall prey to high-tech medicine, that almost all pain can either be eliminated or substantially alleviated, support for killing by doctors as a legitimate response to serious illness or disability generally plummets.

Pain control is not the same as assisted suicide. Assisted suicide advocates often try to create a false moral equivalency between medically controlling pain and so-called mercy killing. The argument goes something like this: Since some people's deaths are hastened by the powerful medications often required for effective palliation and since pain control is unquestionably moral and ethical based on the "principle of double effect," then assisted suicide should also be viewed as proper since the intent of assisted suicide (allegedly) is to alleviate suffering.

There are only two problems with this argument: pain control usually extends life rather than shortens it, and the argument completely misapplies the principle of double effect.

According to ethicist and attorney Rita Marker, the principle of double effect applies to an act that may have both a good effect and a bad effect. Such an act is considered ethical if all of the four following conditions are met:

1. The action taken (in this case, treating pain and relieving suffering) is "good" or morally neutral;
2. The bad effect (in this case, the possibility of death) must not be intended, but only permitted;
3. The good effect cannot be brought about by means of the bad effect; and
4. There is a proportionately grave reason to perform the act (in this case, the alleviation of severe pain) and thereby risk the bad effect.

By these measures, if properly applied pain control accidentally hastens a patient's death, the palliative act remains ethical because the bad effect—death—was not intended. On the other hand, Marker says, "assisted suicide *intentionally causes death* as the means of alleviating suffering. Thus, it fails the second and third requirements of the principle of double effect and therefore remains an immoral and unethical act."[55]

Some people believe that giving large doses of morphine at the end of life—for example, by a morphine drip—is a form of euthanasia. Most of the time it isn't. As pain control specialist and oncologist Dr. Eric Chevlen told me, "When morphine is used properly in the last hours of life, it eases anxiety and discomfort the patient might otherwise have, but it does not hasten death."[56] In most cases, large morphine doses provided at the end of life do not actually cause death—the underlying disease does—but are necessary to ensure that the patient remains pain-free to the end. Moreover, as stated above, providing appropriate palliation, even at the risk of the side effect of dying, is a proper and ethical application of medical expertise. Still, there is no denying that a few doctors intentionally overdose dying patients with pain-killing drugs with the intent to end their lives. But that does not make killing right or necessary. Pain can be controlled at the late stages of life without rushing nature.

Assisted suicide would not be limited to people who are terminally ill. Advocates of assisted suicide are well aware that in early legalization advocacy, popular support for assisted suicide evaporates when legalization proposals include chronically ill, elderly, depressed, or disabled people. Thus, they generally say in public that they want assisted suicide limited to the terminally ill, and their current legislative proposals generally limit access to assisted suicide to people diagnosed with a terminal illness. The truth is, however, they have a hidden agenda containing more grandiose plans. You might even say these goals are hidden in plain sight.

In December 1997, in the immediate wake of the Oregon assisted suicide law going into legal effect, Compassion in Dying (CID) of Washington, an offshoot of the Hemlock Society originally formed to surreptitiously assist suicides,[57] mailed a fundraising letter to its supporters during "the holiday gift-giving season." A key participant in legalizing assisted suicide in Oregon, CID stressed in its public advocacy that doctor-induced death would be absolutely limited to people who are terminally ill. But now with a big victory under its belt in Oregon, the advocacy group was feeling its oats and ready to admit, at least to its own members, that it had a far broader agenda. Supporters were urged to send a donation because "We have expanded our mission to include not only terminally ill individuals, but also persons with *incurable illnesses* which will eventually lead to a terminal diagnosis. The need for increased funding is even more crucial."[58] (Emphasis added.)

"Incurable illness that will eventually lead to a terminal diagnosis" covers a far broader array of maladies than does the term terminal illness, possibly including asymptomatic HIV infection, multiple sclerosis, diabetes, emphysema, early-stage cancer, asthma, and myriad other diseases.

Similarly, on July 27, 1998, the Hemlock Society, perhaps the nation's largest assisted suicide advocacy group, issued a press release calling for the legalization of assisted suicide for people with "incurable conditions." Similarly, the executive director of Hemlock, Faye Girsh, supporting Kevorkian's murder of Thomas Youk, wrote in *USA Today*, "The law must change to permit an exemption to murder for doctors who provide a peaceful death to a suffering, irreversibly-ill adult who makes a competent, repeated request for an assisted death."[59] The use of the words "incurable" and "irreversible" rather than "terminal" was intentional. When people see the former terms in the context of the assisted suicide debate, they generally think "terminal," even though the terms are not synonyms. Arthritis is both incurable and irreversible, but not terminal. Many disabilities are too, such as paraplegia, quadriplegia, and hearing impairment caused by nerve damage.

The true breadth and scope of the assisted suicide movement's agenda came into rare focus in October 1998, when the World Federation of Right to Die Societies—an organization comprising the world's foremost euthanasia advocacy groups—issued its "Zurich Declaration" after its biannual convention. The declaration urged that people "suffering severe and enduring *distress* [should be eligible] to receive medical help to die."[60] (My emphasis.) Finally, the true goal of the assisted suicide movement is revealed; it is "rational suicide" squared: doctor-induced deaths for anyone with more than a transitory desire to die.

The Supreme Court of Canada imposed just such a regimen on that entire nation in a 2015 decision, conjuring a Charter right to "termination of life" for anyone who has an "irremediable medical condition" and wants to die.[61] The scope of the judicial fiat was most definitely *not* limited to the terminally ill; the ruling grants competent adults a right to be made dead if they have an "illness, disease, or disability that causes enduring suffering that is intolerable to the individual," which, it should be noted, specifically includes "psychological pain."

Even these broad words inadequately describe the truly radical social policy the Supreme Court unleashed upon Canada. For example, *a treatable condition* can qualify as "irremediable" if the patient chooses not to pursue available remedies. Hence, an *"irremediable condition" that permits life-termination may actually be wholly remediable*, except that the patient would rather die than receive care.

Here is a hypothetical that clearly would apply: Sally has diabetes that can be fully controlled by medication (or HIV, heart disease, neuropathy, early-stage cancer; the list could go on and on). She decides she wants to die (for whatever reason) and claims that available treatments are "not acceptable" to her. Presto chango, *her theretofore treatable illness is transformed through the sheer power of word alchemy into an irremediable condition*. Ditto Harley, who becomes clinically depressed after his business fails—a diagnosable "illness, disease, or disability"—and refuses psychiatric treatment in order to seek death.

Guidelines do not protect against abuse. Canada's broad death license is well within the mainstream of assisted suicide/euthanasia advocacy and laws around the world. But that doesn't prevent advocates in the US and their media apologists from continually trotting out the old trope that "guidelines" will protect against abuse. Painful experience clearly demonstrates that the promise of protection is specious. Indeed, once a society widely accepts the fundamental premise of euthanasia—that killing is an acceptable answer to the problem of human suffering—like the universe, the euthanasia license never stops expanding.

We need only look to the experience of the Netherlands and Belgium to see what scant protection protective guidelines actually provide. Euthanasia wasn't technically legal in the Netherlands, but doctors were promised that they would not be prosecuted for lethally injecting or assisting in patients' suicides if they followed the guidelines first established by courts and then the Parliament, and reported such deaths to the coroner. Then, despite the steady expansion of euthanasia over decades—euthanasia first became acceptable in the early 1970s— euthanasia was formally legalized in 2001 under legal guidelines such as the necessity of repeated patient requests, unbearable suffering for which there are no reasonable alternatives other than killing (a guideline that does not exist in Oregon or in most US legalization proposals), and the requirement that doctors obtain second medical opinions before dispatching their patients.

In actual practice, these guidelines are ignored routinely and they have been expanded by court interpretation to the point where they are utterly ephemeral. The inadequacy of actual protection has been known for many years. For example, a 1999 study published in the *Journal of Medical Ethics* revealed a full 59 percent of euthanasia and assisted suicide deaths were not reported as then required, meaning that euthanasia in the Netherlands was even then "beyond effective control."[62]

The guidelines also did not prevent the categories of people killed by doctors from expanding steadily since euthanasia publicly entered Dutch medical practice in 1973. Today, in the Netherlands, not only are terminally ill people who ask to be killed euthanized, but also so are chronically ill, the elderly "tired of life," and those with mental illnesses. So too are people with emotional or mental problems who are not even physically ill (i.e., "rational suicide").

That Dutch doctors and psychiatrists practice "rational suicide" is not a matter of interpretation or difference of opinion—it is fact. For example, a pro-euthanasia Dutch documentary, played in the United States on PBS, told the story of a young woman in remission from anorexia. She was so worried about returning to food abuse that she asked her doctor to kill her. He did so without legal consequence.[63]

The landmark Dutch court case opening the door to the killing of depressed people involved a psychiatrist, Boutdewijn Chabot, who assisted in the suicide of Hilly Bossher, a middle-aged woman who had lost her two children, one to suicide and the other to illness. On the day her second son died, she failed in her attempt at suicide. Hilly then became obsessed about being buried between her two dead children. She bought a burial plot, moved her children's bodies to the plot, and left a space between them for her own body. She then attended a Dutch Euthanasia Society meeting and met up with Dr. Chabot.

Chabot took Hilly as a patient but did not attempt to treat her because Hilly feared that treatment would "loosen the bonds with her deceased sons."[64] After four meetings with Hilly over a period of about five weeks, the psychiatrist helped kill her. Chabot was tried, not for the intent of punishment, as would occur in US courts, but to establish a precedent to guide future cases. The psychiatrist's attorney, Eugene Sutorius, told me, "He [the prosecutor] sees that this is not criminality in the normal sense. He is trying to create a precedent.... He wants to make sure these things are done decently."[65]

At Sutorius's urging, the Dutch Supreme Court validated Chabot's act, ruling that suffering is suffering, whether physically or mentally caused, and that Hilly's killing was acceptable medical practice. With the precedent now set in Dutch law by its highest courts, psychiatrists and doctors may kill depressed, suicidal patients, even if patients refuse treatment that might help them overcome the suicidal fixation.

Meanwhile, Dutch psychiatrists have been urged in professional journals to increase their participation in the euthanasia regime. An article published in the Dutch-language *Journal of Psychiatry* (*tijdschrift voor psychiatrie*) in 2011 explicitly advocated assisted suicide a treatment for mental illness: "Assisted suicide, as a last resort in psychiatry, legally admissible since 2002, recently legitimized in practice. The midwife [of] Death is now appropriate for psychiatric reach patients, representing an emancipation of the psychiatric patient and psychiatry itself."[66]

This is killing of the mentally ill depicted as "emancipation" of both patient *and psychiatrist*! Refusing to assist in the suicide—remember, we are discussing mentally ill patients—denigrated as a "failure of the autonomy of psychiatric patients." Thus collapses the last line of defense for profoundly disturbed people. (Psychiatrists apparently heeded the call for greater participation in euthanasia. In 2012, fourteen mentally ill patients were euthanized by their psychiatrists. In 2013, that number tripled to forty-two.)[67]

And lest we forget, as discussed more fully in the last chapter, terminally ill and disabled infants are euthanized in their cribs without legal consequence, a clear violation of Dutch law. Demented patients who feared future decline have also been euthanized with the subsequent approval of Dutch prosecutors.[68]

Infants are not the only children who are eligible for euthanasia in the Netherlands. Pediatric oncologists have provided a *hulp bij zelfoding* (self-help for ending life) program for adolescents since the 1980s, in which poisonous doses of drugs are prescribed for minors with terminal illness.

Moreover, children who want physician-assisted suicide or euthanasia may be able to receive it without parental consent.[69]

Many Dutch doctors also practice non-voluntary euthanasia; that is, they kill patients who have not asked to be killed. The exact number of such killings is hard to quantify definitively and is a matter of some dispute. According to several Dutch studies conducted during the last decade, Dutch doctors kill approximately 1,000 people who have not asked to be euthanized each year because the *doctor's values* dictate that their deaths should be hastened. But that horrific number may underestimate the actual toll of non-voluntary killings. According to a 1991 Dutch government study known as the Remmelink Report, an additional 4,941 patients who had not asked to die were killed by doctors in 1990, by means of massive morphine overdose in which death, not palliation, was the intended result. That means that approximately 6,000 Dutch patients who had not asked to die were killed by doctors in 1990, nearly 5 percent of all Dutch deaths that year.[70] This was considered so significant by the US Supreme Court that the statistic was referenced in its 1997 decision declaring that there is not a constitutional right to assisted suicide.[71] (A more recent study found that non-voluntary killing by morphine overdose continues in the Netherlands, albeit at a lower level.) In 2010, the Dutch government reported 310 cases of "termination without request or consent," clear violations of Dutch law that were not prosecuted and went unpunished.[72] How many went unreported will never be known.

If the Netherlands slid down the "slippery slope," Belgium jumped off the cliff headfirst. Belgium legalized euthanasia in 2002. The very first euthanasia death of a multiple sclerosis patient violated the then-new law's guidelines.[73] No matter: Guidelines are meant to provide assurance more than they are to restrict medicalized killing. Indeed, since 2002, the country has experienced a crescendo of increasingly radical medicalized killings and/or permissions to kill that demonstrate the logical consequences of accepting the premise that killing is an acceptable answer to human suffering. Here are just a few examples:

Joint Euthanasia Deaths: At least three elderly couples who didn't want to face the prospect of future widowhood died together in joint euthanasia killings. The first was in 2011—the couple was not seriously impaired and their joint euthanasia was carried out with the full knowledge and apparent approval of their community. They even made their final arrangements at the local mortuary before being lethally injected.[74] The second known joint euthanasia took place two years later when an elderly couple who had been married sixty-four years—both seriously ill, in this example—were euthanized surrounded by their children and grandchildren.[75] The third joint euthanasia termination—of a still-healthy couple who "feared the future"—was performed by a doctor procured by the couple's own son, who told the *Daily Mail* that his parents' deaths was "the best solution," since caring for them properly would be "impossible."[76] Most societies consider joint suicides by elderly couples to be tragic. In Belgium, apparently, they are seen as a legitimate solution to the problems associated with eldercare.

There have also been joint euthanasia deaths of siblings in Belgium. From the *Telegraph* story:

> Identical twins were killed by Belgian doctors last month in a unique mercy killing under Belgium's euthanasia laws. The two men, 45, from the Antwerp region were both born deaf and sought euthanasia after finding that they would also soon go blind. The pair told doctors that they were unable to bear the thought of not being able to see each other again. The twin brothers had spent their entire lives together, sharing a flat and both working as cobblers. Doctors at Brussels University Hospital in Jette "euthanized" the two men by lethal injection on 14 December last year.[77]

In a morally sane society, the death doctors would lose their licenses and be tried for homicide. But Belgium no longer fits that description.

Euthanasia After Sexual Exploitation by Psychiatrist: "Ann G." was a suicidal anorexia patient who publicly accused her previous psychiatrist of persuading her into sexual relations. When the psychiatrist—who admitted the charge—was not severely disciplined, Ann went to a second psychiatrist for euthanasia. She died at age forty-four.[78]

Euthanasia for a Botched Sex Change: Nathan Verhelst underwent a sex change surgery from woman to man and then was euthanized because of despair over the result. From the *Daily Mail* story: "A Belgian transsexual has chosen to die by euthanasia after a botched sex change operation to complete his transformation into a man left him a 'monster.' Nathan Verhelst, 44, died yesterday afternoon after being allowed have his life ended on the grounds of 'unbearable psychological suffering.' ... In the hours before his death he told Belgium's Het Laatse Nieuws: 'I was ready to celebrate my new birth. But when I looked in the mirror, I was disgusted with myself.'"[79] So, Dufour—the same doctor who killed the disabled twins, described above—agreed to provide a lethal injection.

Words rarely fail me. But they do here.

Euthanasia for Mental Illness: As in the Netherlands, Belgian psychiatrists now use euthanasia as a treatment for suicidal desires caused by mental illness. Indeed, *Humo* magazine reported in 2015 that about fifty mentally ill patients are euthanized a year. Wim Distelmans, chairman of the federal commission for euthanasia, explained:

> Manic-depressive patients, in their manic moments, do the most improbable things in that state: plunder their bank account, stay for weeks in a five-star hotel, buy numerous cars in one day. At that stage they are not mentally competent, that is obvious. But come in moments of depression they back their exhaustion to the baseline, and they are indeed competent. Then they can say, for example: "I live for thirty years crazy highs and lows, I've tried everything to break that infernal cycle, including psychiatric hospitalization, but now I'm back on the baseline, and I know I have a few weeks left before I go back for a dip in the depth or a jump in height." These are people who are eligible for euthanasia.[80]

The story fails to mention that Belgian doctors have coupled euthanasia with organ harvesting—including of the mentally ill, the details about which we will explore in chapter 5.

Assisted Suicide for Children: Belgium legalized assisted suicide for children in 2014 with no lower age limit. The *Associated Press* explained: "Children will have to be interviewed by a pediatric psychiatrist or psychologist, who must determine that the child possesses 'the capacity of discernment,' and then certify that in writing. The child's physician must meet the parents or legal representatives to inform them of the outcome of the consultation and ensure they are in agreement with the child's decision. The request for euthanasia, as well as the agreement by parents or legal representatives, must be delivered in writing, and the child and family must be given psychological care if wanted."[81]

I can't imagine asking a child to write a note requesting poison pills. But the way these things go, it won't be long until the supposedly strict guidelines controlling child euthanasia will sink beneath the waves like other supposed protections in Belgian law. What are we to make of the history of euthanasia in the Netherlands and Belgium? Theo Boer, a Dutch ethicist who once served on a euthanasia review panel as a supporter of euthanasia, believed that opening the door to medicalized killing need not lead to the kind of death inflation we have addressed here (and could have spent many more pages detailing). But after years of watching the constant expansion of the killing license, he came to realize that his initial optimism was misplaced, writing explicitly that guidelines *do not protect against abuse*:

> I used to be a supporter of legislation. But now, with twelve years of experience, I take a different view. At the very least, wait for an honest and intellectually satisfying analysis of the reasons behind the explosive increase in the numbers. Is it because the law should have had better safeguards? Or is it because the mere existence of such a law is an invitation to see assisted suicide and euthanasia as a normality instead of a last resort? Before those questions are answered, don't go there. Once the genie is out of the bottle, it is not likely to ever go back in again.[82]

That, of course, suits the world's euthanasia advocates just fine, since the actual purpose of guidelines isn't to protect vulnerable people so much as to provide false assurance and the appearance of control to the greater population.

Events in Oregon lend credence to this premise. When Patrick Matheny committed assisted suicide, his brother-in-law claimed to have had to "help" him die because Matheny's ALS prevented him from swallowing the prescribed poison he received a few months before via Federal Express.[83] If true, this was a blatant violation of Oregon's assisted suicide law, not that it mattered. A cursory investigation by the local district attorney, *in which the brother-in-law wasn't even questioned*, quickly concluded that no illegalities had occurred.

What happened next confirmed opponents' predictions about where the legalization of assisted suicide would eventually lead. Oregon Deputy Attorney General David Schuman claimed in a letter to a state senator that to avoid "discrimination" against disabled people, Oregon might have to offer "reasonable accommodation" to people like Matheny who wanted to commit assisted suicide but could not self-administer their prescribed lethal drugs. (The requirement of self-administration is one of the core protective guidelines of the assisted suicide law.) What might the term reasonable accommodation mean? If one has a "right" to be made dead and due to disability they are unable to make themselves dead, then somebody is going to have to do the deed for them; in a word, killing. Active euthanasia may just be a lawsuit away in Oregon, despite the repeated promises of proponents to the contrary.

The Kate Cheney case, reported in the (Portland) *Oregonian*, provided another disturbing glimpse of how easily supposedly protective guidelines are circumvented.[84] Cheney, age eighty-five, was diagnosed with terminal cancer and sought assisted suicide. But there was a problem: Cheney was probably in the early stages of dementia, raising significant questions about her mental competence. So, rather than prescribe lethal drugs, her doctor referred her to a psychiatrist.

Her daughter, Ericka Goldstein, accompanied Cheney to the psychiatric consultation. The psychiatrist found that Cheney had a loss of short-term memory. Even more worrisome, it appeared that her daughter was more interested in Cheney's assisted suicide than was Cheney. The psychiatrist wrote in his report that while the assisted suicide seemed consistent with Cheney's values, "she does not seem to be explicitly pushing for this." He also determined that she did not have the "very high capacity required to weigh options about assisted suicide." Accordingly, he nixed the lethal prescription.

Advocates of legalized assisted suicide might, at this point, smile happily and say that this is the way the law is supposed to operate. But that isn't the end of Kate Cheney's story. According to the *Oregonian* report, Cheney appeared to accept the psychiatrist's verdict but her daughter most explicitly did not. Rather than accept the refusal, she went doctor shopping.

Goldstein's demand for another opinion was acceded to by Kaiser Permanente, Cheney's HMO. This time, the consultation was with a clinical psychologist rather than an MD psychiatrist. Like the first time, the psychologist found that Cheney had memory problems. For example, she could not recall when she had been diagnosed with terminal cancer. The psychologist also worried about familial pressure, writing that Cheney's decision to die "may be influenced by her family's wishes." Still, despite these reservations, the psychologist determined that Cheney was competent to commit suicide.

The final decision to approve the death was made by a Kaiser HMO ethicist/administrator named Robert Richardson. Dr. Richardson interviewed Cheney, who told him she wanted the poison pills not because she was in irremediable pain but because she feared not being able to attend to her personal hygiene. After the interview, satisfied that she was competent, he approved the lethal prescription.

In short, once the doctor has prescribed poison, patients may be on their own.

What happened next in the Cheney case illustrates the problems that can arise. Cheney did not take her poison right away. She first asked to die when her daughter had to help her shower after an accident with her colostomy bag, but she quickly changed her mind. Then Cheney was sent to a nursing home for a week so that her family could have some respite from caregiving.

The time in the nursing home seems to have pushed Cheney into wanting immediate death. As soon as she was brought home she declared her desire to take the pills. Her grandchildren were quickly called to say their goodbyes and Cheney took the pills. She died with her daughter at her side, telling her what a courageous woman she was.

If she was depressed, there was no doctor to diagnose it. If she was coaxed (which was not contended in the *Oregonian* story), there were no witnesses from outside the family to protest. The Oregon legal guidelines cease to protect patients once the lethal prescription is written.

This is the awful truth about protective guidelines: Once killing is redefined as "good" instead of "bad," as the experience of the Netherlands and Oregon demonstrate, guidelines cease to be honored as protections against harm but are instead looked upon as obstacles to be overcome. As a consequence, they are attached, ignored, or reinterpreted while potential violations are essentially not investigated—to the point where they become utterly irrelevant.

The Cheney story also reveals that assisted suicide is not working as was expected when voters legalized the practice. Despite being sold to Oregon voters as a way of taking a surreptitious practice "out of the darkness and into the light," assisted suicide operates behind an iron shroud of state-imposed secrecy. What little we do know comes from press releases of assisted suicide advocacy groups, family tip-offs to media—as in the Cheney case—and studies published in the *New England Journal of Medicine (NEJM)*[85] that purported to shed light on the law's actual workings.

Assisted suicide advocates claimed that the *NEJM* reports validate their cause. But a close reading reveals that the worries of assisted suicide opponents were entirely justified. For many years, we have been told repeatedly by assisted suicide advocates that killing is to be a "last resort," applied only when nothing else can be done to alleviate "severe, unrelenting and intolerable suffering."[86] Yet it would appear that few, if any, of the nearly 1,000 Oregonians who have committed assisted suicide as of this writing were in that profoundly desperate a condition. Fear of future pain was a factor in only a few cases. The reason for assisted suicide in the overwhelming majority of these deaths were worries about requiring assistance with daily living (loss of autonomy), being upset about an inability to pursue enjoyable life activities, and fears of being a burden. These are important issues that should be addressed by caregivers, of course. But they do not require suicide as the only choice. Thus rather than being a limited procedure performed out of extreme medical urgency, assisted suicide in Oregon has become a replacement for legitimate medical treatment.[87]

Over the years, it has become clear that whatever guidelines exist in Oregon to protect patients end with the writing of the prescription; the state does not enforce them. Indeed, the system relies substantially on physician self-reporting, and the Oregon Public Health Division (OPHD) has not only no budget to fund investigations of legal violations but also no controlling legal authority to undertake them.

Besides, once the prescription is written, there are no further protections. At no point does the law require to be at the bedside. Nothing needs to be done to ensure that the patient is competent or to prevent coercion. And the psychiatric referral requirement is almost totally ignored.

Not that these referrals necessarily are worth the paper on which they are written. In 2008, psychiatrist Herbert Hendin, an expert on suicide prevention, and Kathleen Foley, perhaps the country's best palliative care physician, studied the practice of legal assisted suicide in Oregon. Writing in the *Michigan Law Review*, they described the experience of Joan Lucas, an ALS patient referred for a mental health evaluation by the death doctor to "cover my ass"[88]; it turned out to be more of a cruel joke than a serious exploration of her mental and emotional health:

> The doctor and the family found a cooperative psychologist who asked Joan to take the Minnesota Multiphasic Inventory, a standard psychological test. Because it was difficult for Joan to travel to the psychologist's office, her children read the true-false questions to her at home. The family found the questions funny, and Joan's daughter described the family as "cracking up" over them. Based on these test results, the psychologist concluded that whatever depression Joan had was directly related to her terminal illness, which he considered a completely normal response.... The psychologist's report in Joan's case is particularly disturbing because without taking the trouble to see her, and on the basis of a single questionnaire administered by her family, he was willing to give an opinion that would facilitate ending Joan's life.[89]

How many other such cases are there? No one knows, and there is no evidence that bureaucrats at the OPHD, tasked with "oversight" of assisted suicide, very much care. No wonder Hendin and Foley concluded that the OPHD "does not collect the information it would need to effectively monitor the law and in its actions and publications acts as the defender of the law rather than as the protector of the welfare of terminally ill patients."[90]

Oregon is not Belgium or the Netherlands—yet. But the state has started down the same destructive path previously blazed by the Netherlands. Thus rather than alleviating concerns that "it can't happen here," Oregon demonstrates that assisted suicide is not only bad medicine but also even worse public policy.

The Money Connection: Ethical values often follow our pocketbooks. That which makes a buck—even if unethical and utterly immoral—is often tolerated and may be even rationalized as a positive good. Profit incentives have thus led to truly evil public policies, epitomized by the "peculiar institution" of American slavery.

This unfortunate fact of life is pertinent in today's debate over assisted suicide. Today's health care system, as previously noted, is no longer predominately fee-for-service but managed care, typified by a health maintenance organization (HMO). In an HMO, profits are not earned by providing services but rather by cutting costs; a penny saved is quite literally a penny earned. Cutting costs is also a key issue in the always-volatile policy debates over how to fund and administer government-funded health insurance such as Medicare, Medicaid, and veterans' hospitals. These economic questions present very real threats to medically marginalized people and, as we shall discuss in more detail later, promote the medical culture of death.

Opponents of legal assisted suicide warn that should killing be redefined as a legitimate medical practice, in the end the ultimate driving force toward hastened death will not be "choice" but money. True, legalized assisted suicide would begin primarily as a phenomenon of white, upper-middle-class people—the kind of people who most tend to support legalization. But once the public became desensitized to doctors directly causing death, the practice could become a cost-cutting tool to shore up strained government health budgets and put extra dollars into the bottom line of for-profit HMOs.

This paradigm has already formed in Oregon, the only state to legalize assisted suicide. Oregon explicitly rations health care to its Medicaid recipients, some of whom are unable to access life-extending chemotherapy that is not expected to extend life for a lengthy period. But assisted suicide is never rationed. Indeed, the Oregon Public Health Division (OPHD), which administers both the rationing regime and the assisted suicide law, published the following statement when removing assisted suicide from the rationing list in 2014: "STATEMENT OF INTENT 2: DEATH WITH DIGNITY ACT. It is the intent of the Commission that services under ORS 127.800-127.897 (Oregon Death with Dignity Act) be covered for those that wish to avail themselves to those services. Such services include but are not limited to attending physician visits, consulting physician confirmation, mental health evaluation and counseling, and prescription medications."[91]

Thus while Oregon will pay for poor citizens to kill themselves, it sometimes will not pay for the far more expensive treatment of some life-threatening conditions, such as a few late-stage cancers and premature birth. That is why many advocates for the poor nationwide, such as the Coalition of Concerned Medical Professionals and Western Service

Worker Associations, denigrate assisted suicide as "death squad medicine" and have commenced grassroots to organize against it.

These attitudes have already claimed victims. Barbara Wagner had recurrent lung cancer, and Randy Stroup had prostate cancer. Both were on Medicaid, the state's health insurance plan for the poor that, like some NHS services, is rationed. The state denied both treatment but told them it would pay for their assisted suicide.

Wagner told ABC News: "It was horrible. I got a letter in the mail that basically said if you want to take the pills, we will help you get that from the doctor and we will stand there and watch you die. But we won't give you the medication to live."[92] "It dropped my chin to the floor," Stroup told Fox News. "[How could they] not pay for medication that would help my life, and yet offer to pay to end my life?"[93] (Wagner eventually received free medication from the drug manufacturer. She has since died. The denial of chemotherapy to Stroup was reversed on appeal after his story hit the media.)

How real is the threat that money will be the ultimate driving force behind legalized euthanasia? That's hard to tell. One study was published that attempted to measure the impact legalization of assisted suicide would have on the economics of medicine: the July 16, 1998 *New England Journal of Medicine* study, undertaken by assisted suicide opponent Ezekiel J. Emanuel, MD, and proponent Margaret P. Battin, PhD.[94] They concluded that the actual financial impact would be approximately $600 million per year. But that study was faulty: it assumed that assisted suicide would be very narrowly applied, a highly unlikely outcome of legalization. (Battin herself has argued elsewhere for a broad use of "rational suicide," for example, by elderly people who require expensive care as a "self sacrifice based on altruistic reasons"—hardly a prescription for restraint.[95]) The study also assumed that virtually all assisted suicides would occur within four weeks of natural death, a most dubious assumption.[96] Indeed, the study itself acknowledged that if 7 percent of people who die in the US committed assisted suicide within two months of deaths, the yearly financial savings would be in the billions.

There is a crucial omission from the Emanuel/Battin study that limits its value, even if their data and conclusions were otherwise correct: the role that personal and family financial issues would play in assisted suicide decision making. The authors did not discuss the issue, they claim, because there were insufficient published studies with which to "quantify these savings." Yet it is here, at the micro level, that money could play the most crucial role of all in the "choice" for assisted suicide.

Extended illness or disability can devastate family finances. In a society that increasingly discounts the inherent moral worth of the lives of sick and disabled people, in light of this unfortunate reality, failure to "choose" assisted suicide could quickly be perceived widely as selfish and insensitive to other family financial obligations. ("Gee, Grandma, because we have to care for you, Timmy can't go to college.") This could, in turn, lead to overwhelming societal pressures favoring hastened death—the so-called duty to die already under active discussion in bioethics literature—not to mention the risk of coercion by relatives hungry for inheritance. Indeed, the Ninth Circuit Court of Appeals in its 1994 ruling declaring a constitutional right to assisted suicide (later overturned by the Supreme Court) stated that it would be proper for dying and disabled people to take "the economic welfare of their families and loved ones" into consideration when deciding to be killed.[97] Similarly, Derek Humphry, cofounder of the Hemlock Society, wrote that avoiding family burdens would be a splendid reason to commit assisted suicide:

> A rational argument can be made for allowing PAS in order to offset
> the amount society and families spend on the ill, as long as it is the
> voluntary wish of the mentally competent terminally ill adult.... There
> is no contradicting the fact that since the largest medical expenses are
> incurred in the final days and weeks of life, the hastened demise of
> people with only a short time to left would free resources for others.
> Hundreds of billions of dollars could benefit those patients who not
> only *can* be cured but who *want* to live.[98] (Emphasis within the text.)

If assisted suicide were ever permitted to become a legitimate and legal part of medical practice, it could become less about "choice" than about profits in the health care system and cutting the costs of health care to government and families. An assisted suicide only costs about $1,000, including the doctor's fee. It could easily cost $100,000 to provide the caring support that would make a patient not want assisted suicide. The financial force of gravity is obvious.

Assisted Suicide Is Not "Death with Dignity": The primary "medical acts" death doctors take when committing Oregon-style assisted suicides are to diagnose the patient with an illness that he or she reasonably expects to cause death within six months—a highly uncertain matter, at best—and to prescribe the poisonous agent. (The doctor is also supposed to refer the patient to a mental health professional if he or she suspects depression that "distorts judgment." But that means little in real life and induced death, especially in a mental health milieu where many professionals have embraced "rational suicide.") Once the prescription is issued, the doctor's duties are officially done. The patient is left on their own to take the poison.

This leaves many suicidal patients at material risk not only for death but also for serious injury. According to none other than Derek Humphry, approximately "25 percent of assisted suicides fail."[99] A 1998 study in the *Journal of the American Medical Association* puts the figure at 15 percent, even though that study involved an analysis of assisted suicides committed by oncologists.[100] More recently, a report published in the pro-assisted suicide *New England Journal of Medicine* revealed that in the Netherlands, despite nearly thirty years of assisted suicide/euthanasia experience, "complications occurred in 7 percent of cases of assisted suicide, and problems with completion in 16 percent of cases complications and problems with completion occurred in 3 percent and 6 percent of cases of euthanasia, respectively."[101] What does "failure" or "complications" mean in the context of physician-induced death? It could mean vomiting, convulsions, coma, or an extended death over several days, or a combination of these.

The "Humphry cure" for a failed assisted suicide is for someone to place a plastic bag over the head of the suicidal person: death by suffocation, hardly a dignified end. In the Netherlands, the cure is for the doctor to give a lethal injection. Demonstrating the corrosive nature of the medical culture of death, the late Yale University's Dr. Sherwin Nuland opined that better medical school training in killing is the answer to failed doctor-induced death[102]—this at a time when doctors are inadequately taught proper pain control techniques and the best methods of providing their patients end-of-life care.

Of even greater concern than failed assisted suicides is the life-devaluing nature of assisted suicide and the crassness with which assisted suicide is often practiced, once the initial jitters and queasiness are past and killing becomes relatively routine. A revealing book, written a few years ago by a Dutch doctor, Bert Keizer, tore the curtains off the supposed compassion of assisted suicide. Keizer works in a nursing home, where he cares for—and sometimes kills—disabled, elderly, and dying people. He looks upon euthanasia as a necessary and proper, albeit distasteful, part of his job. As depicted in the book, so do his colleagues, patients, and their families.

Keizer's book, *Dancing with Mr. D*, demonstrates the dehumanizing effect euthanasia has upon medical practice and civilized society. Keizer is brutally honest. The lives of frail and dying people are depicted as pointless, useless, ugly, grotesque. Those with whom Keizer interacts all seem to share these views, including his colleagues, family members of patients, and the patients themselves. This allows them to be killed without consequence, other than Keizer having a few bad dreams.

And kill patients Keizer does, again and again. One man he euthanizes probably has lung cancer, but the diagnosis is never certain. A relative tells Keizer that the man wants to be given a lethal injection, a request later confirmed by the patient. Keizer quickly agrees to kill the man. Demonstrating the utter uselessness of "protective guidelines," Keizer never tells his patient about treatment options or how the pain and other symptoms of cancer can be palliated effectively. He never checks to see if the man has been pressured into wanting a hastened death or is depressed. Keizer doesn't even take the time to confirm the diagnosis with certainty. When a colleague asks why rush and points out that the man isn't suffering terribly, Keizer snaps:

"Is it for us to answer this question? All I know is that he wants to die more or less upright and that he doesn't want to crawl to his grave the way a dog crawls howling to the side walk after he's been hit by a car."[103]

Keizer either doesn't know or doesn't care that with proper medical treatment, people with lung cancer do not have to die in such unmitigated agony. The next day, he lethally injects his patient, telling his colleagues as he walks to the man's room to do the deed, "If anyone so much as whispers cortisone [a palliative agent] or 'uncertain diagnosis,' I'll hit him."[104]

Another of Keizer's patients is disabled by Parkinson's disease. The patient requests to be killed, but before the act can be carried out, he receives a letter from his brother, who uses a religious argument to urge him to change his mind. The letter causes the man to hesitate, upsetting Keizer, who writes, "I don't know what to do with such a wavering death wish. It's getting on my nerves. Does he want to die or doesn't he? I do hope we won't have to go over the whole business again, right from the very start."[105] Keizer involves the nursing home chaplain to assure the man that euthanasia will not upset God. The man again thinks he wants to die. Keizer is quick with the lethal injection, happy the man has "good veins," and the man expires before his uncertainty can disturb his doctor's mood again.

The book is rife with such stories. In Keizer's world, his patients' lives are inherently undignified. Medical professionals view those in their care with disdain. Family members are mostly selfish, greedy, stupid, and unloving.

Keizer consults with a patient who wants to commit assisted suicide because he has Lou Gehrig's disease. But Keizer objects—not because he values the man's life and wants to convince him to find a better way to deal with his disease—but, fearing the man will botch his own death, he wants to do the killing personally. So Keizer involves a social worker, a longtime acquaintance of the distraught man, who tells him coldly, "Your life is one of the most terrible things I know of and I do believe that it would a great relief to you if it would end. But I cannot believe that you will have the strength to take the overdose in the event the doctor will hand it to you."[106]

Where is the compassion? Where is the valuing of the lives of sick and disabled people? Where is the "dignity" that death advocates yell so much about?

At a key point in his book, a colleague asks Keizer whether he should love his patients, "if only a little." Then, in an illuminating passage, Keizer replies: "I think it's good for the profession if I heave a deep sigh now and declare my heartfelt assent [to the question posed]. And there are situations that do upset you. But love?" Keizer muses, "I doubt it."

Voluntary Stop Eating and Drinking: VSED, what's that? In euthanasia advocacy parlance it means "voluntary stopping eating and drinking" and is taught by some advocacy groups as a way to commit suicide without fears that the law will intervene.

Suicide is not technically illegal, although it is not a right: The authorities may prevent suicides forcefully, if necessary. As we have also seen, patients depending on life support may refuse this treatment, even if it means they are likely to die. This includes the right to remove ANH—not as a right to make someone dead but to refuse unwanted medical intervention.

But euthanasia advocates want more. They argue that people who don't require medical treatment to remain alive should also have a "right to die." Already, Oregon, Washington, California, and Vermont allow assisted suicide: Doctors may prescribe lethal drugs for competent patients expected to die within six months. Belgium, the Netherlands, Luxembourg, Canada, and Colombia (in the latter two examples, because of decisions by the countries' supreme courts) allow active euthanasia.

But these laws (at present) mostly require a serious medical diagnosis, and most legal jurisdictions still outlaw assisted suicide and euthanasia. That leaves those such as the suicidal elderly "tired of life," those with less severe disabilities, and those who are chronically ill who want to die with no legally assisted means to become dead.

That's where assisted suicide organizations like Compassion and Choices (formerly known as the Hemlock Society) promote VSED as a method of suicide. Here's how Compassion and Choices describes the situation in an online booklet teaching people how to commit suicide by self-starvation:[107]

> Some call us because they feel overwhelmed by the symptoms of chron-
> ic and progressive illnesses that fill their days with misery and suffering.
> There are also those who may not be seriously ill but are simply "done."
> After eight or nine decades of life, they want information about ways
> to gently slip away in a peaceful and dignified manner. Regardless of
> their clinical circumstances, these individuals share a common desire to
> maintain autonomy over their own end-of-life decisions. They want to
> die as they have lived, making the important decisions that affect their
> lives with collaboration and support from trusted healthcare providers,
> family members and other caregivers.[108]

A person commits VSED by refusing all sustenance. To ensure that death is not impeded, the suicidal person leaves instructions explicitly refusing any medical intervention to nourish them, which prevents forced feeding or ANH. Because VSED can cause agonizing symptoms, advocates suggest that the suicidal person find a sympathetic doctor or hospice to provide pain relief. (It is important, as with ANH, to distinguish between VSED and the point that may occur in the natural process of dying when a patient stops taking food and drink. This is not suicide, and starvation is not the cause of death. Indeed, in such cases, it is medically inappropriate to force food upon the dying patient.)

The promotion of VSED for the elderly and other non-dying people by the most prominent assisted suicide advocacy organization in the United States proves the lie that the "right to die" will ever be limited permanently to the terminally ill. Indeed, it amazes me that so many people still believe that oleaginous false assurance.

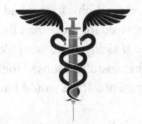

CHAPTER 4

CREATING A DUTY TO DIE

Baby Ryan Nguyen was born in Spokane's Sacred Heart Hospital on October 27, 1994. He was very premature, at just twenty-three weeks' gestation. Ryan's kidneys were not working well, so doctors put him on dialysis. But when the doctors determined that Ryan was not a good candidate for kidney transplantation, they decreed that continuing his treatment was futile. His father was told, "The time has come for your baby to die," and his dialysis was discontinued.

Ryan's parents vehemently objected and retained an attorney who quickly obtained a temporary court order compelling doctors to continue his treatment. Unhappy that its will had been thwarted, hospital administration reported Ryan's parents to child protective services, accusing the Nguyen's of "physical abuse" and "physical neglect" for obtaining the injunction.[1] When that tactic didn't fly, administrators and doctors fought the parents in court, swearing under oath that "Ryan's condition is universally fatal," that the infant had "no chance" for survival, and that treatment could not "serve as a bridge to future care." Based on these contentions, Ryan's doctors urged the judge to permit them to cease his continued treatment as futile and a violation of *their* integrity, values, and ethics.[2]

The court never decided who had ultimate say over Ryan's care—his parents or medical professionals—because his treatment was transferred to Emmanuel Children's Hospital in Portland, Oregon, under the care of a different doctor who did not view Ryan Nguyen as a futile patient. The new doctor, not the original physicians, had it right. Ryan was soon weaned off dialysis and survived for more than four years, a time in which he was a generally happy, if sickly, child who liked to give "high-fives." Had his original doctors successfully imposed their futile care philosophy on their patient and his parents, Ryan would have died before he had a chance to live.

In 2011, a similar struggle between doctors who believed a baby's time had come and heartbroken, loving parents wanting their seriously ill child to experience all that life could offer hit the headlines. Joseph Marraachli was diagnosed with a terminal and progressively debilitating neurological disease at age ten months. Joseph was cared for in a London, Ontario, hospital ICU when doctors told his parents, Moe Marraachli and Sana Nader, that they were going to withdraw all life-sustaining care.

Moe and Sana disagreed with the decision and a bitter dispute erupted with hospital doctors and administrators over continuing Joseph's care. There were two separate areas of disagreement: first, stated intention to end all life-sustaining treatment. Then when Moe and Sana asked doctors to perform a tracheotomy so Joseph could be taken home and cared for by them there, doctors again refused—claiming such a procedure was medically and ethically unwarranted.

Litigation ensued. The bitter impasse was broken when the American nonprofit organization Priests for Life paid to transfer Joseph to a hospital in St. Louis that was willing to perform the surgery. The operation was a success, and Joseph was brought home, where he died peacefully in his sleep five months later.[3]

Princeton bioethicist Peter Singer—whose utilitarian views we have already explored—criticized the money spent on giving Joseph's parents more time with their baby:

Here's the irony. According to the most rigorous charity evaluation agency in the country, GiveWell.org, you can save a child's life for about $1,000. All you have to do is give the money to their top-rated charity, Village Reach, which delivers vaccines and other urgently needed medical supplies to rural areas in developing countries. If Priests for Life were really serious about saving lives, instead of "rescuing" Joseph so he can live another few months lying in bed, unable to experience the normal joys of childhood, let alone become an adult, they could have used the money they have raised to save 150 lives—most of them children who would have gone on to live healthy, happy lives for 50 years or more.[4]

In other words, Singer believes the money spent on Joseph would have been put to better use for children who were not terminally ill.

Consider the facts of this tragic case: Moe and Sana were proved correct *medically* about their son benefiting from the tracheotomy. They said the surgery would allow Joseph to go home in the loving care of his parents. They said the surgery would enable them to manage his care. It all came to pass.

Why were they resisted so vociferously and criticized publicly for wanting medicine to extend Joseph's life? The case was one battle in an increasingly bitter conflict over contesting moral values and worldviews now playing out in the public health, policy, and medical arenas. The doctors sought to *impose* their belief that it would be pointless, expensive, and cruel to maintain Joseph's life. Moe and Sana believed that Joseph was immeasurably precious, and they wanted to love and care for him for as long as he breathed, and moreover, as his parents, they believed strongly that the final decision should be theirs.

Whether Joseph *should* have had those extra months isn't akin to solving a math equation or determining the chemical makeup of a molecule; rather it depends on one's worldview. The simple conundrum thus presented—and it is one we will face increasingly as society generally and the medical system specifically grow more technocratic—was and is *whose values* should prevail in such disputes: the Singer-style utilitarian/quality of life ethic or a morality that accepts the equal importance of all, including sick, disabled, or dying patients.

FUTILE CARE THEORY

The medical tyranny in which the families of Baby Ryan and Baby Joseph became ensnared exemplifies the bioethics-driven policy known as "medical futility," or, as I call it, "futile care theory." FCT authorizes doctors to refuse or withdraw *wanted* life-sustaining medical treatment over the objections of family and patients when the doctors believe that their patient's quality of life is not worth living—or, lurking in the subtext, worth the resources.

To illustrate how dramatically medical futility departs from the autonomy-based medical decision-making model, whose triumphs in the 1960s and 1970s so improved medicine, assume you are dying of cancer and do not want CPR at your death. You instruct your doctor to place a "do not resuscitate" (DNR) order in your medical chart. Your wishes will be honored because the principle of autonomy gives you the right to refuse unwanted treatment. Should your heart stop, you will be allowed to die naturally without medical intervention.

Assume again that your spouse is seriously injured in an auto accident and sustains catastrophic brain damage. Your beloved requires a feeding tube to survive. Time passes, and you decide he or she would not want to live in such a profoundly cognitively disabled condition. You make a hard decision. You instruct the doctors to remove your spouse's feeding tube. As we discussed previously, your decision will be honored by the medical profession and respected at law as encompassed by the so-called "right to die."

Now return to the first scenario, only instead of eschewing resuscitation, you tell your doctor that you *want* CPR in the hope that will gain you a few extra weeks or months of life. In the second case, instead of instructing doctors to remove your spouse's feeding tube, you insist that it be maintained. Or, more vividly, think of Terri Schiavo, but instead of her husband and family fighting over whether to remove her feeding tube, they agree it should remain, but doctors refuse. Under FCT, doctors/bioethics committees should have the right to deny CPR or remove the feeding tube over the objections of family—*even over instructions in the patient's advance medical directive.*

FCT is defended by "futilitarians" (if you will) as upholding the bioethics principles of non-maleficence and/or "distributive justice," and protecting the "integrity" of health care professionals, whom they claim are "demoralized" by having to treat hopelessly ill people. In the words of Susan Fox Buchanan, former executive director of the Colorado Collective for Medical Decisions (CCMD), a bioethics think tank, the issue is about "facing limits on our mortality, on our technology, our community relationships with each other and our responsibility for stewardship of shared resources."[5]

All of this begs the question: What is futile care? That is a matter that bioethicists and other members of the medical intelligentsia are still debating after decades of disputation over the details and the procedures for nationwide implementation. But, like a photo downloading on an old-fashioned dial-up computer modem, a rough bioethical consensus has slowly come into focus.

In May 1994, Dr. Marcia Angell—then the executive editor of the *New England Journal of Medicine* and a big assisted suicide proponent—editorialized that patients diagnosed as permanently unconscious be refused medical treatment so that "demoralized" caregivers would not be forced to provide care they believe is futile or which wastes "valuable resources." How? One way suggested by Dr. Angell would be to change the definition of "death" to include a diagnosis of permanent unconsciousness, a proposal, as we will see in the next chapter, many bioethicists view as a splendid way to increase the number of available organs for transplant. Realizing the PR difficulties inherent in declaring a breathing body a corpse, Dr. Angell declared that she would also accept the creation of mandatory time limits on providing medical treatment for unconscious people after which the care would be withdrawn regardless of family objections. Her third and preferred approach would be to flip the usual legal presumption in favor of life and thereby force families with the "idiosyncratic view" that their loved ones be provided treatment to prove in court that the patient would want such care.[6]

By the time Angell's editorial was published, Daniel Callahan, one of the godfathers of bioethics, offered several rather vague definitions of futility in his 1993 book, *The Troubled Dream of Life*. It exists, he wrote, when:

- "there is a likely, though not necessarily certain, downward course of an illness, making death a strong probability";
- "successful treatment is more likely to bring extended unconsciousness or advanced dementia than cure or significant amelioration";
- "the available treatments for a potentially fatal condition entail a significant likelihood of extended pain or suffering"; or

- "the available treatments significantly increase the probability of a bad death, even if they promise to extend life."[7]

In such cases, Callahan urges that a presumption against medical treatment, other than comfort care, be created and that people who insist on these futile treatments be required to pay for it themselves.

The American Thoracic Society entered the fray early, issuing a policy statement that declared that treatment should be considered futile "if reasoning and experience indicate that the intervention would be highly unlikely to result in a *meaningful* survival for the patient" (their emphasis); it further opined that a "health care institution has the right to limit a life-sustaining intervention without consent."[8]

Specificity has always been the bane of futile care analysis. Thus, in 2011, an article in *Health Care Ethics* proposed a "third generation approach to medical futility" that remains maddeningly vague:

- G. Lack of agreement. If agreement cannot be reached about withholding or withdrawing treatment, an ethics consult should be called and the hospital president or administrator on-call should be notified of the situation. Additionally, attention should now focus on restricting treatment options in light of the patient's best interests with no treatment options being offered to the family that will extend or increase the patient's suffering....

- G1. Offer time-limited trial. If the treatment in question does not extend or increase the patient's suffering and could perhaps achieve its physiological end, the attending/primary treating physician could offer the option of providing the treatment for a time-limited trial. The attending/primary treating physician must delineate the therapeutic goals and the length of time the treatment will be provided to assess the effects of the treatment in light of the goals....

- G2. Discuss alternate care options. If, after the time-limited trial, the treatment is still considered unreasonable or inappropriate, it could be withdrawn provided there is wide agreement among the attending/primary treating physician, other caregivers, hospital president, ethics committee and so on....[9]

So much for patient autonomy, precision, and due process of law.

At this moment, several important points need to be made:

Futility is a value judgment, not a medical determination. Medical futility used to be an *objective* medical determination that a proposed treatment could have virtually no *physiological* benefit to the patient. To illustrate the point with an extreme example: If a patient asked a doctor for an appendectomy to cure an ear infection, the physician is and should be obligated by professional ethics to refuse the request because the proposed surgery would have zero efficacious effect on the ear infection and moreover would harm the patient. This "objective" concept of futility, however, is not what FCT is all about. Rather, when futilitarians use the terms, "medical futility," "inappropriate care," or "non-beneficial treatment," they have entered the realm of *subjective* value judgments. As Dr. Stuart Youngner, a bioethicist and medical professor at Western Reserve University School of Medicine, once put it, "futility determinations will inevitably involve value judgments about: 1) whether low probability chances are worth taking; and 2) whether certain lives are of a quality worth living."[10]

Determinations about futility involve paternalism. "Medical paternalism exists," wrote the late medical ethicist Edmund D. Pellegrino, MD, "when the physician assumes the patient's right to make self-governing decisions and acts to prevent, manipulate, or coerce him or her in the name of the patient's best interests."[11] That was the wrong in hooking people up to medical machines against their will. Now, with futility, a new and more deadly game of "Doctor Knows Best" is being played—and this time, instead of compelling lives to be extended, the doctor decides that the time has come for the patient to die, whether or not the patient or family agree.

The inherent arrogance of strangers imposing futility determinations upon family members and patients was well illustrated in a revealing article in *California Lawyer* written by a former house counsel to Stanford University Hospital. Ethyl had been receiving kidney dialysis at Stanford University Hospital for several years and had entered end-stage renal disease. Ethyl was very ill; she was a diabetic, she had cardiac problems, and she was bloated from fluid buildup caused by her kidney failure.

Ethyl was cared for by her daughter, Mary. Hospital workers noticed that during her treatments, Ethyl seemed "agitated and distressed" but she never "was able to voice any specific complaints or requests."[12] (The article implies that Ethyl was incompetent but does not say so explicitly.) After one dialysis session left Ethyl weak and "unable to move from the dialysis couch to the wheelchair," her urologist decided that the treatment was too difficult for Ethyl. He tried to convince Mary to discontinue Ethyl's dialysis and limit her treatment to comfort care.

Mary did not accede to the doctor's recommendation. A pressure campaign began to convince Mary to cease her mother's life-sustaining treatment. As the months progressed, "Mary became hostile to everyone in the center and threatened legal action if they did not continue her mother's treatments."[13] One can understand why; the staff refused to take no for an answer.

Unable to have his way with Mary, Ethyl's doctor took the issue to the hospital biomedical ethics committee, chaired by a "medical ethicist" with "philosophical and medical training" (i.e., a mainstream bioethicist) and comprising nurses, physicians, case workers, and community representatives. The committee picked apart Mary's motives for wanting her mother to live. It determined that "Mary was a loving and attentive caregiver" but found "no evidence" that Ethyl "had ever expressed her own preferences about medical treatment." Mary had religious beliefs that may have been affecting her decision making, an approach to life some bioethicists disfavor as irrational. "Committee members with training in social services and psychology" asked about Mary's relationship with her mother and were told that she had "few friends" and that Ethyl's death would leave Mary "alone and without a focus."[14]

The ethics committee decided that "Mary's own needs were interfering with her ability to act in her mother's best interest" and "we also agreed that the burdens of Ethyl's treatment more than likely outweighed the benefits." The ethics committee told the doctor to try and transfer care to another physician but, failing that, to stop treatment unilaterally.

A few weeks later, the committee met to discuss Ethyl's case. "To everyone's surprise, Mary had found a doctor willing to continue her mother's dialysis. No one in the committee had expected her to succeed, and we were actually quite dismayed that she had." Thwarted in their desire to impose their values on the situation, one member said bitterly, "The poor woman, her daughter is blind to what is best for her."[15]

Some might call this a happy ending, for it permitted a daughter to decide her mother's care rather than strangers steeped in amoral bioethics training. Frighteningly, as will be described below, the "loophole" Mary used to ensure her mother's continued treatment—getting another doctor to treat in the same facility—has been closed by some hospital futile care policy protocols, which refuse a new doctor permission to render treatment that the hospital ethics committee has proclaimed to be futile.

Futile care decisions will be based on prejudice and bias against disabled patients and other minorities. This may already be happening. The Mayo Clinic has reported that "many physicians' definition of futility includes interventions that might be considered medically reasonable." The report noted that of seventy-five patients whose care was reviewed, "physicians deemed CPR to be futile in 32% despite the probability that survival was 5% or greater and in 20% when the survival probability was 10% or greater." Moreover, the potential for futility decisions being based on prejudice or bias is clearly illustrated when, according to the report, *"CPR was more likely to be considered futile if the patient was not white."*[16] (My emphasis.)

Those most at risk of unequal treatment are people with disabilities, which explains the disability rights community's adamant opposition to granting doctors or hospital committees futile care authority. An article in the *Hastings Center Report* about the "better dead than disabled" mind-set by William J. Peace, the paralyzed author of the *Bad Cripple* blog,[17] amply illustrates the need for concern that "best interests of the patient" medical futility decisions will really be discrimination masked as compassion. When Peace had a serious leg infection that would not heal, his hospitalist (a specialist in the care of hospitalized patients) pushed Peace toward choosing to die under comfort care instead of treating his wound aggressively with antibiotics: "Although not explicitly stated, the message was loud and clear. I can help you die peacefully. Clearly death was preferable to a nursing home care, unemployment, bankruptcy, and a lifetime in bed. I am not sure exactly what I said or how I said it, but I was emphatic—I wanted to continue treatment, including the antibiotics. I wanted to live."[18]

Peace experienced the kind of difficult and expensive recovery predicted by the doctor and cited as the reason to choose death over life. But he is glad to still be alive and remains profoundly alarmed by the doctor's discriminatory attitude that he believed devalued his moral worth as an equal human being:

The fear I felt that night and that gnaws at me to this day is not unusual—many paralyzed people I know are fearful, even though very few express it. Many people with a disability would characterize a hospital as a hostile social environment. Hospitals and diagnostic equipment are often grossly inaccessible. Staff members can be rude, condescending, and unwilling to listen or adapt to any person who falls outside the norm. We people with a disability represent extra work for them. We are a burden. We also need expensive, high-tech equipment that the hospital probably does not own.... Complicating matters further is the widespread use of hospitalists—generally an internist who works exclusively in the hospital and directs inpatient care. The hospitalist model of care is undoubtedly efficient and saves hospitals billions of dollars a year. However there is a jarring disconnect between inpatient and outpatient care, which can represent a serious risk to people with a disability. My experience certainly demonstrates this, as no physician who knew me would have suggested withholding lifesaving treatment.[19]

Peace notes a frightening irony that, in hospitals, disabled people who want to die are quickly supported in their autonomy. "Who is discriminated against?" he asks. "Those people with a disability who choose to live."[20] He concludes with a cogent warning for our discussion of Futile Care Theory: "What I experienced in the hospital was a microcosm of a much larger social problem. Simply put, my disabled body is not normal. We are well equipped to deal with normal bodies. Efficient protocols exist within institutions, and the presence of a disabled body creates havoc. Before I utter one word or am examined by a physician, it is obvious that my presence is a problem. Sitting in my wheelchair, I am a living symbol of all that can go wrong with a body and of the limits of medical science to correct it."[21]

Consider the invidious paradigm in which Peace found himself—and resisted—in an administrative context under which FCT impositions can be imposed by *strangers*. The danger of such an authority to refuse treatment *that is working* (e.g., extending life when that is wanted) should be self-evident.

Futile care empowers strangers to make medicine's most important health care decisions. Deciding whether to accept or reject life-sustaining care is one of the most difficult medical choices patients and families will ever have to make. Indeed, when bioethicists argue that families should be able to discontinue tube-feeding for cognitively disabled family members, they commonly speak of protecting family intimacy and personal values. But under FCT, suddenly such considerations matter less than institutional and professional values, and indeed, when faced with decisions with which they disagree, we are told that patient autonomy must take second place to the values of doctors and bioethics committees.

The trend transforming hospital biomedical ethics committees from mediators of controversies between doctors and patients—a valuable and important role—into quasi-judicial bodies is just one example of medical depersonalization. Another is the emergence of a relatively new medical specialist known as the "hospitalist," the kind of doctor with which Peace contended. Hospitalists are MD specialists who direct and coordinate the overall care of hospitalized patients. They interact with treating specialists, decide when to admit and discharge the patient, and assume all of the duties, which traditionally have been the responsibility of the patient's personal physician. A patient sick enough to be hospitalized will be under the care of a stranger rather than a physician he or she may have known for years, though it is at just such a precarious time that the link of trust forged over time between patient and doctor is most important.

Hospitalists are not paid directly by patients; they are employees of the hospital in which they work or are independent consultants who have contracted to provide hospitalist services. The hospitalist movement was conceived to reduce costs and improve efficiency without compromising quality of care. These are certainly worthy goals. But hospitalists will also become major societal providers of end-of-life care.[22] That could help improve palliation, since pain and symptom control are frequent medical issues at the end of life that hospitalists must be trained to confront. But the emergence of hospitalists is potentially worrisome in the context of FCT: they are virtual strangers to the patient and family, and their primary emotional loyalty, albeit not their professional responsibility, is likely to be to their institution. This could leave marginalized patients at material risk of being written off as futile care cases.

This worry increases exponentially when advocates of the hospitalist movement advocate that practitioners obtain "superb training in biomedical ethics."[23] (According to the pro-medical futility advocate, law professor, and bioethicist Thaddeus Mason Pope, a bioethics committee at Massachusetts General Hospital has been quietly imposing unilateral DNR decisions since 2006.)[24] Making the concern even more acute, futile care legislation has been introduced in some jurisdictions that would permit doctors in hospitals to impose a do-not-resuscitate order on a patient's chart without consent.[25]

In 2015, a joint official policy statement on futile care was issued by the American Thoracic Society, the American Association for Critical Care Nurses, and three other professional organizations that illustrates the points made above. "Responding to Requests for Potentially Inappropriate Treatments in Intensive Care Units" is a frightening document, akin to those signs sometimes seen over a restaurant door: We Reserve the Right to Refuse Service. Three particular points of the position paper illustrate the danger posed by FCT to people with profound disabilities, the elderly, and the dying who want to fight to stay alive:

- First, the statement acknowledges that most futile care controversies *aren't about treatment that is really "futile"* as that word is properly defined. From the statement (my emphasis): "The term 'potentially inappropriate' should be used, rather than 'futile,' to describe treatments that have at least some chance of accomplishing the effect sought by the patient, but clinicians believe that competing ethical considerations justify not providing them."[26]

Think carefully about that: The statement creates an *explicit conflict of interest* with patients by relieving physicians from their fiduciary obligation to each individual patient on the altar of other admittedly important matters, issues that should be of lesser professional concern (such as the cost of care, perceived societal betterment, personal disagreements with patient values, religion, or the doctor's/bioethicists' belief in the quality of life ethic).

- Second, the documents include the usual bromides about effective communication—and I am sure they think they mean it. But realize that *the policy grants the ultimate decision-making power to strangers* rather than the patient or family—including the contents of an advance medical directive. Thus once the talking is done and a treatment conflict becomes intractable, the policy authorizes the following steps:
  1. Offer surrogates the opportunity to transfer the patient to an alternate institution;

2. Inform surrogates of the opportunity to pursue extramural [litigation] appeal; and
3. Implement the decision of the resolution process.[27]

With that power structure firmly in place, communication can quickly devolve into coercion because everyone will know that the most the family/patient can do is *stall* the outcome, not actually prevent the refusal of treatment. Not only that but bioethics committee meetings are held behind closed doors, are confidential, don't keep detailed records such as transcriptions, etc. If (when) it rules that treatment should be stopped, the onus shifts to the very sick patient or overmatched family to take protective action. Notice also that the common sense solution to the conflict of allowing the patient to find another doctor to provide the care in the hospital goes unmentioned, and if Texas is any example, will not be allowed.

- Finally, not content with granting themselves the power to impose these decisions, signators to the policy want their administrative hammer reinforced by the raw power statutory law: The medical profession should lead public engagement efforts and advocate for policies and legislation about when life-prolonging technologies should not be used.[28]

Make no mistake—the policy statement seeks to further the power of the technocracy by enabling government-established cost/benefit panels to make decisions allowing withdrawal of insurance coverage under the Affordable Care Act for efficacious treatments once they are deemed "potentially inappropriate. (We'll consider the hand-in-glove connection between FCT and health care rationing below.)

Futile care theory illustrates the incremental approach with which bioethics corrodes traditional medical ethics. When Dr. Leo Alexander warned of the dangers of utilitarianism in medicine, he had no idea that the bioethics movement would intentionally push the profession away from the values epitomized by the Hippocratic Oath. Nor did he know that the changes he feared would be instituted by deliberate design as incremental "reform." But that is what has happened: A once "unthinkable" practice is rendered debatable by being respectably discussed in bioethics and medical journals. Soon, the new approach will be applied in a few cases—and fought for if those subjected to the new approach object. Eventually, what was formerly controversial becomes a routine part of clinical practice, creating a new ethical paradigm. Finally, the once-unthinkable act or omission may become the required decision.

That was certainly the pattern involving people diagnosed with a persistent vegetative state. First, dehydration, once unthinkable, was promoted as a matter of respecting patient and family choices (i.e., the so-called right to die). Dehydration was applied against a few patients, found legal validation with Nancy Cruzan, and may be seen as the preferred societal approach after the Terri Schiavo case. Today, barely thirty years after the issue first entered the bioethics discourse, patients—both unconscious and minimally conscious—are dehydrated to death throughout the country, and it is deemed a routine and relatively ho-hum clinical practice.

Now, with FCT, hospital protocols could one day require feeding tubes to be withdrawn from PVS patients even *over the objections* of family decision makers and in spite of patient desires expressed in advance medical directives. Indeed, the late Dr. Ronald Cranford, the neurologist/bioethicist, who promoted—and testified repeatedly in support of—dehydrating cognitively disabled people acknowledged that the changes in approach to PVS he advocated "proceeded" in this "logical and incremental way."[29]

Futile care theory has already cut a deadly path through patient and family lives. People have been taken off respirators without consent. Nursing home residents have had DNR orders placed on their medical charts without authorization. Parents have been reported to authorities for child abuse because they have insisted on life support for prematurely born infants. Spouses or relatives have been sued by hospitals to have them removed as decision makers for ill loved ones because they instructed treatment to continue.

One approach futilitarians have taken is to litigate against families unwilling to consent to cutting off life-sustaining care of their loved ones. The first such case, way back in 1990–1991, involved Helga Wanglie, an elderly woman in a permanent coma with multiple organ failure. Helga was dependent on a ventilator for her continued life. Her doctors received permission from her husband to place a DNR order on Helga's chart, but he refused to permit them to withdraw the ventilator.

Dr. Steven Miles, a bioethicist and physician who became the public spokesman for the hospital, sued Mr. Wanglie (technically, he became the petitioner after the original physician withdrew due to a death in the family). Miles told me there were three reasons why Helga's physicians wanted to stop her treatment: "The palliative aspects of her care would not work because she was incapable of feeling the benefit of having the ventilator relieve air hunger; the continued provision of the respirator would not keep open the possibility that she would return to any type of minimally rational life; and the use of the respirator would not allow her to have a relational life in the present." I asked Miles whether her continued life, in and of itself, was considered a benefit to her. "Yes," he replied, "but we did not have a way to help her acquire a quality of life that she herself could value."[30]

For his part, Mr. Wanglie stated that his wife valued life simply for life's sake and that she would want to remain alive under these conditions. The question presented to the court: Whose ultimate moral values should prevail, the husband's/wife's or those of the medical professionals?

After a hearing, the court refused to oust Mr. Wanglie as his wife's medical surrogate, ruling that as her husband of many years, he was the best person to make Helga's health care decisions.[31] The ruling only settled the first part of the case. Still to be decided was whether the doctors had to continue to treat Helga with a respirator despite their view that the treatment was futile. This issue was never adjudicated because Helga died and the matter was dropped.

A similar scenario unfolded in Flint, Michigan, in 1993, where Baby Terry was born prematurely at twenty-three weeks gestation. (The normal gestation for a human infant is thirty-eight to forty weeks.) Baby Terry weighed one pound and seven ounces at birth and was desperately ill. Deprived of oxygen, his brain had been damaged and he required a respirator to stay alive.

Doctors at Hurley Medical Center advised Terry's parents, Rosetta Christle, age twenty-one, and Terry Achtabowski, age twenty-two, that Terry's life support was futile. But Christle and Achtabowski disagreed. They weren't ready to give up. Their baby had gained a pound and successfully resisted a bacterial infection, and they wanted him to have every opportunity to fight for his life.

The parents' refusal to accept treatment termination was unacceptable to Baby Terry's doctors and the hospital administration. They called in the Michigan Department of Social Services, which quickly brought court action to strip the young parents of their right to make decisions over their son's medical treatment. (Such drastic action is usually taken only when parents refuse needed medical treatment for their children.) A hearing was convened and testimony elicited. The physicians were unanimous in their desire to terminate care, testifying that Terry was in pain, although relieved by morphine; that his bodily systems were slowly breaking down; and that he had no chance of long-term survival. The Hurley Hospital ethics committee weighed in on August 9, 1993, opining that removing the parents' insistence on continued treatment "would be contrary to medical judgment and to *moral and ethical beliefs of physicians* caring for the patient."[32] (My emphasis.) In other words, when it came to choosing between the values of Baby Terry's parents, based in large part on their religious faith, and the values of doctors and the hospital, the state argued that only the latter opinions mattered.

Solely on the basis of their refusal to permit treatment to end, Judge Thomas Gadola of the Genesee County Probate Court found Christle and Achtabowski unfit to make proper health care decisions for their baby and stripped them of their rights as parents. He then awarded temporary custody of Baby Terry to his maternal great-aunt, who had previously stated her willingness to obey the doctors and cut off life support.

Legal wrangling continued. Before the case concluded and a final decision was made as to who should have final authority over Baby Terry's care—his parents or his doctors—the infant died in his mother's arms, aged two-and-a-half months. Lawyers for Christle and Achtabowski still wanted a formal court decision overruling the trial court. But the court of appeals dismissed the case as moot.

A case in Canada reveals a threatening tendency in futility cases. Some doctors have taken it upon themselves to cut off care without bothering to get court permission.

"Dad wanted to stay alive long enough to see his estranged brother," George Krausz, of Montreal, Canada, told me.[33] Unfortunately, doctors at the Jewish General Hospital did not allow George's father, Herman Krausz, age seventy-six, that reasonable last wish. Over fifteen hours, they slowly turned off his respirator against the family's wishes and, George contends, against his father's stated desires.

Herman was dying of a respiratory infection, complicated by a burst vein in one lung. He required a respirator to maintain his life. He was conscious, alert, and mentally competent. As it became clear that Herman would die, his doctors began to pressure their patient and the family to remove the respirator. They also put a DNR order on Herman's chart, George claims, without consulting Herman or the family.

Herman's doctors said that his refusal to have treatment stopped was more equivocal. They later claimed at a coroner's inquest, which was called to investigate the circumstances of Herman's death, that they were "unconvinced" that their patient had "indicated his intentions [to continue treatment] clearly."[34] Still, if they truly weren't sure what Herman wanted or didn't want, they didn't seem to take the time to determine unequivocally their patient's desires. Instead, they simply turned down the respirator against his family's wishes. It took less than a day for Herman to die.

Herman's death made headlines in Canada. At the coroner's inquest, George and others testified that Herman's physicians were consistently instructed to continue his treatment, including through gestures and head nods from Herman. One of the doctors, Dr. Denny Laporta, testified, "I clearly stated that we had nothing else to offer him. I said, 'Do you understand?' He nodded his head." That is hardly the same thing as consenting to refuse continued life-sustaining treatment. Indeed, Dr. Laporta admitted that Herman never directly expressed consent to being weaned off the respirator. He did claim that Herman did not object to ending the treatment. But Herman was unable to speak. He had tubes in his mouth.[35] Another doctor was even more blunt about what happened. Dr. Patricia MacMillian testified that she did not believe Herman's physician needed Herman's or the family's consent to stop his care.[36]

George is bitter and resentful at what he considers a profound betrayal of his father's welfare and autonomy. "They treated my father like an object, not a person," he told me. "He had some discomfort, but he wasn't in pain. He wasn't suffering terribly. But they said they wanted the bed. When we tried to protect him, they resorted to trickery and continually pressured us to permit them to do what they wanted: let him die. We were double-teamed, triple-teamed. And when we wouldn't comply, they did what they wanted anyway. It was an awful, distressing experience."[37] (The coroner's report recommended that "independent mediators" be appointed when, as in the Krausz case, families wish to continue life-sustaining treatment and physicians wish to call it quits. That may sound good, but there is a potential problem: these mediators are likely to be trained in the philosophy of mainstream bioethics, the mainstream view of which is supportive of futile care theory.)

Some families whose loved one died after a futile-care cutoff of treatment have sued. But this remedy is generally of limited substantive value. The deceased patients were usually elderly or very ill—which means that, under the law, their lives are not worth much in monetary damages. In addition, juries tend to be reluctant to gainsay the decision making of physicians. Thus, the threat of after-the-death litigation provides scant deterrence against doctors and hospitals imposing futility decisions on patients and families.

This pattern held true in the death of Catherine Gilgunn. Catherine, a woman in her early seventies, was in extremely poor health. She had undergone a mastectomy for breast cancer a few years prior to the events described here; she had diabetes, heart disease, and chronic urinary tract infections. She had also not fully recovered from the effects of a stroke. Then, in June 1989, she fell and broke her hip—for the third time.

Catherine's desire to live was not dampened by her many maladies, however. She instructed her doctors and family that in the event of a catastrophic condition, her treatment was to continue, even if the only benefit of treatment was to prolong her life.

Several days after being hospitalized for the broken hip, Catherine had several seizures, and she became comatose. A DNR was placed on her chart over the family's objections. Under pressure from the family, the attending physician removed the DNR order, after which he was taken off the case by the hospital. The hospital's Optimum Care Committee urged the new physician to place the DNR order back into her chart because its members believed CPR would be "inhumane and unethical."[38] (CPR is a very rigorous procedure that can result in the patient's ribs being broken.)

Not only did the doctor comply, but he began to wean Catherine off the ventilator without the family's consent. This wasn't to determine whether she could breathe on her own, but—as the physician later admitted in court—so that Catherine "would go out with some dignity and ... not be on a respirator at the time she died."[39] Three days later Catherine expired.

The surviving Gilgunns sued. But the jury did not value Catherine's wishes or those of her family. They decided that the doctors and hospital had done nothing wrong.

In the current environment, the only effective protection for vulnerable patients in futility disputes with doctors and hospitals is litigation *before* death occurs. As we saw earlier, that was the strategy of the parents of Baby Ryan when doctors told them, "The time has come for your baby to die," and unilaterally removed him from kidney dialysis over the strenuous objections of his father.

Another family was forced to go to court to obtain wanted treatment in a more recent case in Winnipeg, Canada. Andrew Sawatzky, seventy-nine, had late-stage Parkinson's disease and had experienced debilitating strokes. His doctors decided to place a DNR order on his chart over the objections of Helene, Sawatzky's wife. When Helene could not get the doctors to remove the DNR order off the chart, she sued and eventually prevailed.[40]

In England, the courts sided with doctors in a futility case when parents sought similar relief, with very frightening implications for the most weak and vulnerable members of British society. David Glass, age twelve, was a developmentally and physically disabled boy who was blind and quadriplegic. He was also greatly loved by his parents and siblings, who cherished him as an integral part of his family.

In October 1998, David was admitted to St. Mary's Hospital in Portsmouth with respiratory failure. Instead of trying to save his life, doctors unilaterally withdrew curative treatment and injected him with a palliative agent, telling the parents their son was dying and that nature should be allowed to take its course.

The parents refused to stand by and watch their abandoned son die because doctors did not perceive his life to be worth living. They instituted resuscitation on their own and saved David's life. One doctor later testified that he objected strenuously to the parents' actions because their action "had prevented him from dying."[41] Clearly, if family members could save David without the expertise of formal treatment, the refusal of care was more a matter of physician bias than compassionate allowing of nature to take a sad but inevitable course.

David's parents sued to prevent such awful abandonment from being repeated. Unexpectedly, they lost. Clearly, the issue in the case wasn't whether David's life was beyond saving *but whether it was worth saving*. Shockingly, the trial and appellate courts supported the doctors, ruling that in the UK, doctors—not patients or parents—have the final say as to who should live and who should die.

Litigation is also something that doctors and hospitals seek to avoid. To protect their right to make futile care determinations without interference from judges, efforts are underway to protect physician/hospital prerogatives through creating internal administrative processes for the resolutions of these kinds of controversies. The primary approach toward this end—let's call it "process futility"—employs a bureaucratic procedure to empower doctors to refuse wanted life-sustaining treatment.

As described in the August 21, 1996 issue of *Journal of the American Medical Association* (*JAMA*), hospitals in Houston created a collaboration of area hospital ethics committees with the intent that "professional integrity and institutional integrity" would serve as a counterbalance "to patient autonomy." The protocol involved an eight-step "conflict resolution mechanism"—essentially a quasi-adversary system between doctors and patients—to resolve disputes in which patients or family members refuse to accept a doctor's decision that continued treatment (other than comfort care) is "inappropriate." Once one ethics committee issued its decision, the matter was settled and would be honored by other hospitals.[42]

Many in Texas were alarmed that hospitals would, like Napoleon crowning himself emperor, empower themselves to impose such life and death decisions on patients. When attempts to outlaw the practice failed, Texas passed a compromise law that substantially followed the Houston hospitals' protocol but allowed dissenting patients/families more time to find another institution.[43]

This proved a profoundly dangerous development. Hospital biomedical ethics committees were originally created to help create hospital ethics protocols give informal advice in difficult ethical situations and to mediate disputes between patients, families, and professional caregivers. Because they were not created to be quasi-judicial determiners of treatment disputes, ethics committees have few checks or balances placed upon them, a necessary precaution to any meaningful exercise of power and due process of law. Membership in the committees is anonymous. Deliberations are confidential. There are no uniform criteria member qualifications and no standardized training or education. No written record is kept of committee deliberations, and decisions are usually not included in medical charts. There are no performance reviews. There are no formalized methods for objective oversight. There is no appeals process. Individual members generally cannot be questioned later in court about their assessments.

In practical terms, Texas's ten-day rule has generally been a death sentence. The economics of medicine have changed from the old fee-for-service days. Today, extended care in ICUs is usually a money loser for hospitals, meaning that families find it almost impossible to find a facility willing to accept the transfer of expensive patients whose care has been declared "futile."

There have even been reported cases of desperate families looking *out of state* for a facility willing to provide treatment for a loved one about to be pushed out of the lifeboat by a Texas hospital. The most notable example was the Andrea Clarke controversy. Clarke suffered a serious brain injury during heart surgery and required a ventilator and life support to remain alive. She was not unconscious and, from all reports, wanted to continue to fight for life. Regardless, an ethics committee at St. Luke's Hospital in Houston decreed that she should die. Indeed, after a closed-door hearing, it ordered all further medical efforts to sustain her life while at St. Luke's to cease. As a consequence, Clarke's life support, required because of a heart condition and bleeding on the brain, was to be removed unilaterally, even though she was not unconscious and her family wanted treatment to continue.

Clarke's family threatened to sue and sought publicity in the media. The controversy went viral, with both liberal and conservative policy activists coming to her defense.[44] The family desperately attempted to find another hospital in Texas, without success. Finally, a potential locale was identified in faraway Illinois. St. Luke's turned on the pressure. Jerri Ward, the family's lawyer, told me in an interview for an article I wrote about the controversy for *National Review* that, at one point in the controversy, St. Luke's offered to pay the $14,806 transportation costs to transfer Clarke to Illinois if made within a day—more than 1,000 miles away! But if the decision to transfer was not made until the next day, the hospital would only pay half the cost of transportation. Thereafter, it would pay nothing.[45]

Eventually, under the public pressure of bad publicity, St. Luke's agreed to continue Clarke's care. She died on May 8, 2006. Clarke's sister, Melanie Childers, bitterly noted that the futile care imposition attempt forced her family to spend Clarke's last days fighting for continued treatment rather than focusing on loving Andrea. She wrote:

The fact that we had to fight this battle is both frightening and a sad commentary on the so-called "ethics" now being practiced in medical facilities in this state. The battle for life is a difficult one, in the best of situations, but when a family is put through what we had to go through at such a time, it is especially agonizing. We wish so much that we could have spent more time at our sister's side, when she was living and fighting for her life, rather than having to visit our attorney's office, give interviews to radio and television stations to let the public know of the atrocity about to befall Andrea, and literally stand outside the hospital and beg them not to kill our sister. In attempting to deprive Andrea of the most basic of her human rights—life—St. Luke's Hospital managed to deprive her family and her of that which is most dear to us all, when we are faced with the death of a loved one: a proper goodbye.[46]

Such bitter controversies and profound public distrust will become a regular feature of health care if futile care theory becomes as routine as has dehydrating the cognitively disabled.

I have had personal experience dealing with the question of medical futility and the intimidating power of a doctor insisting on withdrawing life-sustaining treatment when representing the wife of an Alzheimer's patient pro bono before an HMO ethics committee. My client had agreed to a do-not-resuscitate order and to withhold antibiotics if her husband contracted an infection. But that wasn't enough for the doctor in charge of the case—who, despite never having met my client's husband before the man became incompetent, angrily insisted on pulling the man's feeding tube.

My client had her husband's health care power of attorney. She refused this fatal step, leading to a very angry dispute with the doctor over several months that culminated in a dramatic confrontation in front of the committee. Even I—*an experienced trial lawyer*—was somewhat daunted to be sitting alone with my client in front of about twenty members of the facility's bioethics committee—all of whom, including the doctor in question, chatted happily together before the meeting was convened.

We spent about thirty minutes reviewing the case, with the doctor pushing hard for dehydration. After I threatened (in a dramatic fashion) to sue the HMO should the committee authorize removal of the feeding tube—perhaps because this committee only had mediating powers under California law rather than the quasi-judicial authority of Texas law—it instead agreed to my suggestion to change doctors. And that was the end of the controversy.

My client's husband died three years later. She was so grateful that he died in his own time instead of having death imposed by a committee of strangers. But if that committee had possessed the legal power to make a unilateral decision, as such institutional boards do in Texas, I doubt I could have attained such a positive outcome for my client.

Follow the Money: In December 1998, I wrote an article in the political magazine *Weekly Standard* criticizing futile care theory and warning of its dangerous potential.[47] In the article, I asserted my view that the issue is ultimately money driven. In response, Daniel Callahan wrote me a courteous but critical letter in which he claimed that my article had done bioethics "a serious injustice" because futility was not about saving medical resources but meant to be "utterly patient centered." Callahan also opined that while patients have the right to refuse unwanted treatment, they do not have the right to demand care that doctors do not believe should be rendered. "Doctors have to maintain their professional integrity," Callahan wrote, "they are not to be likened to plumbers."[48]

I mention Callahan's comments because they concisely summarize the usual defenses made by defenders of FCT within bioethics and in the pro-futility position statements published by various medical associations. But do these defenses hold water? It is true, of course, that doctors are professionals. But that status does not grant them carte blanche to direct the treatment of patients. Indeed, ending that kind of "paternalism" was what all the fuss over patient autonomy was all about. Moreover, *possessing the status of professional creates a greater duty of care*, not a lesser one. Like other licensed professionals—for example, attorneys—physicians are duty-bound to devote their unswerving loyalty to the patient, as long as they do not act unethically or unlawfully. That may even include performing services with which they might not personally agree, as it does sometimes with attorneys on behalf of clients. But if the hard-won doctrine of informed consent is to remain robust, the "goals of the patient discussed with a doctor, and not the doctor's assessment of efficacy, should control decision making."[49] This is particularly true when you consider that the life-sustaining treatments doctors wish to cease over patient objections in futility disputes are the very treatments that patients couldn't get some physicians to remove under the old paternalistic approach to medical care.

A doctor's obligation to fully disclose the reasons for recommending that treatment cease, of course, involve crucial medical issues (e.g., the physical burdens that treatment will likely cause, the likely medical outcome of continued care). But the ultimate decision is, in the end, a value judgment. Refusing a doctor's recommendation to cease life support is not the same as a patient gainsaying a doctor's diagnosis of an ulcer as the cause of a stomachache by claiming it is cancer and then demanding radiation therapy. But futile care decisions occur in a different realm, one of personal values rather than medical expertise.

Callahan's demurrer notwithstanding, it seems clear that FCT is driven by a profoundly dangerous assumption in bioethics; that by refusing desired treatment for some people, we can save resources for use by other people whose lives are considered more worth living and/or who now have inadequate access to health care. In other words, the sickest who want to live are to be sacrificed to promote "distributive justice."[50]

The opinions of the influential bioethicist Robert M. Veatch, one of the movement's pioneers, illustrate the point. Veatch once was an autonomy absolutist. But once the principle became well entrenched in medical ethics, he began exploring the areas in which autonomy should not predominate because of money and other concerns. "It is often believed," Veatch wrote, "that resource scarcity drives the futility debate," and thus, "it stands to reason that care deemed 'futile' would be an obvious candidate for limitations. Health care inevitably must be rationed; it is wise to ration first care deemed futile."[51]

Additional evidence that the futility movement is ultimately money driven can be found in a commentary published in the *Archives of Internal Medicine* urging that CPR be denied to "certain groups of people" who are near death and that "CPR no longer be considered part of standard care for these patients." The author, Thomas J. Murphy, MD, a leader in the futility movement, admitted that, "The policy ... would limit individual patient autonomy" and "result in earlier death for some patients who would have wanted CPR and who would have survived as a result of CPR." The reason for instituting a change in CPR protocols? Admitted Murphy, "The major rationale for this policy change is cost control."[52]

The Consensus Statement of the Society of Critical Care Medicine's Ethics Committee regarding futile care, among other issues, specifically addresses the role money plays in the futility debate. The statement reads, in part:

It will not be possible for communities or institutions to set limits on treatments, unless there is legal recognition that communities have a legitimate need to allocate resources. Thus, when communities develop such policies in consultation with interested parties, the standards established in these policies should be recognized by the courts. Organizations controlling payment have a profound influence on treatment decisions and should share moral and legal accountability for the outcome of those decisions.... *Given finite resources*, institutional providers should define what constitutes inadvisable treatment and determine when such treatment will not be sustained.[53] (Emphasis mine.)

Dr. Steven Miles wrote about the Wanglie case in the *New England Journal of Medicine*, in which he stated that Helga's continued treatment was wrong in part because she took more than her "fair share of resources that many people pooled [through their health insurance policies] for their collective medical care."[54] Indeed, Miles told me Helga's care cost her insurance company $800,000, after which he added, "I have often thought that maybe we should add a retroactive autonomy provision [to insurance policies] that increases all costs."[55] It is important to note that this incident occurred when most health insurance remained fee-for-service and before cost cutting the mantra of health care.

Dr. Miles has also implicitly acknowledged that resources play a vital part in the futility debate in another article he wrote shortly after the Wanglie controversy: "Medical futility is a psychologically tolerable way of speaking about the most difficult end-of-life decisions with families and our community. It provides a framework within which the value of life, the inevitability of death, professional responsibility and remorse and social justice can be reconciled. Were futility demolished in the name of 'truth,' it would likely be replaced by explicit, politically imposed decisions about *which lives were not worth expending the resources*. Without futility, medically supported life would be a commodity whose span is meted by dollars rather than bounded by natural mortality."[56] (Emphasis mine.) In other words, futility is fundamentally about dollars and cents and, as Miles views the issue, is a well-intentioned subterfuge to the reality of what the movement represents: a surreptitious form of health care rationing founded upon discrimination against those deemed to have a low quality of life.

In recent years, promoters of FCT have pitted sick patients against each other in a contest for limited resources. Thus, in 2014, a study published in *Critical Care Medicine* argued that by providing "futile" life-sustaining treatment, other patients received delayed care.[57] That message has also been communicated in the popular media with increasing frequency in recent years. Similarly, wellness author and health care "outcomes consultant" Al Lewis wrote in the *San Francisco Chronicle* that futile care policies in hospitals could "be a surefire way to save significant money on health care," which should include "the treatment assumption that terminally ill patients want to die naturally with dignity and comfort" rather than receive aggressive life-sustaining or extending care.[58] Thus, Lewis argues, the terminally ill should be required to opt in for aggressive life-sustaining treatment rather than the existing policy that allows such patients to opt out in advance medical directives or on POLST forms.

The passage of the Affordable Care Act—which centralizes cost-benefit decision making into the federal government and focuses intensely on saving resources—will surely increase the pressure on hospitals and other institutions to impose FCT on unwilling patients. This pattern already unfolded in the UK under its socialized National Health Service. Dr. Norman G. Levinsky wrote presciently in the *New England Journal of Medicine* back in 1984 that if "physicians are pressed to balance [economic] needs" against patient welfare, they may do so by making decisions based on money and then "rationalize them as in the best interest of the individual patient." He further wrote, "This phenomenon may be occurring in Britain where physicians 'seem to seek medical justification' for decisions forced on them by limited resources. Doctors gradually redefine standards of care so that they can escape the constant recognition that financial limits compel them to do less than their best."[59]

In my view, this is precisely the path now being taken by futile care theorists here. This is very dangerous and will lead to the victimization of the most medically defenseless whose lives will be cut short due to "justified" medical abandonment. As futilitarian Dr. Donald J. Murphy told me in a 1996 interview concerning FCT and the Baby Ryan case, "There are no questions that there are risks. And there's no question that those with less power will be at greater risk. There are going to be Baby Ryans. There are going to be nursing home patients who would have survived and who wanted to accept their quality of life. But by shifting our priorities, we will be able to do a better job for more people."[60]

The futile care controversy threatens to provoke a profound crisis in medicine and seriously undermine the trust people have in their own doctors. Worse, if the principle is ever established that doctors, hospitals, health insurance companies, and/or "the community" can dictate who must have desired treatment withheld, the door will be thrown wide open to medical decision making based on hierarchies of human worth and the exercise of raw political power. If that occurs, the process of de-individualizing medicine that has begun with FCT will not end there. Like a cancer metastasizing, the category of patients subject to treatment termination will spread steadily throughout our health care system, endangering ever-growing categories of vulnerable patients. Indeed, such radical systemic changes in medicine are already in the planning stages.

PUSHING HEALTH CARE RATIONING

The little-spoken truth in the futility debate is that FCT in and of itself will not save enough money to control health care costs significantly. An early study published by the *New England Journal of Medicine* in 1994 demonstrated that reducing such treatment both voluntarily through the use of advance directives and by imposing futility decisions would likely save only about 3.3 percent of "national health care expenditures."[61] Moreover, while a significant amount of Medicare spending comes at the end of life, the total percentage of health care costs at the end of life have not risen from the year this book was first published in 2001 until the present—coming in at about 10–12 percent.[62] As bioethicist—and health care rationing proponent—Ezekiel Emanuel noted in a 2013 column in the *New York Times*, "The roughly 6 percent of Medicare patients who die each year do make up a large proportion of Medicare costs: 27 to 30 percent. But this figure has not changed significantly in decades. And the total number of Americans, not just older people, who die every year—less than 1 percent of the population—account for much less of total health care spending, just 10 to 12 percent."[63]

But that isn't all. As a 2012 study published by the National Institute for Health Care Management pointed out, whether a particular treatment will be efficacious to prevent death or fail and add to the costs at the end of life often cannot be predicted before the event: "Managing high spending at the end of life can also be problematic. Not all persons with high spending will die soon, and predicting timing of death and distinguishing between care that may extend life in a meaningful way and care that does little good is something that is often accomplished only in retrospect."[64] Moreover, as Dr. Joann Lynn, one of the foremost experts in the country on the issue of end-of-life care testified before the United States Senate Finance Committee, "Very few dying persons now have resuscitation efforts or extended stays in intensive care."[65]

Futile care theorists know this, of course. But the actual level of cost savings is only a small part of the point. The primary benefit, from their standpoint, would be the creation of the principle that rationing medicine is both ethical and necessary. Seen in this light, futility is quite literally the foot in the door that would begin a step-by-step descent from a health care system based on Hippocratic principles to a medical regimen in which access to treatment is restricted to some but open to others. Thus, futile care disputes do not represent the finishing line of this important ethical and legal struggle but merely the starting gate of a far longer race, increasing our system's already existing propensity to function in a manner that former Surgeon General C. Everett Koop denigrated as "political medicine."[66]

In 2009, during the debate over the Affordable Care Act—sometimes called Obamacare—former Alaska Governor and 2008 Republican vice presidential candidate Sarah Palin made a provocative charge, writing on her Facebook page, "Who will suffer the most when they ration care? The sick, the elderly, and the disabled, of course. The America I know and love is not one in which my parents or my baby with Down syndrome will have to stand in front of Obama's 'death panel' so his bureaucrats can decide, based on a subjective judgment of their 'level of productivity in society,' whether they are worthy of health care. Such a system is downright evil."[67]

Supporters of the legislation—and most of the media—were apoplectic over the charge that Obamacare would deploy death panels to control costs. For example, Politifact called it the "Lie of the Year" for 2009.[68]

It is true that the ACA did not authorize the immediate implementation of health care rationing; however, it did authorize the federal bureaucracy to promulgate regulations to assess and promote control over health care costs and to create national treatment standards. Thus, for all the screaming by pundits and the white-hot criticism of Palin, her charge resonated deeply with the public, so deeply, in fact, that the term "death panels" entered the political lexicon. Indeed, it has been central to the ongoing debate over health care cost controls generally and the wisdom of the ACA specifically, ever since.

Moreover, there can be no question that many supporters of the ACA among bioethicists and public pundits have wanted to go there for a long time. Take former Colorado Governor Richard Lamm, now the co-director of the Center for Public Policy and Contemporary Issues at the University of Denver. Lamm has long called for the dismantling of the Hippocratic tradition of medicine, compelling medical professionals to give their loyalty to each individual patient. He told me, "States can't take a 'do no harm' approach. Approximately 50 percent of health care is paid with public funds. That means that policy makers have a duty to buy the most public health for the most people with the funds. There is something fundamentally unethical about keeping an anencephalic baby alive [an infant born with much of its brain missing]. Public money should not be dissipated on marginal procedures. You are going to have to ration. It is much better to ration procedures than people."

"How do you decide what marginal medicine is?" I asked Lamm.

"Kaiser Permanente of Southern California [a nonprofit HMO] asked me how to buy the most health care with a defined pot of money. To me, that is the right moral question. We should give women prenatal care before we give people transplants. What do you do with somebody who has sclerosis of the liver and a bleeding esophagus? You can treat a lot of alcoholics for the amount of money it takes to treat those conditions. It is a public policy decision."[69]

In other words, the Hippocratic tradition would be replaced by a new regimen of political medicine that would reflect the values of the politically strong at the expense of those with less power. Thus, in 1994, Robert M. Veatch wrote in apocalyptic tones, "The era of health care rationing is upon us!" Veatch urged rationing via "global budgeting," in which "an administrator of a state health plan, a hospital, a specific hospital department, or a health maintenance organization would be given a fixed pile of money." The amount would not be "enough for every physician to do everything for every patient." How would this money be allocated? By "the community," guided by "religious and philosophical traditions"—in other words, bioethicists—"drawing on its common wisdom to work out a compromise between utility and equity."[70]

The first casualty of such a plan, Veatch asserted, would be the "Hippocratic Ethic," which Veatch urged we discard because it "specifies in its most crucial central principle that the individual physician should benefit the patient according to the physician's ability and judgment." Veatch castigated Hippocratic medicine as the reason "we are in such serious economic trouble today." Thus, under rationing in a global budgeting plan, the individual medical needs of patients would be subservient to the priorities of rationing authorities. That would mark the end of the principle of informed consent because doctors would not be able to offer some medically beneficial treatments to patients.

Daniel Callahan, one of bioethics' founding fathers and a longtime advocate for health care rationing, has written extensively on the topic in professional literature and in at least two books. In *False Hopes: Why America's Quest for Perfect Health Is a Recipe for Failure*, Callahan calls for a radical reshaping of our health care system to achieve "sustainability." A sustainable health care system, he asserts, is one that is both "affordable and equitable." Sounds good until you look at the fine print. Rationing, as Callahan envisions it, would intentionally turn away from further medical progress in the pursuit of what Callahan labels a "steady state."[71]

Callahan's prescription for maintaining this steady state is worse than the disease he seeks to cure. Traditional medical ethics are out the door. Private medical decisions between patient and doctor would be severely curtailed. "The aim," Callahan writes, "is to overcome the present assumption that health care should be tailored to individual needs."[72] Doctors' loyalty would be divided between patients and their duty to "the community," which would be empowered through political decision making (undoubtedly under the guidance of bioethicists) to decide what could and could not be prescribed under various circumstances. Little if anything would be done to increase average life expectancy or find new ways to help prematurely born babies survive. Research into the causes and cures of terrible illnesses such as cancer, AIDS, heart disease, and other afflictions would be reduced through negative financial incentives intended to dissuade private enterprise from investing in medical research. Funding to pay for acute medical care would be drastically cut to restrict treatment options for sick and disabled people. And if, despite the heavy hand of government policy, new "diagnostic and therapeutic technologies" were discovered, only those demonstrating in advance that "50 percent of patients will show a significant improvement"[73] would be permitted for clinical use.

The funds that once went into health research and treatment would be diverted by what Callahan himself calls "a drastic reallocation of resources"[74] to fund a bureaucracy charged with public health education. These new health care policies would include "social coercion" to persuade people to live healthy lifestyles, which Callahan justifies as "good for them and good for the rest of us."[75] Universal participation in "health promotion programs and health risk monitoring" would also be required. "Such practices now are ordinarily voluntary," Callahan writes breezily. "There is no reason, save for employee protest, why they should not be made mandatory."[76]

Rationing protocols would be strictly enforced, with doctors required to deny individual patients beneficial treatment to serve their higher obligation to "the community." Treatment provision or restriction would be based on patient characteristics such as age, disability—so much for Helen Keller—and even lifestyle choices. "High technology medicine would be scarce for the elderly, limited for babies and children, and limited for all other age groups."[77] After the age of "sixty-five to seventy years," the "highest priority for medicine should become not to avert death but enable people to live as comfortable and secure a life as possible."[78] Since the system would be based on collectivism—"solidarity" is the term Callahan employs—"the overriding aim will not be to meet each and every health and medical need, but only those that are most common."[79] The "lowest priority" would be "given to those conditions that affect comparatively few people and require significant expenditures or technology."[80]

Callahan admits that the policies he advocates would "lead to harm or death to some portion of the population at risk."[81] But preventable death inflicted on some individuals is the price that must be paid to achieve distributive justice and medical affordability. Rather than demand excellence in medicine, the ethical standards of medical treatment would be reduced to the level of providing "decent care."[82] According to the bioethicist, "a sustainable medicine can do no other than accept this unpleasant reality."[83]

The societal benefit that would justify such a radical restructuring of medical ethics and the limitation of individual freedom it would introduce into American life, Callahan asserts, would be health coverage for everyone. That is the real false hope. A universal but significantly limited basic health plan would work fine for the young, healthy, and vital, but it would be of marginal benefit to people who are elderly, seriously ill, or disabled. If you doubt that, consider the dire consequences of the implementation of a Callahan-style rationing policy: people with renal failure, ALS, cancer (especially if the patient smoked), or AIDS could have desperately needed medical treatment denied. So might the multiple sclerosis patients and the patient with spinal cord injury who needs years of rehabilitation. The eighty-year-old who needed a hip replacement might have it denied while the sixty-year-old would receive it, while prematurely born children with guarded prognoses, whose lives might be saved, would instead receive only palliation and be allowed to die. People with significant brain injury, elderly people with congestive heart disease, and people with debilitating mental illnesses might be denied basic medical treatment based on "inappropriate care" protocols. For many, the only significant medical treatment obtainable would be palliation. Any health care system that systematically denied treatment to the people who need it most—a common feature of most bioethics-inspired rationing schemes—by definition does not "cover" everybody. Worse, it is a prescription for medical despotism.

With the Affordable Care Act's passage, advocacy for health care rationing has accelerated—even as some of these same advocates deny Palin's death panel warning. The bioethicist Ezekiel Emanuel, for example, held a very high post at the National Institutes of Health during ACA's crafting and passage. Emanuel has supported health care rationing, at least in theory (for example, if based on democratic deliberation and, apparently, "quality of life" criteria), writing in the *Hastings Center Report*:

This civic republican or deliberative democratic conception of the good provides both procedural and substantive insights for developing a just allocation of health care resources. Procedurally, it suggests the need for public forums to deliberate about which health services should be considered basic and should be socially guaranteed. Substantively, it suggests services that promote the continuation of the polity—those that ensure healthy future generations, ensure development of practical reasoning skills, and ensure full and active participation by citizens in public deliberations—are to be socially guaranteed as basic. *Conversely, services provided to individuals who are irreversibly prevented from being or becoming participating citizens are not basic and should not be guaranteed. An obvious example is not guaranteeing health services to patients with dementia.* A less obvious example is guaranteeing neuropsychological services to ensure children with learning disabilities can read and learn to reason.[84] (My emphasis.)

A high-profile adviser to the Obama administration was even more explicit. Writing, "We need death panels" in the *New York Times*, a former Obama Treasury Department adviser named Steve Rattner opined, "Well, maybe not death panels, exactly, but unless we start allocating health care resources more prudently—rationing, by its proper name—the exploding cost of Medicare will swamp the federal budget." Rattner doesn't mince words:

> No one wants to lose an aging parent. And with price out of the equation, it's natural for patients and their families to try every treatment, regardless of expense or efficacy. But that imposes an enormous societal cost that few other nations have been willing to bear. Many countries whose health care systems are regularly extolled—including Canada, Australia and New Zealand—have systems for rationing care. Take Britain, which provides universal coverage with spending at proportionately almost half of American levels. Its National Institute for Health and Clinical Excellence uses a complex quality-adjusted life year [QALY] system to put an explicit value (up to about $48,000 per year) on a treatment's ability to extend life.... We may shrink from such stomach-wrenching choices, but they are inescapable.[85]

Recall from our discussion in the first chapter that the acronym QALY stands for "quality adjusted life year." It is a health care rationing system that gives greater value to the lives of some patients than to others, invidious distinctions used in a formula to determine whether the cost of care is worth the benefit desired. The ACA does not permit QALY rationing. This does not sit well with the *New England Journal of Medicine*, which editorialized in favor of instituting a QALY-form of health care rationing under Obamacare.

> A ban on valuing life extension presents its own ethical dilemmas. Taken literally, it means that spending resources to extend by a month the life of a 100-year-old person who is in a vegetative state cannot be valued differently from spending resources to extend the life of a child by many healthy years.... As the country searches for ways to curb health care spending, consideration of the cost-effectiveness of health interventions will unavoidably be part of the health care debate.... The use of explicit, standard metrics such as cost-per-QALY ratios has the advantage of transparency and can help direct our resources toward the greatest health gains. These kinds of analyses will therefore endure as a rough benchmark of value and as a normative guide to resource-allocation decisions. It would be unfortunate if the ACA created a barrier to their development and use.[86]

Some rationing advocates try to hide the wolf of rationing behind the sheep's clothing of eliminating waste and inefficiencies. Writing in the *New England Journal of Medicine*, well-known bioethicist and physician Howard Brody shifted the lexicon to hide the reality of his call for increased futile care impositions and blatant rationing. From "From an Ethics of Rationing to an Ethic of Waste Avoidance": "Bioethics has long approached cost containment under the heading of 'allocation of scarce resources.' Having thus named the nail, bioethics has whacked away at it with the theoretical hammer of distributive justice. But in the United States, ethical debate is now shifting from rationing to the avoidance of waste. This little-noticed shift has important policy implications."[87]

Brody would include futile care theory into the concept of avoiding waste. Even though the concept of medical futility has had a vexed history, this new ethical question is a subcategory of the futility debate. We used to think that the issue of futility arose only when physicians, in keeping with their professional integrity, refused to offer useless treatment, even when patients or families demanded it.

Futile care isn't refused because it is "useless"—recalling my illustration of a patient demanding an appendectomy to cure an earache—but *because it does or may work.* When they impose "qualitative" futility impositions, futilitarians in essence declare the *patient* futile by refusing efficacious treatment precisely because it could extend life they deem not worth living.

People have pushed back against futile care and invidious rationing plans politically. So Brody trots out a new lexicon by which to justify the planned service interruptions that bioethicists intend to impose: "Few tests and treatments are futile across the board; most help a few patients and become wasteful when applied beyond that population. But the boundary between wise and wasteful application will often be fuzzy."[88] Make no mistake—Brody is pushing rationing by a more palatable name:

> In the end, the ethics of rationing and of waste avoidance are complementary, not competing. Perhaps at present, waste avoidance could save enough money to permit both universal coverage and future cost control. As medical technology advances, especially with personalized genomic medicine, we will almost certainly arrive at the day when we cannot afford all potentially beneficial therapies for everyone.... The ethical challenge of rationing care will have to be faced sooner or later, particularly when we confront inequitable distribution of health care resources globally.[89]

Globally? Does that mean across the world continuum or across the USA spectrum? Either way, bioethics is moving strongly toward promoting its version of social justice that will require an ever-growing technocratic sector to implement. Who would be hired to perform most of the arcane bureaucratic studies and sit on the ever-proliferating bureaucratic boards? You guessed it: bioethicists.

Health care rationing would de-professionalize medicine and undermine the proper physician/patient relationship. Currently, doctors owe fiduciary duties to each individual patient, not general society. Changing that focus will sow distrust in the health care system.

More broadly, rationing would exacerbate the already strained social divisions in this country. Once people believed that the level of their own medical coverage was directly dependent upon the cost of treating the illnesses of others, then ill will, hatred, and discrimination against people with "expensive" conditions such as AIDS, significant disabilities, and serious mental illnesses would surely follow. Moreover, different "disease advocacy groups" would struggle bitterly over the allocation of resources made artificially scarce. "What we do in this country [when deciding funding levels] is succumb to the greatest pressure," C. Everett Koop told me. For some diseases, like AIDS or breast cancer, "it is politically correct to fund them" because "groups working on behalf of the victims of these diseases make a lot of noise." Disease categories that are not well organized or that don't take politically confrontational approaches are often left behind.

A rumble broke out in Oregon when instituting its Medicaid health care rationing scheme. The purpose for Oregon's rationing experiment was laudable: to increase access to Oregon's Medicaid insurance plan to the working poor, people who usually do not receive health insurance at work, cannot afford private policies, and who do not qualify for government assistance. Toward that end, in the years before rationing went into effect, the Oregon Health Department created a list of nearly 800 diagnoses and treatments, and then prioritized them on a rationing list. Ailments at or below the cutoff number are covered. Those with numbers higher than the cutoff number are not covered. The cutoff number changes every two years, as do the priority listings.

In the initial proposal, treatment for late-stage AIDS was assigned a higher number (that is, very low on the priority list), meaning that those AIDS patients on Medicaid who wanted treatment would not receive it. AIDS activists were appropriately outraged. They viewed it—correctly, in my view—as abandonment by the state of poor people with AIDS in order to provide other poor people with medical coverage. AIDS activists were determined not to let their comrades be cast aside and agitated politically to make late-stage AIDS a covered treatment in the rationing schedule. They prevailed, and today AIDS patients on Oregon's Medicaid receive care. However—as we saw with terminal cancer patients Barbara Wagner and Randy Stroup, denied chemotherapy but offered payment for assisted suicide—other dying people without such political clout did not fare as well.

There is a crisis in health care funding that requires political will to ameliorate. But health care rationing, whether as envisioned by Veatch, Callahan, the Oregon Health Plan, or other methods of mandating limits in individual medical treatment based on predefined patient categories or characteristics, is not an equitable answer. Rationing would reduce societal comity by pitting people with different diseases against each other in a mad scramble for resources that have been intentionally limited: AIDS versus cancer, multiple sclerosis versus head injury, healthy children against premature infants. It would allow the ongoing corporatization of the American health care delivery system, and the resulting diversion of health care dollars into corporate profits and reduced levels of charity care, to go virtually unchallenged. It would unjustly sacrifice the most medically vulnerable among us, thereby transforming the term "distributive justice" into an oxymoron. The winners in any rationing regimen would be the politically powerful and the influential, the losers, the weak and exploitable. As Dr. Norman G. Levinsky wrote in *The Lancet* about age-based rationing, "People with wealth, social standing, education, and the ability to appeal to the media will work the system to get the care they need. The poor, the uneducated, and the socially disadvantaged will bear most of the burden...."[90]

THE DUTY TO DIE

Even as most bioethicists have promoted the false premise that health care rationing is inevitable and unavoidable, bioethics has more quietly also been debating an even more oppressive approach to coping with the financial and emotional "burdens" of caring for elderly, disabled, chronically ill, and dying people. The question presented is this: What moral duties do people who need continuing care have toward their families, society, and themselves? The awful answer, according to some bioethicists, is that they have a "duty to die."

Richard Lamm, the former governor of Colorado and rationing proponent, first came to widespread public notice when he was widely criticized for asserting in 1984 that "old people have a duty to die and get out of the way," an accusation that sticks to Lamm like flypaper to this very day. Lamm pleads not guilty to the charge, strongly contending that his remarks were taken out of context and his meaning substantially misunderstood.

The offending quote came in a speech Lamm made while still governor, to the Colorado Health Lawyers Association. Lamm questioned the wisdom of spending large sums of money on medical treatment for people with serious medical conditions, a position that has since hardened in Lamm's mind into explicit support for health care rationing. He then alluded to an article by Leon R. Kass called "The Case for Mortality." That's when he got into trouble. Here is Lamm's quote as published in the *Boston Globe*: "Essentially [Kass] said we have a duty to die. It's like if leaves fall off a tree forming the humus for other plants to grow out. We've got a duty to die and get out of the way, with all our machines and artificial hearts and everything else like that, and let the others in society, or kids, build a reasonable life."[91]

In fact, Kass's essay is deeply philosophical and reflective. It makes the case that human mortality is "not simply an evil, perhaps it is even a blessing—not only for the welfare of the community, but even for us as individuals."[92] Kass further suggests that death has its proper place in life and that human attempts to overcome it at almost all costs are misguided. Lamm's description of Kass's philosophical point came largely from the following strikingly beautiful and poetic paragraph:

> In perpetuation, we send forth not just the seed of our bodies, but also a bearer of our hopes, our truths, and those of our tradition. If our children are to flower, we need to sow them well and nurture them, cultivate them in rich and wholesome soil, clothe them in fine and decent opinions and mores, and direct them toward the highest light, to stand straight and tall—that they may take our place as we took that of those who planted us and who made way for us, so that in time they, too, may make way and plant. But if they are truly to flower, we must go to seed; we must wither and give ground.[93]

This may be evocative of our organic cycle, but it is by no means a call for old people to die and get out of the way. It would thus seem that Lamm spoke clumsily and did not fully or accurately depict what Kass was writing.

That is what Kass, a friend of Lamm's, believes happened. He told me, "My essay was an argument asserting that the desire of people for ever-longer lives, and in principle for immortality, is a mistake. The human way is to make way for the next generation by living our lives to the full and, when the time comes, letting go gracefully. That by no means translates into bumping off the infirm."[94]

Whether or not Lamm was done an injustice, the contretemps remains relevant more than thirty years later by illustrating how far we have fallen since 1984. Then, Lamm's political career was almost destroyed for allegedly claiming a duty to die. Today, that *very argument* is actively discussed within bioethics as a respectable topic of discourse, and few eyebrows are raised.

The premier advocate for the "duty to die" is an East Tennessee University philosophy professor named John Hardwig. Hardwig takes the ongoing deconstruction of the Hippocratic tradition to a new level, asserting "it is sometimes the moral thing to do for a physician to sacrifice the interests of her patient to those of non-patients—specifically to those of the other members of the family."[95] According to Hardwig, there are "many cases [when] ... the interest of family members often ought to *override* those of the patient.... Only when the lives of family members will not be importantly affected can one rightly make exclusively or even predominantly self-regarding decisions."[96] (Emphasis in the original.)

Hardwig's approach is explicitly utilitarian. He worries that some family members will decide to sacrifice their own interests to help another needy member, thereby reducing overall happiness. He writes:

> If a newborn has been saved by aggressive treatment but is severely handicapped, the parents may simply not be emotionally capable of abandoning the child to institutional care. A man whose wife is suffering from multiple sclerosis may simply not be willing or able to go on with his own life until he sees her through to the end. A woman whose husband is being maintained in a vegetative state may not feel free to marry or even to see other men again, regardless of what some revised law might say about her marital status.[97]

To avoid the societal degradation that Hardwig acknowledges would develop should people "lose their concern" for loved ones "as soon as continuing to care began to diminish the quality of their own lives," Hardwig urges that doctors refuse treatment when it would harm the interests of the family. "Physicians would no longer be agents of their patients and would not strive to be advocates for their patients' interests," Hardwig wrote. "Instead, the physician would aspire to be an impartial adviser who would stand knowledgeably but sympathetically by ... and discern the treatment that would best harmonize or balance the interests of all concerned."[98] Thus, if the continuing life of the woman with MS, in Hardwig's example, would harm her husband's life, the physician would cease treatment so that she could die and the husband could get on with his life without the guilt of having abandoned her.

This may sound like fringe thinking, but it is disturbingly close to the mainstream—if not always explicitly, certainly as an implicit consequence of many bioethics proposals. Moreover, the article quoted above appeared in the *Hastings Center Report*, one of the foremost bioethics journals in the world.

In 1997, Hardwig further developed his idea about a duty to die in an essay, which was featured on the cover of the *Hastings Center Report* entitled, aptly, "Is There a Duty to Die?" Not surprisingly, Hardwig concluded that there probably is, if continuing to live will constitute a burden upon one's family. Hardwig proposes nine circumstances when the duty might arise, including:

- "A duty to die is more likely when continuing to live will impose significant burdens—emotional burdens, extensive caregiving, destruction of life plans, and yes, financial hardship—on your family and loved ones. This is the fundamental insight underlying a duty to die."
- "A duty to die becomes greater as you grow older.... To have reached the age of say, seventy-five or eighty without being ready to die is itself a moral failing, the sign of a life out of touch with life's basic realities."
- "A duty to die is more likely when you have already lived a full and rich life."
- "There is a duty to die if your loved one's lives have already been difficult or impoverished."
- "A duty to die is more likely when your loved ones have already made great contributions—perhaps even sacrifices—to make your life a good one."
- "A duty to die is more likely when the part of you that is loved will soon be gone or seriously compromised."

- There is a greater duty to die to the extent you have lived a relatively lavish lifestyle."[99]

The response to Hardwig's article in the *Hastings Center Report* was telling. Several correspondents agreed wholeheartedly with Hardwig, although they believed, like Hardwig, that the duty should not be mandated legally due to the importance of autonomy. (Recall, however, that same thing was once said about dehydrating people in PVS. Now, futile care protocols may require it.) One correspondent, a self-described family practice physician, suggested that when the duty arises, elderly people should not only refuse intensive medical treatment but ordinary care. "This refusal of available medical care could include no longer receiving annual influenza vaccinations nor periodic pneumococcal vaccinations and declining antibiotics for all infections."[100] Hardwig himself goes further. He told me that someone with a duty to die should seriously consider suicide.[101]

Some bioethicists dissented. Daniel Callahan was "appalled and embarrassed" that Hardwig quoted his book, *The Troubled Dream of Life*, a book about the desirability of "good deaths" in support of the duty-to-die thesis. "I believe it is unwise and unrealistic not to be ready to die by the time one reaches old age," Callahan retorted, "but I see nothing whatever immoral about that: everything unwise is not immoral."[102] Hardwig's rejoinder to Callahan, precisely and succinctly stated a major thesis of this entire chapter. "My claim," he wrote, "is not that Callahan endorse(s) my view; it is that [he] may have trouble avoiding it, given the logic of [his] position."[103]

Hardwig is only partly right. The duty to die does not spring from the arcane nuances of individual advocacy. It springs logically and inescapably from the utilitarian ideology and underlying implications that are the hallmarks of the bioethics movement.

Of perhaps greater concern, it appears that society may be moving in that general direction. In recent years, family-supported suicides have made the news with increasing frequency. As I related earlier, in Belgium elderly couples have been euthanized together because they preferred immediate death to the prospect of future widowhood. In one case, the death doctor was procured by the couple's son, even though his parents were not ill![104] Similarly, the English conductor Sir Edward

Downes died with his cancer-stricken wife Joan at a Swiss suicide clinic, a decision quickly endorsed in the media by his children.[105] Similarly, NPR-syndicated radio personality Diane Rehm very publicly supported her husband John's suicide by VSED self-starvation, telling the *New York Times* that they had a pact to help the other die if suffering seriously with a terminal illness. (John had Parkinson's disease.) "There was no question but that I would support him and honor whatever choice he would make," she said. "As painful as it was, it was his wish."[106] Rehm subsequently argued that her experience required assisted suicide legalization.

Is it right or wrong to support a loved one's suicide? This seems to be one of those issues, increasingly prevalent in our society, about which debate is not possible; the answer depends on one's overarching worldview. Some will believe that their duty is to support their family member's choice, come what may. Others, including this writer, believe that supporting suicide is an abandonment that validates loved ones' worst fears about themselves—that they are a burden, unworthy of love, or truly better off dead.

Either way, there is no question that family backing for suicide furthers the normalization of hastened death as a proper response to human suffering. Such normalization, over time, will put increasing pressure on those coping with the infirmities of age and with the debilitations of serious illnesses and disabilities to view their suicides as not only a suitable approach but also perhaps even as an obligation to those they love (e.g., a duty to die).

No, a day won't come when the euthanasia police kick down doors and force unwanted lethal injections upon the sick and elderly. But legal compulsion isn't the only way to push people out of the lifeboat. The more public support families and friends give their ill or debilitated loved ones' suicides, the more culturally legitimate such actions become, the greater the prospect that the elderly, very sick, disabled, and mentally ill will come to believe that they have a duty to die and get out of the way. Moral duty to die will become culturally legitimate.

As Hardwig said to me with a wry smile, "The real question is, does the philosopher espouse a new idea or does he or she merely articulate what is already bubbling up?"[107]

CHAPTER 5

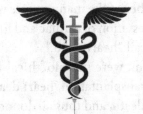

ORGAN DONORS OR ORGAN FARMS?

Dr. Jeffrey I. Frank, director of the Neurointensive Care Unit at the prestigious Cleveland Clinic, was stunned when the Ohio State Board of Pharmacy accused him of being part of a "conspiracy" to "commit homicide so as to obtain organs."[1] The investigators at the board accused Dr. Frank of creating a medical protocol that explicitly "hastened death" of non-terminally ill patients, that did not wait "for the irreversibility of death" before organs were procured, and that demanded "the removal of organs from living people."[2] To put it bluntly, the charges accused Dr. Frank of being a modern-day Dr. Frankenstein.

How had this respected neurologist come under such a dark cloud? Dr. Frank's troubles began two years previously when his colleague at the Cleveland Clinic, Dr. James Mayes, a transplant surgeon and head of the organ transplant service Life Banc, requested him to review a proposed medical protocol intended to increase the number of organ donations at the Cleveland Clinic. Dr. Frank wasn't personally involved in procuring or transplanting organs, but as the director of the Neurosurgical Intensive Care unit, he was required to give his input because all potential organ donors at the clinic were required to have had catastrophic brain injury.

At the time of this incident in 1997, the only eligible organ donors at the Cleveland Clinic were people declared "brain-dead," that is, those with total brain failure, a concept I will define and discuss more fully below. The proposed new protocol sought to add another group of potential donors: a small number of the many people who die each year at the clinic from irreversible cessation of cardiac and lung function, which, for ease of reading, we will call "heart-dead."

Drs. Mayes and Frank were not bioethical trailblazers. Indeed, at the inception of organ transplantation, heart death was the only legally recognized criterion for death, and thus all donors—as few as there then were in the 1960s—died from heart death. Then, around 1970, bioethicists, physicians, and legal academics envisioned brain death, in large part to expand the number of eligible organ donors. Widespread legal and popular acceptance of brain death as a medically legitimate standard for determining when a patient has died followed quickly, significantly increasing the eligible donor pool. Brain-dead donors soon became the primary source of organs throughout the world.

Organs are more easily and successfully procured from brain-dead people than they are from heart-dead people. To remain healthy and viable, body tissues require a constant supply of oxygen and nutrients delivered to the cells by the blood, which also removes waste products. After heart death, organs rapidly lose viability in a process known as "warm ischemia," the medical term that describes the quick deterioration of still-living cells in the organs of the newly dead. Unless preserved medically, organs soon become non-transplantable. In contrast, when a person is declared brain-dead—when death occurs to a catastrophically brain-damaged person being maintained by intensive medical technology—the blood still circulates, keeping the organs healthy and functioning until removal. (People who experience heart death and then become organ donors are known in the transplant community as "non-heart-beating cadaver donors" because their organs are removed after their heart has stopped. Brain-dead donors are known as "heart-beating cadaver donors" because their organs are removed while the heart is still functioning.)

Recent improvements in organ preservation techniques now permit doctors to delay substantially the onset of warm ischemia, thereby allowing organs to remain viable for a longer period after death. This advance has reopened the possibility that a significant number of people who die unexpectedly can have organ preservation procedures applied to their bodies quickly thereafter, as can people who die "planned" deaths in a hospital after having life support removed.

All of this occurs in a high-tech medical milieu in which ever-increasing numbers of patients are waiting for life-saving organs to become available for transplantation. Many of these patients are desperately ill or dying, creating intense pressure to increase the organ supply. Feeling the burden, many organ transplant centers around the country, most notably the University of Pittsburgh Medical Center, had already quietly begun to procure organs from people who expired by heart death. Thus, by updating its own procedures, the Cleveland Clinic hoped to "catch up" with what other organ centers around the country were already doing.

This was (and remains) a delicate business. "The public trust in the system of organ donation is precarious," Dr. James L. Bernat, then the chairman of the ethics committee of the American Academy of Neurology, told me. "It is based on absolute faith that doctors will not take them before the person dies. If that confidence is ever breached, the organ donation system could suffer a terrible blow." As proof, Dr. Bernat points to the unfortunate situation in England some years ago in which a television program reported falsely that some doctors were declaring patients dead who were really alive in order to obtain their organs. "This led to a dramatic and sustained reduction of voluntary donations throughout the UK," Bernat says. "People were really afraid that doctors would want them to die sooner to get their organs. Confidence in this area is so fragile, it doesn't take much to break it."[3]

To prevent the kind of panic that occurred in England, American transplant medicine has long been bound by the "dead donor rule," prohibiting the procurement of all vital or non-paired organs from living patients. An essential aspect of the dead donor rule—let's call it the "do not kill" corollary—requires all organ donors to have died naturally of disease or injury. Strict adherence to these ethical protocols is a literal matter of life and death for people awaiting transplants. If people ever believe that their organs might be taken while they are alive or that they risk being killed or medically neglected to death so their tissues can be obtained, the public's shaky confidence in organ transplant medicine would collapse. The level of organ donations would plummet. Sick people who could have been saved by receiving the "gift of life" would instead die.

Knowing the stakes, and realizing that the public's trust in the ethics of transplantation was perilously thin, Dr. Frank decided upon a conservative approach for the Cleveland Clinic. He devised an eligibility protocol for heart death donors, which he claimed was more stringent than most other such programs. Only people "who have suffered devastating brain injury" and had severe brain stem dysfunction, albeit not brain death, would be considered. A "demonstrated loss of respiratory drive," which would lead to almost certain death within fifteen or twenty minutes after the removal of respiratory support, was also required. Only patients in the care of Dr. Frank or his colleague, Dr. John Andrefsky, would be considered for eligibility, a condition that Dr. Frank told me he placed in the protocol to ensure it would always be conservatively applied.

As with existing heart death organ procurement protocols, the decision to remove life support would have to be made by the family free and clear of any discussions or consideration of organ donation. Even then, no one at the Cleveland Clinic or Life Banc would be allowed to raise the issue of organ donation; patient families would have to bring up the subject themselves.[4] Under the proposed protocol, the date of the deaths of patients/donors, which would occur after life-supporting medical treatment was withdrawn, would be planned. The patient would be prepared for surgery, the family allowed their final goodbye, and then the patient would be moved into an operating room. After life support was removed, the patient would be given two drugs, heparin and Regatine, which would not benefit the patient but instead help protect the viability of his or her organs after death. After life support was removed, if all went as planned, the patient would quickly cease breathing and go into cardiac arrest. Two minutes after the heart stopped, the patient would be declared dead, and the organ removal process would commence. If the patient did not die within one hour, the patient would be removed from the operating room, put back on life support, and brought back to the hospital ward, after which the patient would never again be eligible as a donor.

The Cleveland Clinic adopted the protocol, but before it could be implemented, the roof fell in. A clinical bioethicist named Mary Ellen Waithe worried that the new rules would amount to organ procurement from living patients and/or the killing of patients in violation of the dead donor rule. She also believed that injecting heparin and Regatine would hasten death and thus constituted euthanasia. She reported the matter to the Ohio Board of Pharmacy, which conducted an investigation (without questioning Drs. Frank and Mayes). The board reported its negative conclusions about the matter to the public prosecutor's office, which in turn threatened to indict any doctor who procured organs under the protocol.

The controversy became a media magnet. It was broken wide open when CBS's *60 Minutes* ran a provocative segment in its April 13, 1997 program entitled "Not Quite Dead," in which the Cleveland Clinic, among other transplant centers, was accused of preparing to take organs from patients who were not brain-dead but "neurologically impaired." The *60 Minutes* story mentioned that the hearts would stop before procurement, but correspondent Mike Wallace claimed that the "absence of heartbeat" is "a less precise method" of declaring a person dead than is brain death. (As we shall see, brain death itself remains very controversial.) To back up its thesis, *60 Minutes* showed an edited clip from a staff training video that gave the false impression that organs would be procured before the patient actually died. (I viewed the entire video: Drs. Mayer and Frank made it abundantly clear throughout their presentation that the patients would be heart-dead before procurement commenced. The patients would, however, be prepared for surgery and brought into the surgical suite while still alive, perhaps accounting for the confusion.)

With the prosecutor threatening legal action and the media threatening a feeding frenzy, the Cleveland Clinic scrapped Dr. Frank's proposed heart death donor protocol. Dr. Frank, who left the Cleveland Clinic a few years after these events to create and head a new neurological intensive care unit at the University of Chicago Hospital, was badly shaken by the experience. He told me:

> Dr. Mayes and I were accused of terrible things, outrageous things. We were accused of being in cahoots. Our training video was offered as proof that we were engaged in a conspiracy, otherwise "why would we appear in it together?" People who never bothered to speak with us accused us of being ready to manipulate ethical medical practice in order to get organs. CBS rushed the *60 Minutes* program onto the air and put it on their network news because the *Cleveland Plain Dealer* was going to do a story. I was reported to the state medical board, which

dropped the case, but I could have had my career impacted. And the whole thing was a macabre, sick story and it wasn't even true.[5]

Subsequent to this controversy, the Cleveland Clinic adopted a non-heart-beating donor protocol—now called "donation after circulatory death" (DCD). Indeed, DCD donations now take place regularly throughout the country, usually with a waiting period of between two to five minutes from cardiac arrest.[6] When the DCD controversy struck the Cleveland Clinic, the number of such donors was under one hundred. In 2009, barely ten years later, there were more than 900 reported DCDs in the United States.[7]

Still, DCD remains controversial, and for good reason. Several aspects of typical DCD protocols have the potential to threaten the public's confidence in transplant medicine and need to be explored. For example, is a patient whose heart has been stopped for only two minutes really dead? Does the injection of heparin or other organ-preserving drugs, sometimes administered to patients expecting to die and become donors, constitute euthanasia? Is it moral to inject drugs and perform other invasive techniques that have no therapeutic value to the dying patient but are undertaken solely to protect the organs? Finally, are donor eligibility criteria for heart death donation too loose?

The core concept in determining if death has occurred—whether by cessation of brain or circulatory functions—is "irreversibility." Under the Uniform Determination of Death Act, model legislation from which most state death definition statutes are derived, heart death occurs when there has been an "irreversible cessation of circulatory and respiratory function." The question then becomes: Has a heart that has stopped beating for two minutes irreversibly ceased functioning?

This raises two subordinate issues: 1) Could CPR ever restart the heart after two minutes? and 2) Could the heart restart itself? The answer to the first query, in at least some cases, is clearly yes. Many people are alive today whose hearts were stopped for longer than two minutes before being revived by resuscitative medical treatment. But that isn't the final answer to the question. Patients who will become heart death donors after they die *do not want CPR*, a medical procedure they (or their families) have a right to refuse. To apply the "irreversibility" standard to them in a rigidly literal and sophistic manner would require such patients to lie "dying" without heartbeat for fifteen or twenty minutes—perhaps even longer—before the official declaration of death could be made. That would not only be cruel to families but a pointless legalism that would breed disrespect for medicine while serving no meaningful purpose for the dead patient or society.

But the possibility that a donor's heart might restart spontaneously is a different matter altogether. If the heart is capable of self-resuscitation after two minutes of cardiac arrest, the patient is unquestionably still alive because the heart stoppage is not necessarily irreversible. Unfortunately, medical science cannot apparently answer this question because "the exact point at which auto-resuscitation will not occur in humans" is not known.[8] As late as 2010, a compilation of studies on the subject showed a few cases of the heart starting spontaneously as late as seven minutes after cardiac arrest. But all of these were preceded by cardiopulmonary resuscitation efforts. To me, this is the important finding when considering DCD: "No cases of autoresuscitation in the absence of cardiopulmonary resuscitation were reported anywhere in the world."[9] (The two-minute time period used in heart death organ procurement protocols is based on spontaneous resuscitation studies in animals—not exactly comfort-giving knowledge.) Some have recently suggested shortening the two-minute minimum time limit[10]—a profoundly unwise idea, as it could materially erode the public's confidence that organs were only being procured from those who are truly dead. But as of this writing, the two-minute rule (if you will) remains in place.

Is this merely an academic issue? Dr. Stuart J. Youngner, a psychiatrist and mainstream bioethicist—and also one of the more influential thinkers in heart death organ procurement protocols who was deeply involved in the early ethics debates about DCD—believes the issue of whether death has occurred after two minutes asks the wrong question. The important issue, Youngner contends, is whether the patient is actually harmed. I asked him if he thought the patient was harmed by the protocol. "I don't think so," he answered. "First, they or their families have agreed to donate under these circumstances. Second, at that point in time, the donor is not feeling anything. You are about dead, you are probably dead, you are as good as dead, although you might not be exactly dead. It is an ambiguous state, but the donors themselves are beyond harm."[11]

Justifying the breaking of the dead donor rule with what amounts to a "no harm, no foul" defense was a worrisome sign of the direction that, in the years since my interview with Youngner, increasingly has been advocated to increase levels of organ procurement. As we have seen, modern bioethics is not content to merely tinker around the edges of current medical ethics or health care public policy. Rather, the movement seeks to stretch and even break traditional ethical boundaries and then quickly occupy the new territory in pursuit of radical change. Like a football team known for a good "ground game," bioethicists typically take an incremental approach, moving the ball toward the end zone a few yards at a time. But should a hole open in the defensive line or the chance appear to complete a Hail Mary pass, they can quickly change tactics and go for the big play.

Thankfully, the public does not share bioethicists' zeal for frequently redrawing ethical maps. Whether or not the donor is *actually dead* when organs are procured, a mere two minutes may not "feel" right to average folk. In matters as delicate as this, appearances matter as much as actualities—as the furor over the Cleveland Clinic policy and the panic in Britain described earlier by Dr. Bernat clearly attest. Indeed, even without widespread publicity about heart death donors, many Americans already refuse to sign donor cards, and families refuse to consent to procurement out of fear that their medical care may be compromised in order to garner their organs.[12] Thus unless there is an essential *physiological* reason to declare death in such seeming haste, why not, in Dr. Frank's evocative term, "put a fence of sensitivity around the process" and wait a bit longer before death is declared and organ procurement commences?

A key concern is whether a longer waiting period will destroy the purpose of heart death donation by ruining the organs. Kidneys can withstand the effects of warm ischemia for up to one hour, so little problem there.[13] Other organs, however, are not as hardy. According to some doctors, waiting for the death of brain cells, which takes roughly ten minutes after the heart has ceased beating, could endanger the viability of the liver and pancreas.[14]

Another crucially connected question about the two-minute DCD protocol is whether the donor—whose brain is not "dead" when organs are removed—might feel pain from the procedure. Several reputable neurologists assured me that people who have been without a heartbeat for two minutes are incapable of experiencing any sensation. "There is no perception,"[15] Dr. Frank told me unequivocally. "The EEG will go flat before one to two minutes of no blood flow," agrees UCLA pediatric neurologist Dr. Alan Shewmon.[16] (An EEG measures electrical activity in the brain. A "flat" EEG means an absence of activity.) But what about published reports of heart death donors receiving pain control in the operating room?[17] I was relieved to discover that the palliation efforts described were directed at preventing suffering *during the dying process*, not given to prevent donors from experiencing pain when their organs were removed after they had been declared "dead."

Does Organ Preservation Kill?: In the context of this discussion, the short answer to this question is clearly no. (Advocacy to permit killing for organs is another matter.) But there have been occasional cases that have caused doubt about this ethical concern. For example, a transplant physician was criminally accused of hastening the death of a developmentally disabled man named Ruben Navarro in 2006. Navarro was slated to be a DCD donor. But when he didn't die as expected when life support was removed, the transplant doctor entered the surgical suite and ordered that he be given painkillers and other drugs—even though he showed no sign of pain.[18] It took several hours for Navarro to die,[19] and it made a big news splash when the doctor was criminally charged.

The transplant physician was the author of his own trouble. Under DCD protocols, the transplant doctor is supposed to have nothing to do with the living patient's treatment. When the doctor in question entered the suite and took control of the patient's care, he breached this crucial wall of separation. When the surgeon administered potentially life-shortening drugs instead of returning the living patient to the ward, he invited suspicion. The physician was found not guilty of any crimes, but his breach of these crucial protocols cast an unnecessary pall over organ transplant medicine.

Such rare cases notwithstanding, the public's fear reflects the continuing confusion between ceasing unwanted medical treatment that leads to death and intentional killing. The other source of this fear is that still-living patients may be administered drugs that do not benefit them medically but rather are aimed at organ preservation after death. The drugs increase blood flow to organs so as to slow warm ischemia or prevent clotting. But the dead donor rule is not violated because these drugs do not hasten the death of patients.

This isn't to say that the question doesn't raise a crucial concern. A "basic rule of organ procurement has been that the care of living patients must never be compromised in favor of potential organ recipients."[20] Thus a fixed ethical obligation of transplant medical practitioners has always been that all treatments provided to living patients be administered solely based on their effectiveness in promoting the patient/donor's comfort or longevity. This isn't only essential to respecting the inherent dignity and moral worth of dying patients, but it has a deeply pragmatic purpose in heart death donation: *Some patients don't die after the removal of life support* and thus don't become organ donors. Indeed, there are reports in the medical literature of patient/ donors living ten hours after the removal of life support, requiring their eventual return to their hospital care units.[21]

Defenders of permitting the injection of non-beneficial drugs and insertion of medical tubes into patients expected to become heart death donors argue that these medical actions—they cannot be called treatments—are ethically valid because they are consented to by the patient or the family. This was the justification given by the University of Pittsburgh's ethics committee, represented by Michael DeVita and James V. Snyder, for revising the original protocol's prohibition on performing medically non-beneficial procedures:

> While the heparin would not harm the patient, the treatment would permit an action—organ donation—that the patient or his surrogate wanted.... The [transplant] policy was therefore altered after the first case to allow interventions that would not harm the patient but might improve the probability of organ function post transplant.[22]

Yet consent is not the end-all and be-all of medicine. I could consent to have my nose cut off to spite my face, but no ethical doctor would perform the surgery. The point is the same in this circumstance, although it is more difficult to perceive because, unlike my example, the intended benefit is not frivolous. But to justify what would normally be an act of medical abuse as ethically valid when, boiled down to its essence, it is little more than a rationalization to shift medicine's overriding purpose toward heart death patient/donors away from their individual welfare thereby turns the Hippocratic tradition on its head. Moreover, there is some indication that the drugs in question are not entirely benign to the living patient but have the potential to cause minor harm if the patient survives the removal of life support.[23]

A newer wrinkle to this question was presented with a 2015 proposal published in the *Journal of the American Medical Association* arguing that doctors be allowed to preserve organs in those who died unexpectedly. The idea, proposed by physician Stephen P. Wall and bioethicists Carolyn Plunkett and Arthur L. Caplan, would permit doctors to begin organ preservation in the wake of unexpected and sudden death *before* obtaining actual consent to procure. The hope is that by preserving organs in these sudden and often tragic situations, time would be gained for the family to go through the traumatic process of grappling with the death and subsequent request for organ donation. (I have seen how excruciating this can be: A friend's wife died unexpectedly of a heart attack. After I took him home from the hospital, he received a phone call requesting consent to procure her corneas. I will never forget the look of utter horror on the newly bereaved widower's face, still in shock that the wife he breakfasted with the day before was forever gone.)

Wall, Plunkett, and Caplan propose that "the conversation" with family to permit preservation—again, not procurement—be tailored to whether the deceased was a known organ donor or not:

> One path would be for those who have indicated prior willingness to donate (e.g., joined a donor registry), which more likely would lead authorized persons to permit preservation to effectuate the decedent's wishes. The other path would be for those for whom evidence is absent. In the former, authorized persons can be asked to "affirm" the decedent's intention to donate. In cases in which there is no evidence, family members or authorized persons should be asked to "permit" not donation but preservation.[24]

I actually think that a known donor's organs should be able to be preserved without prior consent of the family. This is a good proposal that does not sacrifice ethics or system trust on the altar of increasing the organ supply. Organs would still only be taken from the truly dead, and there is little likelihood that family members could think their loved one was treated more as an organ farm than a living patient.

Are Donor Eligibility Requirements Too Loose?: At the Cleveland Clinic, Dr. Frank restricted heart death donor eligibility to patients with irreversible and profound brain stem damage who had demonstrated extreme loss of respiratory drive—people who were the most catastrophically injured short of brain death. Yet despite this conservative approach, he was accused falsely of planning to procure organs from living, brain-damaged people.

Contrasting with Frank's conservative approach, most DCD protocols permit much broader eligibility standards that may not restrict heart death procurements to catastrophically brain-damaged patients and terminally ill people. Indeed, some could be construed as applying *also to disabled people who are not dying or brain damaged*, if they are dependent on ventilator support for survival. Thus some DCD protocols unintentionally endanger the lives of depressed, disabled patients who may consider their organs of greater value to the world than their own lives—a perception that could and often does change over time—and whose worst fears about their perceived personal uselessness are validated when they are accepted as eligible donors under the protocol.

The heart death donor protocol was devised in Pittsburgh in part because of just such a case. A ventilator-dependent forty-eight-year-old woman with quadriplegia caused by multiple sclerosis asked to have her treatment stopped and her organs procured. DeVita and Snyder write:

> The medical staff was surprised by her novel decision, but her clear thinking put everyone at ease. The attending physician consulted selected ethics committee members, legal counsel, and the UPMC administration, who all supported the decision. She was weaned from ventilatory support over 20 minutes, but then continued to breathe spontaneously for several hours. After prolonged hypotension and hypoxemia [low blood pressure and insufficient oxygen in the blood] the transplant surgeon, who had not participated in the ICU management–concluded that the organs had become unusable because of prolonged warm ischemia.[25]

Using disabled people as sources of organs in this way is very unsettling. "There is a tremendous amount of prejudice and mistaken assumptions in our culture about what it means to have a significant disability," disability rights advocate Diane Coleman told me. She continued:

> We are so extremely disrespected that many people believe in an ideal world, disabled people wouldn't exist. There is going to be growing pressure on disabled people who are dependent on life support to "pull the plug." Allowing them to believe they are being altruistic by doing so through organ donation will only increase the pressure on disabled people to choose to die in the belief that by giving their organs up their lives can have some meaning. The danger is especially acute for people who are newly disabled, many of whom believe, falsely, that their lives can never be worth living.[26]

Coleman's point is worth heeding. In our cultural milieu, in which the lives of disabled people are increasingly devalued, how easy for medical personnel to believe that the "novel decision" of dying to donate organs would be beneficial for all concerned. How easy to mask implicit and explicit exploitation and abandonment because of disability as benign and compassionate, a mere facilitation of the exercise of altruism and personal autonomy.

THE QUESTION OF CONSENT

Actually being dead isn't the only ethical requirement that must be met before one can donate a vital organ. The second rule is that that the donor—or his/her family—must consent to the procurement. Indeed, in actual practice, even when donors have consented, careful organ transplant professionals may not remove organs unless the family is firmly on board.

The requirement of both death and explicit consent, some claim, has led to lengthening waiting lists for organ transplants. While there is certainly an element of truth to that claim—and indeed, many more sick people need kidneys, hearts, and livers than there are kidneys, hearts, and livers to go around—this organ shortage is actually the result of both decreased supply and increased demand. Why decreased supply? Public safety laws requiring motorists to wear seat belts, motorcyclists to don helmets, and the installation of airbags in automobiles have reduced the number of catastrophic head injuries that often lead to organ donation—good news, to be sure, with an unintended adverse consequence to the organ transplant field. Concomitantly, the science of transplant medicine has advanced exponentially, allowing more people to benefit than ever from organ transplants. This reduced supply, coupled with increased demand, has led to the lengthening waiting lists for transplant surgeries, a problem measured in the number of patients who die while waiting vainly for an organ to become available.

Most of the organ transplant controversies discussed in this book have their genesis here—from the good-hearted desire of bioethicists and transplant medical professionals to reduce the excruciating waits so many people endure while waiting to reach the top of the transplant waiting list.

So how is consent obtained? Most countries—including the United States—have an "opt-in" form of consenting to organ donation, meaning that the donor or his family must specifically consent before organs can be procured. This is often done at the bedside of a dying or brain-dead patient. (We will get to the brain death question below.) But people can also consent to being a donor long before they are in the position of becoming a donor. For example, I checked the "I want to be a donor" box when renewing my driver's license, demonstrated by a red dot on the front of the document. This lets the medical team and my family know my wishes should I die under circumstances that permit organ procurement.

A few countries, most notably Spain and France, reverse the consent presumption. Known as "presumed consent," rather than requiring donors or family to opt in, this system requires anyone not wishing to be a donor to sign a form explicitly opting out. Fail to sign a form, and your organs will be procured upon your death, conditions permitting, with no further inquiries required.

Spain and France saw an increase in the number of donors under the presumed consent system, and similar proposals have been made in the US—although, as of this writing, none have been enacted. This raises an important question: Is presumed consent ethically appropriate for the US? I think not, particularly given the public's broad but very shallow trust in organ transplant medicine.

We are not Europe. People of the United States tend to "value individualism over collectivism, autonomous decision making over the imposed 'greater good.'" Indeed, presumed consent laws could unleash a boomerang effect: many would resent the new approach as government coercion over one of the most intimate decisions anyone can make and protest by taking the opt-out option.

The current societal context must also be considered. The Obamacare debate, with its specter of "death panel" rationing boards and waiting lines, significantly undermined the people's faith in our medical system. Now factor in presumed consent to the popular fears that expensively ill and injured patients will soon be discarded as so much medical waste. Finally, mix in already-existing medical futility policies discussed in the last chapter—such as the law in Texas permitting hospital ethics committees meeting behind closed doors to refuse *wanted* life-sustaining treatment based on "quality of life" or the cost of their care—and you have a perfect prescription for distrust in all things medical. In such a milieu, the temptation to believe that your catastrophically head-injured son could have been saved but died because his organs were deemed more valuable than his life would be, for some, hard to resist.

Finally, there is the issue of integrity. We have become a public policy promise-breaking nation. Think of the many times solemn assurances have been given that reasonable restrictions will be maintained in order to gain popular acceptance of controversial policies and how casually they were cast aside once the deal was sealed. Organ donation received acceptance from a wary public precisely because of the promises, solemnly made, that only the organs of the truly dead would be taken and then only with specific consent. Break either of those promises, and I suspect that the shaky faith people have in the organ transplant system would plummet like a crowbar thrown off a bridge.

If doctors ever start taking organs without explicit permission—even if allowed by law—there will be hell to pay. In this day of cost-cutting and utilitarian "quality of life" judgmentalism, a PC law makes it too tempting for medical personnel to (almost unconsciously) look upon the catastrophically ill or disabled as so many organ farms instead of patients with equal moral value. (Just look at the mess that became of the well-motivated Liverpool Care Pathway in the UK, meant to ensure that the dying receive proper palliation but which actually led to backdoor euthanasia!)

The tens of thousands of sick and dying people waiting desperately for a transplant would be the ultimate victims of changing our laws of consent. Indeed, if we reverse our presumptions, I believe we could end up with fewer donated organs rather than more, with more arguing and increased litigation. It's just not a risk worth taking.

THE BRAIN DEATH CONTROVERSY

Which brings us back to the question of what constitutes "dead" for organ donation purposes? For more than thirty years, "brain death"—the irreversible cessation of all function within the entire brain—has been the primary method of declaring death when organ donation is contemplated. While still controversial, the criteria for brain death has served humanity well, permitting thousands of lives to be saved through organ transplantation; the gift of life. But just as the public had become more comfortable with brain death, some bioethicists began to call the very concept into doubt.

Ironically, the criticism comes from two conflicting and paradoxical perspectives. One view holds that that brain death isn't really dead, a view also held by some pro-lifers. If true, it would mean that organs have been procured from living people for more than two decades, an ethical horror. The other less publicized—but ultimately more dangerous—view rejects brain death for being too narrowly drawn, thereby unduly limiting the supply of organs as potential recipients die waiting for organs to become available. Both challenges have the potential to damage public confidence in organ transplantation.

Is Brain-Dead Really Dead?[27]: In December 2013, an Oakland, California thirteen-year-old girl named Jahi McMath entered Children's Hospital for serious throat surgery to relieve her sleep apnea. She survived the surgery without incident, and after awakening even enjoyed a Popsicle. Then, a terrible complication: Jahi began bleeding profusely and suffered a cardiac arrest. It took many minutes to restore her heartbeat. Too late: Jahi was later declared "brain-dead." Doctors informed Jahi's mother that she had died and that they would soon remove all medical technology that sustained her.*

Jahi's family protested. She was still warm, they noted. Because of medical machinery, air was still flowing into her lungs, and her heart was

---

* Many commentators use the term "Jahi's body" when describing her current circumstance. While I believe properly diagnosed "brain death" is dead—as described below—I don't employ that terminology because it would be so hurtful to Jahi's family.

still beating, pulsing blood through her arteries. Surely, they pleaded in anguish, she is alive.

With hospital administrators and doctors adamant that, tragically, Jahi was dead—and would be so treated—the family went public. The story exploded into international headlines and bitter litigation ensued.

Alameda County Superior Court Judge Evelio Grillo appointed a Stanford University Medical School neurologist to render an independent assessment. When this well-respected physician also determined that Jahi was brain-dead—the third to so conclude—Grillo declared her legally deceased and Alameda County issued a death certificate.[28]

But the judge did not force her off of medical support, as he could have under California law.[29] Rather, he ultimately arm-twisted the parties into a settlement under which the hospital released Jahi to the Alameda County coroner and thence to her family—still on the ventilator. Most expected Jahi's body would deteriorate, but that didn't happen. As of this writing, three years after Jahi's catastrophe, she is being maintained at a New Jersey hospital.[30] Meanwhile, her mother sued in California, claiming that Jahi's condition is no longer consistent with a finding of brain death—which, if true, would be unprecedented—and whether her injuries were caused by medical malpractice.[31]

At about the same time, a similar tragedy made the news in Texas. Marlise Muñoz, fourteen weeks pregnant, collapsed. She received CPR and was rushed to the hospital but never regained consciousness. When she was declared brain-dead, her husband, Erick, requested that her life support be terminated so that the family could make final arrangements.

But John Peter Smith Hospital administrators refused. It wasn't that her doctors disagreed that Marlise was dead; they worried that complying with the request would violate a Texas statute that states: "A person may not withdraw or withhold life-sustaining treatment under this subchapter from a pregnant patient."[32]

Erick sued, claiming that Marlise would not have wanted her body maintained, that her body was deteriorating—as usually happens in such cases—that tests showed the fetus was irremediably damaged by the mother's death, and that the statute did not apply in any event since, as a deceased person, Marlise was not a "patient."

A judge agreed, ruling that the law indeed was not applicable to the facts of the case "because Mrs. Muñoz is dead."[33] The hospital was ordered to remove medical intervention, which came to pass, even though by then the fetus was twenty-two weeks or so along, although the family claimed that the unborn child was also dead. The case was not appealed.

The white-hot McMath and Muñoz controversies reignited public interest in a story that had broken in the *Daily Mail* in November 2013 but that had received little attention at the time. Hungarian doctors reported the birth of a healthy baby from a brain-dead mother: "A baby which was 15 weeks old when its mother was declared brain-dead was delivered by Caesarean section at 27 weeks, after doctors kept the mother alive on life support. The Hungarian doctors who delivered the baby in July believe the birth is one of only three such cases in the world."

The above reporting made a subtle mistake—often seen in stories such as this—which adds to the public's confusion about brain death. As will be described in more detail below, if the Hungarian mother was actually brain-dead, the doctors did not keep her "alive" but rather kept her organ systems functioning long enough for the baby to be delivered. As we shall see, at least legally, that is a distinction with a profound difference. Back to the story:

> In the spring, she had been rushed to hospital, operated on but was declared brain-dead. She was kept on life support and doctors were able to see through an ultrasound that the foetus was moving. "In the first two days we struggled to save the mother's life and it was proven ... that circulation and functions stopped," said Dr. Bela Fulesdi, president of the University of Debrecen Medical and Health Science Centre.

The baby was delivered when, like Muñoz, the mother's body began to deteriorate: "While they were hoping to keep the baby in the womb as long as possible, in the 27th week, the woman's circulation became unstable and doctors decided to deliver the baby because the womb was no longer safe."[34]

The confusion and public debate that erupted around these "brain death" cases shows how little the concept is understood by most people and the media. It also raises important scientific, moral, and ethical questions: Is brain-dead really dead? Why do the bodies of brain-dead people remain viable for a time? Can I decide I don't want my own death to ever be so declared?

"Total Brain Failure": The term "brain death" was coined by French physicians (*coma dépassé*) in 1959, in recognition of how the "profundity of coma, apnea [cessation of breathing] and unresponsiveness exhibited by patients with destroyed cerebral hemispheres and brain stems differed fundamentally from previously described forms of coma."[35]

The condition's existence was an unexpected consequence of the technological revolution in medicine that transformed health care in the middle of the last century. Indeed, because a person who is brain-dead cannot breathe, the condition would not exist at all but for the development of the ventilator and other forms of medical technology that have saved the lives of so many desperately ill and injured people. For some of these patients, high-tech medicine has been the road that led to a full recovery. For others, ongoing high-tech life-sustaining treatment is necessary to prevent death. In contrast, for a relative few—the most catastrophically injured or ill—the functioning of the whole brain was utterly destroyed by the underlying disease or injury, but the medical machinery kept other body systems viable for a time. It was this latter group that came to be known as brain-dead.

The concept of brain death has become inextricably bound with organ donation. Into the early 1960s, most organ transplants were either of single kidneys or liver grafts taken from living relatives or kidneys removed from donors whose hearts had stopped beating. At about this time, a few donors were people who would today be considered brain-dead. But because the concept of brain-dead as "dead" did not exist, medical interventions were ceased so that cardiac arrest would ensue before procurement.

Then, in 1967, the South African physician Dr. Christiaan Barnard electrified the world with a heart transplant taken from a donor declared brain-dead, a concept then accepted in that country. However, even Dr. Bernard did not procure the heart he transplanted until after removing the medical machines from the body and waiting for cardiac arrest.[36]

The question of whether "brain death" was a valid concept moved swiftly to the forefront of medicine, pregnant with possibilities for saving the lives of those needing organ transplants. At that time, organ transplant medicine lacked today's capability to substantially delay the onset of organ decay in those declared dead by standard means (irreversible

cessation of cardiopulmonary function, or "heart death"). As a consequence, many donated organs were rendered unusable.

But if brain death were a biologically legitimate and verifiable condition, the problem of decay could be reduced dramatically, since the
donor's organs would remain in the body and be kept healthy by the
medically maintained circulation of blood until the very moment of procurement. That could save many lives among potential organ recipients
that were then being lost because organs became nonviable.

Organ donation was not the only pressing issue for which the concept
of brain death was seen as potentially providing a solution. These were
the years when many doctors were very reluctant to remove life support
from living patients. But there has never been an obligation in medicine
to treat dead persons. More pragmatically, if brain death were accepted
as deceased in law, no doctor could be charged criminally for turning
off the ventilator of a dead patient—rarely an issue today, but a significant fear at the time. Thus when a committee was convened at Harvard
University in 1968 to determine the criteria that could legitimately be
used to determine when a human being had died, investigating brain
death was high on the agenda.

The Harvard Committee Report concluded that brain death was
physiologically and ethically sound, and a condition for which objective
diagnostic criteria could be developed. The new method to determine
death won quick approval through much of society, including among
widely respected representatives of religious groups (then a more important societal force in public policy matters than now) as well as medical
and legal professional organizations.

Assent was not, however, unanimous. A minority of commenters
worried that brain death was simply a utilitarian expedient to permit the
exploitation of profoundly disabled people for their organs. (Some, as we
shall see, still think that.) But these voices held little sway.

In 1970, Kansas became the first state to formally include brain death
in its statute defining death, and the rest of the nation—and then most
of the Western world—quickly followed suit. Because organs procured
from brain-dead donors were much more likely to function properly after
transplant, the use of heart-dead donors fell substantially out of favor
in transplant medicine until revived some twenty years later—a matter
not without its own controversies, the details of which are beyond our
scope here.[37]

The Uniform Determination of Death Act—which has essentially been adopted in all fifty states—defined brain death as follows: "An individual who has sustained ... irreversible cessation of all functions of the entire brain, including the brain stem, is dead. A determination of death must be made in accordance with accepted medical standards."[38] The American Academy of Neurology similarly defines brain death as "the irreversible loss of the clinical function of the brain."[39]

Brain death is sometimes misunderstood as meaning that there are no living brain cells remaining in the brain. That isn't required for a determination of brain death and, in any event, also isn't true when a person is declared dead because his heart has stopped. In fact, studies have shown that brain cells may remain alive for an extended time after heart death, with one study reporting that viable brain cells were obtained during an autopsy conducted *eight hours* after death.[40]

Part of the continuing intensity of the brain death controversy may have to do with nomenclature. According to a white paper put out by the President's Council on Bioethics in 2008, the term "brain-dead" causes much public confusion. "First, the term (as well as heart death) wrongly implies that there is more than one kind of death: Whatever difficulties there might be in knowing whether death has occurred, it must be kept in mind that there is only one real phenomenon of death. *Death is the transition from a living mortal organism to being something that though dead, retains a physical continuity with the once-living organism.*"[41] (My emphasis.)

Second, describing a deceased person as brain-dead "implies that death is a state of cells and tissues constituting the brain." Rather, "what is directly at *issue is the living or dead status of the human individual*, not the individual's brain."[42] (My emphasis.)

Finally, the council noted that death "is *a clinical state or condition made evident by certain ascertainable signs*"[43] (my emphasis). In other words, there are measurable indicia of life—or its absence—that can be determined in a clinical setting.

The council recommended replacing the term "brain death" with the more comprehensible "*total irreversible brain failure*," or "total brain failure," for ease of wording[44] (my emphasis). This is very helpful and elucidating. Just as a patient has unquestionably died when her heart and lung functions have irreversibly collapsed, so too has the human being ceased to be, *once her brain has totally failed.*

Another useful descriptive is "death declared by neurological criteria." In laypeople's language, all of this means the *entire brain, and each of its constituent parts,* is not functioning *as a brain,* and *never will again.* There is very little or no neural electrical activity; there is no respiratory drive; there is a complete absence of even the most rudimentary brain stem reflexes. For example, the pupils remain at the midpoint, just like the pupils of heart-dead corpses, and they don't react to bright light. The usual gagging response is absent, even when a tube is inserted through the mouth into the pharynx. According to a finding of the American Academy of Neurology published in 2010, there have been "no published reports of recovery of neurologic function [in adults] after a diagnosis of brain death."[45] None.

The popular media also sows confusion about whether brain-dead is dead, sometimes incorrectly using the term when referring to a patient diagnosed to be in a persistent vegetative state (PVS)—such as the late Terri Schiavo. This is a misnomer. Unlike those who have experienced total brain failure, *patients in PVS are unquestionably alive*—both legally and physically. For example, the persistently unconscious have measurable brain activity, some reflex function, and indeed, like Schiavo, can often breathe without medical assistance. In contrast, people who have experienced total brain failure exhibit none of these properties of living persons.

A Never-ending Controversy: Brain death remains heatedly controversial among a minority of observers. As we will see below, many bioethicists want to do away with the requirement of "death" before donation, or expand the definition of death to include patients diagnosed as persistently unconscious. Some pro-life activists reject that brain death is dead, worrying that the concept is actually a subterfuge to permit organ harvesting from severely disabled but still-living people, or see it as an excuse to stop life support for expensive and/or morally devalued patients.

Perhaps the most well known and passionate of these advocates is the neonatologist and pediatrician Dr. Paul A. Byrne, who argues that brain-dead people remain alive *precisely because* ventilator-facilitated respiration works and these people's hearts continue to beat:

> Without respiration and circulation, health of the person deteriorates, ultimately ending in death. This deterioration is manifest in cessation

of vital activities and structural changes of disintegration, dissolution and/or destruction of cells and tissues of organs and systems. These changes can be detected at the microscopic level, but eventually in death, they become evident as decay, decomposition and putrefaction. After true death chest compressions or a ventilator can only move air; there cannot be respiration, because respiration is a function of a living human body.[46]

Byrne also brings religion into his advocacy: "Contrariwise, if such efforts at ventilation and respiration are successful, that can be only because soul and body unity is still present, i.e., because the person is still living, not dead. Respiration, circulation and heart beat can be present only in a living person, not a cadaver."[47]

Souls can't be measured. Moreover, Byrne is factually incorrect: The heart does not require a living body (or presence of a soul) to continue beating. In fact, kept in a proper solution, the heart can continue to beat outside the body for hours because it has independent nerve centers that stimulate its contractions.

Moreover, ventilation requires no intrinsic activity of the lungs. The lungs themselves are inflated with air only if the diaphragm and some chest wall muscles contract. Deflation occurs when those muscles relax, and the natural rubber-like elasticity of the lungs squeezes them down to their former volume. Contraction of the muscles essential for breathing occurs only if a signal descends from the brain to direct that contraction. Unlike the heart, the lungs have no intrinsic nerves to maintain their activity. Thus, when the brain totally ceases to function, there are no signals to the diaphragm to expand and contract, the result of which is that breathing stops.

Byrne's use of the words "ventilation" and "respiration" could leave the misleading impression that they are synonyms. But these are distinct biological activities. Ventilation simply is air moving in and out of the lungs, just as it does in a bellows. In contrast, respiration is the "sum total of the physical and chemical processes in an organism by which oxygen is conveyed to tissues."[48]

Thus, when the brain totally ceases to function, spontaneous ventilation does not occur. Artificial ventilation can put oxygen into the blood, and the intrinsic activity of the heart can make the blood circulate and can maintain respiration throughout the body. Importantly, however, in the case of brain death there is no blood flow to the brain, and therefore *there is no respiration in the brain*. In fact, that is why the brain is dead and will never recover.

The fact that a heart can beat and the lungs function passively after death has been demonstrated vividly by the recent invention of machines that allows both organs to work from the time of removal from a donor's body until they are later transplanted into living patients. (Previously, the hearts and lungs, like other transplantable organs, would be kept cold but inert during this time period.) As one story reported:

> When the lungs are inside the Organ Care System, "they are immedi-
> ately revived *to a warm, breathing state* and perfused with oxygen and a
> special solution supplemented with packed red blood cells," according
> to the UCLA press release.... UCLA is also known for developing the
> "heart in a box," a similar technique that keeps a transplant heart beat-
> ing and warm before transplantation.... In November 2012, a team at
> UCLA successfully completed the first "breathing lung" transplant on a
> 57-year-old patient who had pulmonary fibrosis. Pulmonary fibrosis is a
> disease causing the air sacs of the lungs to be replaced by scar tissue. The
> patient received two new lungs and recuperated properly afterward.[49]

Clearly, then, the heart can beat and the lungs function passively when not inside a still-living person. It is thus hardly surprising that other organs and body functions that don't require direct brain involvement continue to function in the brain-dead. In almost all cases, however, despite technological interventions, even these self-directed capacities will eventually be lost in someone with total brain failure, as medical complications accumulate with the passage of time.

Ah, but not in every case, notes brain death skeptic Dr. Alan Shewmon. The UCLA neurologist, once a believer in the validity of brain death, now asserts that the rare *extended* continuation of bodily function after decla-ration of brain death calls into question the entire concept.

Years ago, Shewmon identified some 175 cases of brain-dead bodies functioning for one week or more. Half of these cases experienced body survival for one month, a third for two months, and 7 percent for one year. One person declared dead by neurological criteria had been kept functioning for more than sixteen years at the time Shewmon wrote his paper.[50]

I am not convinced that these rare anomalies undermine the concept that total brain failure equals death. Maintaining long-term body viability involves much more than artificial respiration. For example, the bodies of those with total brain failure don't manufacture crucial hormones, which therefore must be administered. Blood pressure also becomes a significant issue and needs to be addressed by medical means.

With advances in medical sophistication, it is possible that more of the brain-dead could be maintained long term. But that isn't the same thing as being "alive." As most of the members the President's Council noted in accepting brain-dead as dead:

> [T]he patient with total brain failure is no longer able to carry out the fundamental work of a living organism. Such a patient has lost—and lost irreversibly—a fundamental openness to the surrounding environment on his or her own behalf.... A living organism engages in self-sustaining need-driven activities critical to and constitutive of its commerce with the surrounding world. These activities are authentic signs of active and ongoing life. When these signs are absent and these activities have ceased, then a judgment that the organism as a whole has died can be made with confidence.[51]

A more vivid—if crass—way of describing why total brain failure is dead was made to me many years ago by Dr. Frank as I researched for the original version of this book: "Imagine a person with their head cut off who is somehow kept from losing blood and whose circulatory system is intact. That is the functional equivalent of a true brain death. We can keep the body going for a time through medical technology, but would anyone really consider a headless but functioning body a living person?"[52] For me, that remains the most compelling argument.

What If You Don't Believe Total Brain Failure Is Dead?: Some readers of this discussion may remain unconvinced that total brain failure means that a person is really dead. The question thus becomes: Can anything be done to ensure that they or their loved ones are not declared dead by neurological criteria and/or to ensure medical maintenance in the face of total brain failure?

The simple answer in most states is no. New York and New Jersey allow a religious exception to brain death. But most state laws and/or hospital practices are like those followed in California: If family members object to the finding, their only recourse is that they may have to litigate. In such cases, such as that of Jahi McMath, a judge will often obtain an independent medical opinion. But this will not be a contest about *whether* total brain failure is dead—that is now settled law. Rather, the litigation would primarily contest whether *the condition was properly determined* in the particular circumstance.

It is true that some, like Jahi's family, opt to maintain their loved ones for as long as possible. But with rare exceptions noted above, they don't necessarily have the legal right to so do, and in any event the costs will not be paid for by health insurance or government benefits because the brain-dead person is not legally a living patient.

But what if one refuses to be an organ donor? Will that provide protection against declaration of brain death and the subsequent withdrawal of all medical interventions?

No. The question of organ donation and declaration of death are distinct. The ultimate issue isn't whether a patient will be an organ donor *but whether that patient is alive.* Once death has been declared, by either brain or heart criteria—again, with rare exceptions—the hospital has no legal obligation to continue medical intervention beyond a brief adjustment period. Moreover, as with the Jahi McMath case, a death certificate can be issued.

Brain death controversies get a lot of attention, but the reality of the concept is all but universally accepted in medicine, law, and among general society. It is also acknowledged as bona fide by most religious traditions. For example, the Catholic Church—hardly an advocate of utilitarian medicine—recognizes total brain failure as a valid reason for declaring a person to be legally dead.[53]

Whatever one might believe on an individual basis, here's the hard bottom line: Once a patient is declared brain-dead, legally he or she is no longer among the living but has, as Shakespeare artfully put it, passed "through nature into eternity."

Killing the Dead Donor Rule: My 2005 online debate about the Terri Schiavo case with Florida bioethicist Bill Allen, sponsored by Court TV Online, eventually got down to the nitty-gritty[54]:

Wesley J. Smith: Bill, do you think Terri is a person?

Bill Allen: No, I do not. I think having awareness is an essential criterion for personhood. Even minimal awareness would support some criterion of personhood, but I don't think complete absence of awareness does.

Knowing that this kind of thinking predominates in contemporary bioethics, I decided to move the discussion to the practical consequences of such thinking:

WJS: If Terri is not a person, should her organs be procured with consent?

BA: Yes, I think there should be consent to harvest her organs, just as we allow people to say what they want done with their assets.

Put that in your hat and ponder it for a moment: If organ harvesting from the cognitively devastated were legal today, Michael Schiavo would have been the one, no doubt, who could have consented to doctors "stopping" Terri's heart and harvesting her organs—in other words, killing her as part of the organ procurement process.

Think that's a horrid thought? Starting in the 1990s and accelerating since the publication of the first version of this book, some of bioethics' most prominent voices have advocated just such a course in many of the world's most prestigious medical and bioethics journals—sometimes in the popular media as well.

Many of the articles argue—as Allen did above—that patients diagnosed as permanently unconscious should be considered dead, since they have lost their personhood. For example, Dr. Norman Fost, professor of pediatrics and director of the program in medical ethics at the University of Wisconsin in Madison, made such an argument in a bioethics book chapter about organ donation entitled "The Unimportance of Death." "My contention is that that there is ample precedent in the law and good moral justification for removing organs from persons who are not legally dead," wrote Fost, arguing to permit harvesting patients diagnosed with permanent unconsciousness who are ventilator-dependent. "In such a case, with appropriate consent, kidneys and liver could be removed prior to discontinuation of the ventilator. Such removal would not immediately cause death. The cause of death would be the same as traditionally occurs,

namely respiratory failure leading to irreversible loss of cardiac function."
But what if the patient continues to breathe after discontinuation of the
ventilator, as Karen Ann Quinlan did? Fost doesn't say, but death by organ
failure would be the clear consequence.

The unconscious aren't the only ones Fost envisions as eligible for
vital organ procurement during life. Terminally ill people could also participate in having their organs harvested before they are actually dead "as
part of their care." Fost uses the example of cystic fibrosis patients: "From
a moral perspective, these patients would seem to be ideal organ donors.
Their death is commonly anticipated for many years, allowing ample time
for reflection and truly informed consent, a rare event in organ removal
from brain-dead patients; they could truly be donors."[55]

Another case in point: Published in the January 19, 2012 edition of the
Journal of Medical Ethics, "What Makes Killing Wrong?" was an article
in which the authors argued that death and "total disability" are morally
indistinguishable, and therefore harvesting organs from living, disabled
patients is not morally wrong. Bioethicists Walter Sinnott-Armstrong of
Duke University and Franklin G. Miller from the National Institutes of
Health's Department of Bioethics (which should really get the alarm bells
ringing!) arrived at their shocking (for most of us) conclusion by claiming
that murdering the hypothetical "Betty" isn't wrong because it kills her;
rather, it's wrong because it "makes her unable to do anything, including
walking, talking, and even thinking and feeling."[56]

How do they get from deconstructing the definition of death to
harvesting the disabled? First, they change the scenario so that Betty is
not killed but severely brain-damaged to the point that she is "totally
disabled." But their definition of that term encompasses hundreds of
thousands of *living* Americans who are our mothers, fathers, children,
aunts and uncles, siblings, friends, and cousins—people with profound
disabilities like that experienced by Terri Schiavo and my late Uncle
Bruno toward the end of his struggle with Alzheimer's disease: "Betty
has mental states, at least intermittently and temporarily, so she is not
dead by any standard or plausible criterion. Still, she is universally
disabled because she has no control over anything that goes on in her
body or mind."[57]

Never mind that these diagnoses are often inaccurate; the authors
claim that Betty "is no worse off being dead than totally disabled" and

hence it is no worse "to kill Betty than to totally disable her." Not only that, but according to the authors, "there is nothing bad about death or killing other than disability or disabling," and *since she is already so debilitated, then nothing wrong is done by harvesting her organs,* thereby ending her biological existence. And thus, in the space of not quite five pages, killing innocent human beings ceases to be wrong and the intrinsic dignity of human life is thrown out the window, transforming vulnerable human beings into objectified and exploitable human resources.

Other articles suggest that the dead donor rule be scrapped in favor of "consent" as the primary criterion for donating vital organs. Thus, writing in the *Cambridge Quarterly of Healthcare Ethics,* Canadian University of Calgary bioethicist Walter Glannon argues that death is "morally insignificant" to organ donation; some living patients are beyond "neurological and psychological capacity to be harmed," and thwarting a patient's desire to donate organs because they are alive "defeats their interest in donating organs." Hence:

> What matters is not that the donor is or is not dead, or when death is declared, but that the donor or a surrogate consents, that the donor has an irreversible condition with no hope of meaningful recovery, that procurement does not cause the donor to experience pain and suffering, and that the donor's intention is realized in a successful transplant. These conditions are consistent with the principles of respect for patient autonomy and physician nonmaleficence. None of these conditions requires that donors be dead before organ procurement can proceed.[58]

Please note: There is a great deal of room for *interpretation* in the term "meaningful recovery"; indeed, sufficient space to open the door to killing a wide swath of patients for their organs, not "just" the imminently dying or those believed to be permanently unconscious.

I could go on and on, quoting articles published in such notable journals as the *Lancet, Critical Care Medicine, Nature*—even the prestigious *New England Journal of Medicine*—that explicitly advocated killing for organs: "Whether death occurs as the result of ventilator withdrawal or organ procurement, the ethically relevant precondition is valid consent by the patient or surrogate. With such consent, there is no harm or wrong done in retrieving vital organs before death, provided anesthesia is administered."[59] Whew. At least they don't want the person who dies by homicide to feel any pain.

Advocacy to discard the necessity for actual death before organ harvesting has been generally restricted to professional journals, where they receive little public notice. But lately, advocates have begun to broach the subject to a more general readership. Thus two doctors wrote in the *Atlantic*:

> If medical guidelines could be revised to let people facing imminent death donate vital organs under general anesthesia, we could provide patients and families a middle ground—a way of avoiding futile medical care, while also honoring life by preventing the deaths of other critically ill people. Moreover, healthy people could incorporate this imminent-death standard into advance directives for their end-of-life care. They could determine the conditions under which they would want care withdrawn, and whether they were willing to have it withdrawn in an operating room, under anesthesia, with subsequent removal of their organs.[60]

At this point I think it is important to emphasize that these kinds of harvests *are not yet happening* in our organ transplant medical centers, and that transplant medicine remains an ethical enterprise. If we want to keep it that way, these proposals must not be allowed to germinate. As they say, sunlight is the great disinfectant: the best way to prevent this dark agenda from ever becoming the legal public policy is to expose it in popular media every time it is proposed.

Euthanasia and Organ Harvesting: I first became involved in bioethical issues when my friend Frances committed suicide in 1992 under the influence of Hemlock Society (now called Compassion and Choices) literature that taught how to use lethal drugs and a plastic bag to commit suicide.[61] Frances's suicide led me to write my first anti-euthanasia piece in *Newsweek*, published in 1993, in which I worried:

> Life is action and reaction, the proverbial pebble thrown into the pond. We don't get to the Brave New World in one giant leap. Rather, the descent to depravity is reached by small steps. First, suicide is promoted as a virtue. Vulnerable people like Frances become early casualties.

Then follows mercy killing of the terminally ill. From there, it's a hop, skip and a jump to killing people who don't have a good "quality" of life, perhaps with the prospect of organ harvesting thrown in as a plum to society.[62]

Over the years, I was frequently called an alarmist for predicting that euthanasia would one day be coupled with organ harvesting. But once a society generally accepts that killing is an acceptable answer to human suffering, euthanasia and organ donation move steadily toward each other with gravitational attraction. It's only logical: If people who want to die can save the lives of those who want to live, why not let them?

As the argument over assisted suicide and euthanasia ebbed and flowed, I waited for the organ harvesting shoe to drop. My fear was first realized during Jack Kevorkian's assisted suicide reign of criminality in the 1990s. In 1998, Kevorkian assisted the suicide of Joseph Tushkowski, age forty-five. By then, Kevorkian-assisted suicides had dropped off the front pages. But this death had a macabre twist: Tushkowski's body underwent "a bizarre mutilation," proclaimed Oakland County (Michigan) Medical Examiner L. J. Dragovic. According to the autopsy findings, after lethally injecting Tushkowski to death, in an abattoir-scene the medical examiner called a "slaughterhouse," the mutilators simply lifted up Tushkowski's sweater, did their dirty work, and tied off the blood vessels with twine.[63]

This was not a bizarre plot twist from a new *X-Files* movie. Jack Kevorkian helped commit this despicable and gruesome act. He admitted it proudly in a news conference held shortly after the deed during which he and his lawyer offered Tushkowski's organs for transplant, "first come, first served."

Kevorkian's taking of Tushkowski's kidneys was no surprise. As described in his 1991 book *Prescription Medicide*, organ harvesting from assisted suicide victims was the second in Kevorkian's strategic three-pronged plan designed to give him a free hand to pursue his macabre obsessions. The first phase was to make assisted suicide seem routine and even banal, which succeeded. The second phase was to harvest organs from assisted suicide victims and offer them for use in transplants to make the voluntary killing of despairing disabled and sick people seem beneficial to society—thus the Tushkowski grotesquerie. The third and ultimate goal, which he would have eventually attempted had he not been jailed for Thomas Youk's murder, would have been to use assisted suicide victims as living "subjects" in human experimentation; in other words, human vivisection.

Kevorkian had grounds to believe his plan would work. Less than a year before the assisted killing/mutilation of Tushkowski, Kevorkian and his attorney promised to hold a press conference with medically preserved organs at their side to announce the first assisted suicide/organ harvest.[64] The public was little outraged by the promise, and even more alarmingly, the organ transplant community mostly raised mere procedural objections to the plan. For example, one organ procurement agency director complimented Kevorkian for recognizing the organ shortage and opined that while "his generosity is sincere," organs from a person killed by "carbon monoxide or poison" might not be usable, making Kevorkian's plan "unfeasible."[65]

After the Tushkowski outrage, the organ transplant community's reaction was similarly muted. Instead of erupting in a forceful and unified condemnation of the immoral assisted killing of a disabled man and the attempt to make the slaying publicly palatable via organ harvesting, most—with a few exceptions—focused on Kevorkian's failure to comply with necessary transplant protocols. For example, a president of an organ sharing network told the Associated Press that there would be several hurdles to cross before organs from assisted suicide could be offered, including ensuring the proper place of organ removal (in a transplant center), appropriate organ preservation, packaging, and adequate tissue typing.[66]

Still, other than the Kevorkian eruption and some arguments in bioethics journals, the idea that euthanasia could be coupled *as a matter of public policy* with organ harvesting remained, for most people, an "It can never happen here" prospect. Then came Belgium.

As noted earlier, euthanasia was legalized in Belgium in 2002. In 2008, Belgian doctors announced the first known legal coupling of euthanasia and organ harvesting in the case of a woman in a "locked in" state—fully paralyzed but also fully cognizant. After doctors agreed to her request to be lethally injected, she asked that her organs be harvested after she died. Doctors agreed. They described their procedure in a 2008 issue of the journal *Transplant International*:

This case of two separate requests, first euthanasia and second, organ donation after death, demonstrates that organ harvesting after euthanasia may be considered and accepted from ethical, legal, and practical viewpoints in countries where euthanasia is legally accepted. This possibility may increase the number of transplantable organs and may also provide some comfort to the donor and her family, considering that the termination of the patient's life may be seen as helping other human beings in need for organ transplantation.[67]

It didn't take long for Belgian doctors and bioethicists to promote the conjoining at medical conferences around Europe. Their PowerPoint presentation touts the "high quality" of organs obtained from patients after euthanasia of people with degenerative neuro/muscular disabilities.

This advocacy has clearly been put into practice. A 2011 article in *Applied Cardiopulmonary Pathophysiology* recounts in chillingly clinical detail the euthanasia killings and harvesting of four patients, three with neuromuscular diseases and one with the (ironic) mental illness of self-harming:

> Donors were admitted to the hospital a few hours before the planned euthanasia procedure. A central venous line was placed in a room adjacent to the operating room. Donors were heparinized immediately before a cocktail of drugs was given by the treating physician who agreed to perform the euthanasia. The patient was announced dead on cardiorespiratory criteria by 3 independent physicians as required by Belgian legislation for every organ donor.... The deceased was then rapidly transferred, installed on the operating table, and intubated. The thorax and abdomen were shaved, disinfected and draped. A rapid sterno-laparotomy was performed.... The abdominal team took care of liver and kidney preservation with a rapid flush cooling technique via a cannula inserted into the abdominal aorta. The thoracic team then opened pleural cavities and quickly inspected both lungs before topical cooling with ice-cold saline was started. The pericardium was opened, the main pulmonary artery was encircled and a 24 Fr pulmoplegia catheter was inserted through the right ventricular outflow tract.[68]

The article goes on to celebrate that the lungs taken from euthanasia deaths grafted well into their organ recipients. It also noted that 2.8 percent of all DCD organ procurements came after euthanasia—a number that will almost surely rise as the country grows comfortable with the "plum to society" of harvesting the organs of euthanasia donors.

Not to be outdone by their neighbor, the Netherlands' minister of health announced in 2014 that she believed organ donation following euthanasia was merely a "practical application" of Dutch law and announced plans to promulgate new protocols to govern such procurements.[69] No doubt, Belgium and the Netherlands will be followed by the newest kid on the euthanasia block, Canada, after its sweeping Supreme Court ruling creating a charter right to medicalized killing. Indeed, doctors and bioethicists began debating that very question within months of the ruling.[70]

Some might ask, if these patients want euthanasia, why not get some good out of their deaths? After all, they are going to die anyway.

But coupling organ harvesting with mercy killing creates a strong emotional inducement to suicide, particularly for people who are culturally devalued and depressed and, indeed, who might worry that they are a financial, caregiving, or emotional burden on loved ones and society. People in such anguished mental states could easily come to believe (or be persuaded) that asking for euthanasia so that they could donate organs would give a meaning to their deaths that they believe their lives could never have.

By joining euthanasia with organ donation, Belgium and the Netherlands have already crossed a very dangerous bridge, giving society a *utilitarian stake in euthanasia*. But the acceptance of joint killing and harvesting also sends the cruel message to disabled or mentally ill people: *"Your deaths have greater value than your lives."* In such a milieu, self-justifying bromides about "choice" and the "voluntary" nature "of the process" become mere rationalizations.

Killing for organs—whether by harvesting the cognitively devastated or after euthanasia—turns a very dangerous corner, either making a mockery of the dead donor rule or violating it blatantly. But for some transplant ethicists, that doesn't present a problem, since they believe the dead donor rule itself should be discarded as archaic. Indeed, as far back as 1993, some were preparing the intellectual groundwork to permit just such a path or praising the proposals with nonexistent or faint damnation. In a chapter of the book *Procuring Organs for Transplantation*, discarding the dead donor rule is presented prominently as a way to increase organ supplies. Psychiatrist Youngner and Robert M. Arnold, a physician and medical ethicist deeply involved in organ transplant issues, write in that chapter, "*Killing*, in and of itself, would no longer constitute a harm. Real harms would have to do with suffering, and violations of patient autonomy or interests."[71] (Emphasis within the text.) To what could this lead? The authors are brutally candid in their assessment:

> A ventilator-dependent ALS patient could request that life support be removed at 5:00 p.m., but that at 9:00 a.m. the same day he be taken to the operating room, put under general anesthesia, and his kidneys, liver, and pancreas removed. Bleeding vessels would be tied off or cauterized. The patient's heart would not be removed and would continue to beat throughout surgery, perfusing the other organs with warm, oxygen- and nutrient-rich blood until they were removed. The heart would stop, and the patient would be pronounced dead after the ventilator was removed at 5:00 p.m., according to plan, and long before the patient could die from renal, hepatic, or pancreatic failure.... If active euthanasia—e.g., lethal injection—and physician-assisted suicide are legally sanctioned, even more patients could couple organ donation with their planned deaths; we would not have to depend only upon persons attached to life support. This practice would yield not only more donors, but more types of organs as well, since the heart could now be removed from dying, not just dead, patients.[72]

To say the least, this remains a shocking scenario. But does it represent a widely shared perspective? When I asked co-author Arnold whether he advocated these policies, he replied that he was ambivalent because he believes legalizing assisted suicide would be bad public policy. At the same time, he believes that we should explore exactly why such scenarios disturb us to determine whether our conservatism is justified or merely an excuse for not making the difficult decisions that would move us toward better organ procurement policies.[73]

I also interviewed Youngner, telling him that I believed average readers of my book would be appalled that the idea of discarding the dead donor rule is being taken seriously in bioethics and transplant medicine. Youngner understood the cause for worry but explicitly stated that his primary concern was in expanding the donor pool—even at the cost of crossing long-existing ethical and legal boundaries. He told me:

> We have already taken organs in ways that are more or less uncontroversial in society. So, in expanding the donor pool, we are moving into areas that are controversial. The question is; how do we make that move? Do we make it by continuing to gerrymander the line between life and death [as in heart death protocols]? Or would it be better to have a public discussion and say that maybe there are circumstances where we can take their organs before they are dead. If we do it that way, we can make sure they are not feeling pain. We can do it at their request. So that is a more honest way to do it. Society does evolve. People ought to be aware that we are going in a certain direction.[74]

Of course, not everybody within bioethics is either ambivalent or in favor of tossing aside the dead donor rule and the "do not kill" corollary. Sociologist Renée Fox, an especially forceful critic, worries that "zeal-ridden strategies for augmenting the number of donated organs"[75] threaten the morality of the entire organ transplant enterprise. Expressing similar concern, Dr. Bernat warned me, "The utilitarian perspective works in an incremental fashion. Each year they push policies a little further, and it may be difficult to defend against an individual shift. But when you add it all up, you end up where you do not want to be."[76] Meanwhile, the prominent bioethicist Arthur Caplan remains adamant in his opposition to making such radical changes in transplant medical ethics.[77]

Still, the dark scenario painted years ago by Youngner and Arnold illustrates what I believe is a slowly building consensus quietly nudging the organ procurement community toward taking what (for now) seem to be drastic measures to countervail the chronic shortage of donated organs. Evidence of this emerging reality can, once again, be illuminated by quoting Youngner and Arnold:

> The irresistible utilitarian appeal of organ transplantation has us hell-bent on increasing the donor pool. Giving up the dead donor rule, however, raises the question of how far we are willing to go to procure

more organs—and some point out, save more lives. Are we headed for the utilitarian utopia espoused by Jack Kevorkian, where organ retrieval and scientific experimentation are options in every planned death, be it mercy killing or execution? ... If a look into such a future hurts our eyes (or turns our stomachs), is our discomfort any different from what we would have experienced 30 years ago by looking into the future that is today? ... Given the difficulties our society is likely to experience in trying to openly adjudicate these disparate views, *why not simply go along with the quieter strategy of policy creep? It seems to be getting us where we seem to want to go*, albeit slowly. Besides, *total candor is not always compatible with the moral compromises that inevitably accompany the formulation of public policy*.[78] (My emphasis.)

CHAPTER 6

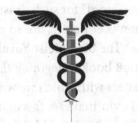

BIOLOGICAL COLONIALISM

Never in human history has suffering been more readily relieved than today. And yet, paradoxically, we have never been more afraid of suffering.

Our forebears would find this very odd. For them, horrendous suffering was ubiquitous, the bane of rich and poor alike. Pain was an integral part of life: If a man suffered appendicitis, he died in agony. If a woman contracted bone cancer, she died in agony. If a child became infected with tuberculosis, he or she died in agony. Then there were the nonterminal illnesses and injuries, like gout, carbuncles, migraines, arthritis, and broken limbs. Suffering was the hard price one often paid for simply being alive.

Happily, those bad old days are mostly long gone, at least in the developed world. Thanks to tremendous breakthroughs in modern medicine, suffering has been pushed largely into the shadows. Surgeries no longer kill from the pain as they once did. Hospice and palliative care offer tremendous relief for even the most painful chronic and terminal diseases. Organ transplantation saves thousands of lives. Medical breakthroughs and improved methods of social support help people live lives of greater quality and fulfillment.

Ironically, our many medical triumphs and the consequential receding of serious suffering from everyday experience created a concomitant terror of travail that threatens the morality of society, many of which are issues discussed in this book. That paradox used to make me wonder: *Why now*, when there is less "need" for such drastic action such as euthanasia and a duty to die than ever before, are so many of us accepting of "culture of death" agendas? The bioethicist Yuval Levin provided a very plausible answer in his 2008 book, *Imagining the Future*—a discussion of the stem cell debate, matters with which we will not concern ourselves here. But along the way, Levin makes a fascinating observation about suffering and modern culture: "The worldview of modern science sees health not only as a foundation but also a principal goal; not only as a beginning but also an end. Relief and preservation—from disease and pain, from misery and necessity—become the defining ends of human action, and therefore of human societies."[1]

This is a crucial point, because, as Levin also notes, "Any society's understanding of the foundational good necessarily gives shape to its politics, its social institutions, and its sense of moral purpose and direction."[2] And therein we face a significant ethical menace: Once avoiding suffering becomes the *primary purpose* of society, it too easily mutates into a license for *eliminating the sufferer* or exploiting the weak and defenseless.

We've already discussed issues involving euthanasia and the threat to the bodily integrity of the cognitively devastated. But the prevent-suffering-at-any-cost attitudes—suffering that includes emotional pain caused by normal human limitations or unwanted circumstances, such as the inability to have children, in addition to illness—are increasingly expressed in other culturally corrosive ways.

Take what I call "biological colonialism." Colonialist imperialism of nations is dead, but a new form of resource hegemony is aborning. Rather than exploiting natural resources such as copper deposits and timber forests, the new colonialism seeks to harness human biological capacities, parts, and substances. Indeed and alas, as science gains an ever-greater understanding of how to extend life and overcome biological dysfunction, the living human body is quickly becoming one of the world's most valuable commercial commodities.

Kidneys for Sale?: April 10, 2020: The financial report on the Investor's Reporting Network is routine: "The price of human kidney futures dropped two points today. Insiders attributed the downturn to the expected increase in supply caused by the ripple effect the recession is having on the economy. With the number of people out of work and/or deeply in debt growing, it is expected that more will sell a kidney to make ends meet. Greater supply means lower prices, thus the drop in the price of futures."

A paranoid fantasy? Perhaps. But such a scenario isn't as far-fetched as it might at first seem. Some bioethicists and government officials advocate harnessing marketplace economics to human organ donations in the hopes of increasing supplies.

The prospect of buying and selling human organs raises very serious ethical and moral issues. If organs can be bought and sold, which is currently against the law almost universally, then the only sellers of organs will be the poor and the buyers will be the rich. In such a crass, materialistic milieu, the potential for exploitation is as obvious as it is gruesome. Indeed, as the world grows increasingly market oriented—and, perhaps not coincidentally, socially Darwinistic—outrages involving the purchase and sale of human organs have already been reported.

In 1990, two British doctors had their medical licenses revoked after they brought two impoverished Turkish men to England, removed a kidney from each, and paid the clearly desperate men $3,400 apiece.[3] As we will discuss in detail below, China has been repeatedly accused of selling the organs of its prisoners around the world. "It's a moneymaking operation," Dr. Ronald Guttmann, a transplantation expert and an adviser to the International Transplantation Society, told *ABC News.* "They are in business. It is an industry. They are moving it around the world."[4] A European trade in children's organs was alleged to exist after a boy was found dead in Italy with a kidney removed. The suspected victims of the suspected trade were destitute Albanian children who fled from their impoverished nation to Italy. The going price of organs was unknown, but the going price for the purchase of whole children reportedly was 20,000 British pounds apiece.[5] Trafficking in human organs of the poor to benefit the rich has gotten so bad around the globe, in fact, that organizations such as Human Trafficking.org have been created to help fight against the growing scourge.[6]

The desire to create financial incentives to induce organ "donation" may be tinged by a racial motivation. According to CSU bioethicist Arthur L. Caplan, an opponent of organ markets, "The primary targets of financial compensation in many of the [marketing] plans ... are African Americans. Studies show that blacks do not donate organs at the same rate as whites and have not for some time. Proponents of fiscal rewards argue that since minorities are more likely to be poor, financial incentives are likely to be more attractive to them." In this regard, Caplan, director, Division of Medical Ethics at NYU's Langone Medical Center, notes correctly that, "A public policy of money for body parts is inexcusably indifferent to the history of African Americans and slavery in this and other countries."[7]

The specter of buying and selling human vital organs also threatens the ethics and morality of medical decision making involving poor people. Imagine a poor family that wants expensive life-supporting treatment for a loved one faced down by doctors and clinical ethicists who insist that treatment end based on futility theory or ad hoc health care rationing. Amid the cajoling and pressure, including perhaps threats to unilaterally cease the treatment, an offer of compromise is made: Permit us to terminate treatment and put your son into a heart-death procurement organ protocol and your son's children will receive a $10,000 scholarship. Allowing such a transaction would be to quite literally put a price tag on human life, thereby transforming the "worth" of living human beings into the going market price of the sum of their parts. Renée Fox puts it well when she writes, "Treating organs as if they were a commodity, or property, is demeaning. The symbolic implications just carry us toward a very dangerous, slippery slope."[8]

Making matters worse, the offer of financial incentives for access to poor people's organs might be induced as much by profit motive as by the altruistic desire to save lives. Organ procurement is often very remunerative for organ distribution organizations, transplant surgeons, hospitals, and others within the organ transplant industry. Thus, those who procure or transplant organs often do quite well by doing good. When organs are donated, this fact of organ transplant medicine is of lesser concern morally because the supply chain is not influenced by commercialism. But when money incentives enter the picture, the risks to vulnerable patients increase. In this sense, opening the door to organ selling could easily distort proper medical decision making for the seriously ill and disabled poor, leading slowly but perhaps inevitably, to a presumption in favor of non-treatment and organ "donation." Indeed, society's very perception of the exploitable poor could undergo a deleteriously dehumanizing shift; rather than viewing them as people of equal moral worth, they might instead be viewed, in the prophetic words of Paul Ramsey, as "precadavers" best suited to be scavenged for their parts. Thus Caplan, who is not known for his dogmatic opinions, writes, "Calls for markets, compensation, bounties, or rewards should be rejected because they convert human beings into products, a metaphysical transformation that cheapens the respect for life and corrodes our ability to maintain the stance that human beings are special, unique, and valuable for their own sake, not for what others can mine, extract, or manufacture from them."[9]

Since this book was first published, the push to permit contracts for the purchase and sale of kidneys and nonlethal surgeries (e.g., removing a slice of liver) has accelerated. For example, writing in the *Wall Street Journal*, Nobel Prize laureate in economics Gary S. Becker and economics professor Julios J. Elias computed the amount they thought it would take to induce people to sell their kidneys:

> We have estimated how much individuals would need to be paid for kidneys to be willing to sell them for transplants. These estimates take account of the slight risk to donors from transplant surgery, the number of weeks of work lost during the surgery and recovery periods, and the small risk of reduction in the quality of life.... Our conclusion is that a very large number of both live and cadaveric kidney donations would be available by paying about $15,000 for each kidney. That estimate isn't exact, and the true cost could be as high as $25,000 or as low as $5,000—but even the high estimate wouldn't increase the total cost of kidney transplants by a large percentage.[10]

The authors suggest that kidney markets would do much to alleviate suffering by dramatically reducing the waiting list for cadaveric organs. Perhaps. But that shouldn't be the only consideration. Who would do the selling for such a small amount? It won't be members of the ruling class like the authors, that's for sure! *That's for desperate people*, easily exploitable. But that's okay with the economists:

Though the poor would be more likely to sell their kidneys and other organs, they also suffer more than others from the current scarcity. Today, the rich often don't wait as long as others for organs since some of them go to countries such as India, where they can arrange for transplants in the underground medical sector, and others (such as the late Steve Jobs) manage to jump the queue by having residence in several states or other means. The sale of organs would make them more available to the poor, and Medicaid could help pay for the added cost of transplant surgery.[11]

We'll get to the organ black market below. There is no question that such immoral practices and loopholes that allow the legitimate system to be gamed (like in the case with Jobs) need to be stopped. But we should not add *another wrong* on top of those already engaged—even if a few poor people might benefit from the exploitation of their selling peers. Indeed, *our real focus should be on the immorality of the buyers and the medical professionals who make it possible*, not slouching toward greater inequities in the organ transplant system.

The poor aren't the only targets of this advocacy. In 2011, writing in the *British Medical Journal*, a former member of the United Kingdom's Unrelated Live Transplants Regulatory Authority compared kidney selling to paying prisoners for their labor or footing the expenses of human research subjects—as she extolled kidney selling as a splendid way to allow university students to pay off onerous tuition debts:

> But there are other models that it's time we looked at. We have the wage payment model, for services supplied by participants in medical research, who often are admitted to hospital for a fortnight or more and undergo unpleasant, sometimes risky procedures. We have compensation models, for criminal, worker, and military injuries, which have agreed tariffs, such as £2,500 for a fractured coccyx and £22,500 for the loss of one kidney.... It would not be such a big step to move towards regulated paid provision for live donors' kidneys. This would be far different from the illegal organ market that exists now in several countries, and we must not make the mistake of ruling out a properly regulated system because of the depredations of the current illegal market. The standards of care before and after operation would be as

good as they are now for kidney donors in the UK. The kidneys would be allocated in the same fair way as they are now.... One reservation that many people express about such a proposal is that it might exploit poor people in the same way the illegal market does now. But if the standard payment were equivalent to the average annual income in the UK, currently about £28,000, it would be an incentive across most income levels for those who wanted to do a kind deed and make enough money to, for instance, pay off university loans.[12]

Not all kidney-selling proposals crassly propose the direct exchange of money. The psychiatrist and fellow of the American Enterprise Institute Sally Satel became one of the most vocal proponents of establishing organ markets after the writer Virginia Postrel made an altruistic living kidney donation to Satel, probably saving her life. Satel argues that rather than direct buying and selling, an organization should be established to purchase kidneys for fair distribution throughout the population:

> To make a real impact on kidney shortage, we have to find ways to persuade more healthy young and middle-aged people to give a kidney to a stranger.... Here is a plan to do just that. Donors would not get a lump sum of cash; instead, a governmental entity, or a designated charity, would offer them in-kind rewards, like a contribution to the donor's retirement fund, an income tax credit or a tuition voucher.... Meanwhile, imposing a waiting period of at least six months would ensure that donors didn't act impulsively and that they were giving fully informed consent. Prospective compensated donors would be carefully screened for physical and emotional health, as is done for all donors now.... These arrangements would screen out financially desperate individuals who might otherwise rush to donate for a large sum of instant cash and later regret it.[13]

Just what we need: more bureaucracy. And what makes Satel think that once the program is up and running, the "protective guidelines"—so easily promised—won't soon be reinterpreted into meaninglessness, as so often happens in the real world?

Thankfully, it is unlikely that kidney buying will be permitted, at least over the short term. Buying organs remains deeply controversial and bioethics remains deeply divided about the issue. As seen above, one of the strongest opposing voices is Arthur Caplan, one of the most prominent commentators to the general public on bioethical issues, with whom I have often disagreed, particularly about the Terri Schiavo case. But we are of one accord when it comes to this issue. Writing in a book published by the Hastings Center, Caplan made a powerful point against turning kidneys into commodities: "In a market—even a regulated one—*doctors and nurses still would be using their skills to help people harm themselves solely for money.* The resulting distrust and loss of professional standards is too a high price to pay to gamble on the hope that a market may secure more organs for those in need."[14] (My emphasis.)

I asked Caplan to expand on the danger of merchandizing human organs. He told me:

> Markets are morally problematic because they will almost certainly exploit the poor—they offer no chance at regular earning through a job.... In nations such as India, there is no evidence that the poor who sell a kidney work their way out of poverty as a result. They pay a debt but remain poor.... Markets also create two track systems, since they really only apply to kidney sales, imperiling the altruism needed to obtain livers, hearts, lungs and other body parts.... Markets also increase the motivation to lie about the seller's health, making transplantation more dangerous. And markets violate the prohibitions against the sale of the body held by many religions—thereby risking their withdrawal from organ donation altogether and perhaps leaving those in need with fewer organs.... Lastly, it is very hard to regulate organ markets, leaving sellers at great risk of being maltreated.[15]

I wrote earlier that organ buying is "almost universally" illegal. The word "almost" was necessary because one country has created a bazaar in living human kidneys: Iran.

Some believe we should follow the Iranian theocracy's lead and permit organ sales. In *The Kidney Sellers: A Journey of Discovery in Iran,* Sigrid Fry-Revere applauds Iran for allowing poor Iranians to ameliorate financial difficulties in an open and transparent system of kidney selling, proposing a pilot project that would pay America's poor $50,000 to "give a leg up in life" to "those out of work, those behind on their mortgages, those who need help paying for an education, or those who want to start a business." Not doing so, she writes, both prevents the saving of some lives and sacrifices "justice on the altar of altruism." In the end, manipulating the poor is a price worth paying: "We must simply overcome our natural objections to exploiting the unfortunate because we need their organs" so as to stop feeding the black market that "covertly discriminate[s] against poor prospective donors and recipients alike."[16]

But other observers see a contrary lesson in the Iranian approach, arguing that the country's experience demonstrates the corrupting power of allowing desperate poor people to sell—and desperate rich people to buy—organs. For example, once money starts exchanging hands, corruption soon follows, including line cutting by rich foreigners, even though the system is supposed to be reserved exclusively for Iranians. From a July 26, 2014 *Payvand Iran News* story:

> On Sunday July 20, CASKP chief Mostafa Qasemi told the Fars News Agency: "These patients enter the country with false documents; doctors do not examine their documents and are paid millions to carry out a kidney transplant for them." In Iran, kidney donation to foreign nationals is illegal, but according to Qasemi, in recent years intermediaries have been producing fake National ID Cards and Birth Certificates and procuring Iranian kidneys for non-Iranians ... Qasemi referred to two "Saudi patients" who travelled to Iran recently for kidney transplants, noting that one of the patients died during treatment.[17]

Let the finger-pointing begin:

> The Ministry of Health supervisory board says any report of misconduct in kidney transplants has been dealt with severely by the ministry and the only violations reported have involved private hospitals.... The ministry has blamed physicians for failing to adequately scrutinize patient documents. According to the Ministry of Health: "Physicians have been sloppy in the examination of patient documents, even though it is very easy to recognize if they are treating an Arab or Afghan foreign national. Physicians are not complying with the law and are readily accepting fake documents."[18]

Why is anyone surprised? Organ buying will always lead to official and purveyor corruption because *it involves frantic people on both sides of the transaction.* And it is worse for the destitute, who put their health at risk for the relative pittance they receive.

Here's my bottom line: Kidney removal is serious surgery. It can be dangerous, attendant with all the risks of side effects of any invasive procedure. Rarely—but it happens—people die donating a kidney.[19] Beyond that, we have the redundancy of two kidneys for a reason. If one goes bad, we still have the other. Later in life, a donor's remaining kidney could become injured, cancerous, or otherwise dysfunctional, and they would then wish very much that they still had their sold organ.

Utilitarianism can be appealing. People who need organs are understandably desperate to increase the organ supply, which is a very worthy goal. But the lives and well-being of the healthy matter as much as those of the sick. Those, like Postrel, who out of deep empathy want to give a sick person a kidney should be allowed to so do. But organ markets are a very bad idea that would open the door to a terrible potential for exploitation.

THE BLACK MARKET IN ORGANS

And that is precisely what happens every day in the black market for kidneys: naked exploitation. Despite ongoing advocacy among some intellectuals, we in the West currently have little to fear from a commodities market in human organs. Not so the destitute living in the developing world or political prisoners in the tyranny that is the People's Republic of China. In dreadfully poor places such as Turkey, Peru, Bangladesh, and other poor nations around the world, desperate destitute people are persuaded by fast-talking organ brokers and their own dire circumstances to sell a kidney to "organ tourists," seeking to avoid waiting lists for ethically legitimate surgeries. Meanwhile, brokers profit from the desperation on both ends of the transaction.

Sometimes these blood contracts have deadly consequences. Bloomberg's Michael Smith wrote an excellent investigative piece, "Desperate Americans Buy Organs from Peru Poor in Fatal Trade," about this. From the story:

> Luis Picado's mother remembers the day her son thought he had won
> the lottery. He came home to their tin-roofed cinder-block house
> in a Managua, Nicaragua, slum and said he'd found a way to escape

poverty and start a new life in the United States. An American man had promised to give Picado, a 23-year-old high school dropout who worked as a construction laborer, a job and an apartment in New York if he'd donate one of his kidneys.... He jumped at the deal, his mother says. Three weeks later, in May 2009, Picado came out of surgery at Managua's Military Hospital, bleeding internally from the artery doctors had severed to remove his kidney, according to medical records. His mother, Elizabeth Tercero, got on her knees next to her son's bed in the recovery room and prayed ... "I told my boy not to worry, that I would take care of him," Tercero, 49, says. "But it was too late." Picado bled to death as doctors tried to save him, according to a coroner's report. "He was always chasing the American dream, and finally, it cost him his life," she says.[20]

Biological organ colonialism is a growing problem, as Smith reported:

In the illegal organ trade, brokers scour the world's slums, preying on the poor with promises of easy money and little risk in exchange for a kidney. Inside hospitals, people are injured or killed by botched surgery as doctors place money above ethics, criminal investigators say. In Colombia, 321 foreigners got transplants from 2005 to 2010, according to the country's National Health Institute. Juan Lopez, a doctor who oversees Colombia's organ transplant system as director of the NHI, says many of these surgeries are driven by profit for hospitals, doctors and brokers. "I don't want my country to be a Mecca for transplant tourism," Lopez says.[21]

Part of the problem is that too many of us are indifferent to the suffering of poor people half a world away. Some of us even celebrate the exploitation. Take the 2009 book *Larry's Kidney*,[22] written by Daniel Asa Rose, recounting the author's biological colonialism in China—buying a kidney for his cousin Larry. Rather than wait in line like everyone else, Larry and Rose flew to China to purchase a kidney on the illegal—but blatant—black market. After a series of mishaps and complications, Larry got his new organic blood filter. Oh, joy for Larry!

But it almost certainly was not a good thing for the "donor." Many sold organs in China—which include vital organs—are harvested from persecuted Falun Gong practitioners and other political and criminal prisoners. The case hasn't been wholly proved—the China tyranny has never permitted a full and transparent investigation—but human rights campaigner David Matas and former Canadian member of Parliament David Kilgour have spent years pursuing stories of organ harvesting butchery in China against Falun Gong and other political prisoners. The duo issued a detailed and chilling report in 2006 alleging that Falun Gong practitioners were systematically imprisoned, tissue-typed, and killed for organs, to great profit by Chinese organ marketers.

"Report into Allegations of Organ Harvesting of Falun Gong Practitioners in China"[23] simply boggles the mind. Indeed, the authors recoil from their own conclusions, stating that "the very horror [of the findings] makes us reel back in disbelief.... But that disbelief does not mean that the allegations are untrue." In forty-four grueling pages, plus appendixes, Matas and Kilgour meticulously build a strong case "that there has been and continues today to be large scale organ seizures from unwilling Falun Gong practitioners"[24] in China. Much of the evidence is circumstantial rather than the proverbial smoking gun. For example, the report states that "there are many more [organ] transplants" in China—about 10,000 per year—than there are "identifiable sources" for the organs that were procured. But China is an opaque society, and even though the organ-procurement numbers do indeed seem woefully insufficient to support the number of reported transplants, this fact alone would not support their charge.

If each particular bit of evidence does not convince, the cumulative effect of the entire case effectively persuades. For example, the authors compare the numbers of total organ transplants in China in the six years before the crackdown on Falun Gong began with the numbers reported in the six years after the sect was outlawed. The figures startle: Between 1994 and 1999, there were about 18,500 organ transplants in China. Since the government initiated its Falun Gong pogrom—between 2000–2005— there have been about 60,000 transplants, representing an increase of 41,500 from the previous six-year period. "Where do the organs come from for the [additional] 41,500 transplants?" the authors ask pointedly. "The allegation of organ harvesting from Falun Gong practitioners pro- vides an answer."[25]

Matas and Kilgour acknowledge that this dramatic increase "does not establish that the Falun Gong allegations are true. But it does put the onus on China to disprove its claim. Indeed, it would be easy for the Chinese government to put this matter to rest simply by identifying the organ sources for these extra 41,500 transplants. It has not done so."

There's more. Several surviving family members of Falun Gong who died in detention reported seeing their loved ones' bodies with "surgical incisions and body parts missing." One witness—not a Falun Gong member—told the investigators that her surgeon husband "told her that he personally removed the corneas from approximately 2,000 anaesthetized Falun Gong prisoners." According to this hearsay evidence, none of the prisoners survived and all of the bodies were cremated.

There were also taped telephone conversations presented to Matas and Kilgour that support the allegations. (The transcripts were verified by an independent Mandarin translator.) On June 8, 2006, for example, "Mr. Li," an official at the Mishan City Detention Center, was recorded having the following conversation with a Falun Gong member, given the pseudonym "M," who posed as a potential organ customer:

M: Do you have Falun Gong [organ] suppliers?...
Li: We used to have, yes.
M: ...what about now?
Li: ...Yes....
M: ...How many [Falun Gong suppliers] under age forty do you have?
Li: Quite a few. ...
M: Now, for...the male Falun Gong, how many of them do you have?
Li: Seven, eight, we have [at least] five, six now.
M: Are they from the countryside or from the city?
Li: Countryside.[26]

An even more explicit conversation was taped on May 22, 2006, between M and a Mr. Lu, who works at Nanning City Minzu Hospital in Guangzi Autonomous Region:

M: Could you find organs from Falun Gong practitioners?
Lu: Let me tell you, we have no way to get them. It's rather difficult to get it now in Guangzi. If you cannot wait, I suggest you go to Guangzhou because it is very easy for them to get the organs. They are able to look for them nation-wide...
M: Why is it easy for them to get?

Lu: Because they are an important institution. They contact the judicial system in the name of the whole university.
M: Then they use Falun Gong practitioners?
Lu: Correct.[27]

M then asks Lu how Falun Gong were selected when Lu's hospital did have access to prisoners:

M: …what you used before (from Falun Gong practitioners), was it from detention centers or prisons?
Lu: From prisons.
M: …and it was from healthy Falun Gong practitioners…?
Lu: Correct. We would choose the good ones because we assure the quality in our operation
M: That means you choose the organs yourself?
Lu: Correct…
M: Usually, how old is the organ supplier?
Lu: Usually in their thirties…
M: Does the person know his organs will be removed?
Lu: No, he doesn't.[28]

As shocking as these conversations are, the most compelling evidence of systemic wrongdoing in Chinese organ-procurement practices is the stunningly brief time purchasers wait to receive a properly matched organ—a wait so short the authors worry that it means "there are a number of people now alive who are available almost on demand as sources of organs."

For context, the authors contrasted the waiting periods for American and Canadian organ recipients with those then apparently in force for organ buyers in China. Citing websites from various Chinese hospitals—long since scrubbed—the investigators write:

The wait times for organ transplants for organ recipients in China appear to be much lower than anywhere else. The China International Transplantation Assistant Centre website says, "It may take only one week to find out the suitable (kidney) donor, the maximum time being one month…" It goes further, "If something wrong with the donor's organ happens, the patient will have the option to be offered another organ donor and have the operation again in one week." … The site of the Oriental Organ Transplant Centre in early April, 2006, claimed that "the average waiting time (for a suitable liver) is 2 weeks." The website of the Changzheng Hospital in Shanghai says: "… the average waiting time for a liver supply is one week among all the patients."[29]

Matas and Kilgour then make a telling comparison: "In contrast, the median waiting time for a kidney in Canada was 32.5 months in 2003 and in British Columbia it was even longer at 52.5 months [citing the Canadian Institute for Health Information]."[30]

Adding weight to the evidence that Falun Gong "donors," like so many lobsters in a restaurant aquarium, were being kept alive until their tissues could be matched with an organ customer, the report alleges:

> This website as of May 17, 2006 indicated in the English version … that the centre was established in 2003 at the First Affiliated Hospital of China Medical University "…specifically for foreign friends. Most of the patients are from all over the world." The opening sentence of the site 29 introduction declares that "Viscera (one dictionary definition: "soft interior organs … including the brain, lungs, heart etc.") providers can be found immediately!" On another page 30 on the same site is this statement: "…the number of kidney transplant operations is at least 5,000 every year all over the country." So many transplantation operations are owing to the support of the Chinese government. The supreme demotic court, supreme demotic law—officer, police, judiciary, department of health and civil administration have enacted a law together to make sure that organ donations are supported by the government. This is unique in the world.[31]

The authors didn't need the deductive genius of Sherlock Holmes to reach their reasonable conclusion: "If as indicated the survival period for a kidney is between 24–48 hours and a liver about 12 hours, the presence of a large bank of living kidney-liver 'donors' must be the only way China's transplant centres can assure such short waits to customers.

The astonishingly short waiting times advertised for perfectly-matched organs would suggest the existence of both a computer matching system for transplants and a large bank of live prospective 'donors.'"[32]

China has repeatedly denied the charges and promised reforms to prevent the bloody organ harvest from happening in the country. But as the old rock 'n' roll song put it, the beat goes on. A 2014 opinion column published in the *American Journal of Transplant Medicine* by physicians affiliated with Doctors Against Forced Organ Harvesting[33] reached a depressing conclusion:

> Organ procurement from executed prisoners in China is internationally condemned, yet this practice continues unabated in 2014. This is despite repeated announcements from Chinese authorities that constructive measures have been undertaken to conform to accepted ethical standards. While there is unanimous agreement on the unethical nature of using organs from executed prisoners, due to its limitations on voluntary and informed consent, there is insufficient coverage of forced organ procurement from prisoners of conscience without consent. Strategies to influence positive change in China over the last few decades have failed to bring this practice to an end. While organ donation and transplantation services in China have undergone considerable structural changes in the last few years, fundamental attempts to shift practice to ethically sourced organs have floundered.[34]

China is almost surely the only country where political prisoners are systematically killed for their organs as a means of making money, but it is certainly not the only place where the organ black market profitably exploits the powerless. Organ traffickers operate all over the world. In 2011, the government of Bangladesh busted a kidney trafficking gang, as described by the *Herald Sun*, in an especially impoverished village; there were 200 victims, people who sold a kidney for as little as USD $1,900.[35] In fact, organ tourism became such an acute problem that Pakistan outlawed all organ buying and live-organ donations (other than to close family members). For the same reason, the Philippines legally prohibited noncitizens from undergoing kidney transplant surgeries in the country. The Philippine effort to stem the kidney trade proved successful, as transplants fell in that country from 1,046 when the organ market was thriving to 511 in 2010, all bona fide ethical surgeries.[36]

The organ exchange is now apparently spreading to developed countries like South Korea. From a *Korea Times* story:

> A 35-year-old man from Incheon, surnamed Lee, is one of those who decided to sell his kidney to repay part of his debts, after suffering from financial difficulties for years. "My online shopping mall business went bankrupt three years ago, leaving me massive amounts of debt," he said, adding the sale of his organ was the only way to earn a substantial sum of money at one time.[37]

Biological colonialism also exists in the United States. A few years ago, a "matchmaker" paid poor Israelis to travel to the US to sell their kidneys. Levy Izhak Rosenbaum bought the organs for $10,000 and sold them for as much as $150,000. Part of his service involved making up stories to convince hospitals and doctors that the donations were altruistic. Rosenbaum was eventually sentenced to two and a half years in prison for his felonious scheme.[38]

The world remains a cruel place. The World Health Organization recently reported that there are 10,000 black-market kidney transplants each year.[39] It's clear that the corruption bred by biological colonialism extends well beyond the criminal class—medical professionals, for instance, are necessary participants in every black market organ transaction. And there's a lot of money to spread around; a "donor" may receive $5,000 for his organ—if he is lucky—for which the buyer may pay up to $200,000.

How to stop it? The United Nations called for a binding treaty in 2009, but we're still waiting. The Declaration of Istanbul, issued in 2012 after a summit convened by the Transplantation Society and International Society of Nephrology, unequivocally condemned organ trafficking but was woefully short on remedies, mostly urging action to increase ethical donations, banning advertising that solicits organ selling, and passing penalties for acts "that aid, encourage or use the products of organ trafficking or transplant tourism."[40] Still, the declaration was credited with helping crystalize an international consensus "that these practices are unacceptable."[41]

More concrete proposals have been made in the wake of the exposés of the China atrocities. These include:

- National legislation to prohibit citizens from receiving illegal organs in any country;
- Prohibiting reimbursement of transplants performed anywhere around the globe involving illegal practices or the organ trade; and
- Denial of entry visas to individuals who have engaged in illegal organ procurement in any country, in any capacity.

Organ transplant medicine saves lives. But the wealthy sick should not be able to save their own hides at the expense of the healthy poor. Buying an organ should be just as illegal as traveling overseas to sexually exploit a trafficked child. Some organ tourism opponents might thus say we should prevent recipients of illegal transplants from being cared for medically in their home countries. But that would be a death penalty and go too far. However, we should require doctors to report patients who received an illegal organ, relieving them of the duty of strict confidentiality in the same manner as we do when doctors see signs of spousal abuse or diagnose certain infectious and venereal diseases. Then those who obtained the illegal organs should be prosecuted and publicly named and shamed.

Laws can only do so much. In the end, it is up to each of us. For example, we should stop validating and supporting those who—like Daniel Asa Rose—enable this loathsome mercantilism as customers. When *Larry's Kidney* received good reviews rather than universal condemnation, we demonstrated that our society doesn't much care about the political prisoners exploited for their organs. But if we let people who are considering entering the organ black market know that we would break friendships over it, that if family members promise to support and love their ailing loved ones in illness but to shun them in biological colonialist exploitation, perhaps we could blunt the growth we see in human organ futures. In other words, we need to apply the power of peer pressure in these difficult circumstances to promote character and integrity, even in times of direst crisis.

RENT A UTERUS

The commercialization of women's uteruses and gestational capacities in India is big business, providing another vivid example of biological colonialism, sometimes with lethal consequences. An Indian woman named Premila Vaghela died at age thirty-six when she gave birth prematurely. Although she carried the fetus for eight months, Vaghela wasn't considered the mother of the baby, who survived. She was merely a paid "gestational carrier"—the dehumanizing term coined by the in vitro fertilization (IVF) industry to keep surrogate mothers from being perceived as "mothers"—who rented her uterus to a Western couple.[42] That decision resulted in Vaghela's own two children having to grow up without their mother. But at least there was some good news (he said sarcastically): "Three days later, it was an emotional scene at Arpan Newborn Care Centre in Navrangpura as Helen—the biological mother of the boy Vaghela delivered prematurely—saw her son for the first time on Thursday. Onlookers said Helen looked tired and gloomy after her flight, but when she saw the baby in the incubator tears welled up in her eyes."[43]

Biological colonialism can extract a terrible cost to those not involved in the actual surrogacy transaction. Another case of an Indian woman dying while giving birth to surrogate children involved a Norwegian couple. The baby was taken home, leaving a distraught and ill widower in India with no one to look after him. So he turned to Norway for help:

> An Indian man whose wife died after giving birth to a Norwegian couple's surrogate child may sue the Norwegian state for damages within days, Dagsavisen has reported. Naeem Qureshi's wife Mona entered a surrogacy programme to pay for his medical treatment, but suffered fatal complications during the birth. One of the twins she was carrying died shortly after birth but the other is now in Norway with its parents.... Norwegian lawyer Shahzad Nazir, who is giving Qureshi free legal aid, said he hoped the state would provide help without his client having to go to court. "We have sent a request to the Ministry of Foreign Affairs (MFA) and the Ministry of Children, Equality and Social Inclusion (BLD), asking them to provide financial and medical assistance to my client," he said. "He is seriously ill and is constantly at the hospital." In the letter, Nazir argues that the state is liable because although surrogacy is illegal in Norway, it provides a loophole allowing Norwegian couples to use it abroad.[44]

So, Norway does not allow its poor women to be exploited by commercial surrogacy—the proper policy, in my view—but is perfectly

fine with allowing Norwegians of means to exploit the women of other
nations. And a woman is dead, leaving a sick widower without support.
How is that different from a powerful nation expropriating a poor nation's
natural resources and engaging in bad environmental practices it would
never countenance within its own borders?

There has been growing reportage about the social injustice associated with international surrogacy. "Outsourcing a Life," a 2013 investigative
report published by the *San Francisco Chronicle* into India's surrogacy
industry, revealed the high cost paid by women so poor they are willing
to gestate others' babies for pay. This includes the surrogates forced or
fooled into medically unnecessary caesarian sections:

> On a mattress in her room at the clinic, Manisha struggled through
> the early stages of recovery. Even eating and sitting hurt, thanks to the
> incision on her abdomen. Her cesarean section, Dr. Patel said, had
> been a last resort when she determined the baby was too big to deliver
> vaginally.... But the surgical nurse who had fetched Manisha from her
> room two hours before the birth, and another who helped prepare the
> delivery room, both said they were readying her for surgery from the
> start. Manisha trusted the doctor's judgment. After all, her baby was
> the 649th born to a surrogate at the clinic, and Dr. Patel had delivered
> virtually every one. But unknown to Manisha and the Kowalskis, *close
> to three-fourths of them had been delivered by cesarean, an extremely
> high rate.*[45] (My emphasis.)

The story is accompanied by the photo of a woman recovering from
such surgery lying on a cot, writhing in pain because she received inadequate (or no) pain control. This is the face of biological colonialism.

It gets worse. According to the story:

- Women sign contracts requiring them to abort on demand of the
  biological parents;
- Women are forced to leave their families for months and live in
  crowded dormitories with other pregnant surrogates;
- Women are maneuvered into having medically unnecessary
  caesarean sections. Seventy-five percent of the surrogates in the
  clinic discussed in the story deliver surgically;
- There may be adverse social consequences for the surrogate, who
  may become isolated by a disapproving family or culture.

An Indian study published in 2012 similarly revealed the many profound wrongs associated with the commercial surrogacy industry in India, "including sex selection, parents refusing to take the child after birth, and surrogates being paid a pittance, with most money going to so-called baby brokers."[46] The report also found that surrogate mothers sometimes "feel attached to the babies even they were not biologically their own children." Of course they do. Such feelings are a natural biological process associated with gestation. That's part of biological colonialism's intrinsic cruelty.

The personal and medical welfare of the surrogate also take a backseat to that of the baby they are carrying. For example, the report found that surrogate contracts rarely address issues related primarily to the well-being and health of the surrogate mother: "It is only [when] health issues related to the fetus [arise] when the health of the surrogate mother becomes a priority."[47] And, as we have seen, Indian surrogates have died giving birth to other people's babies, orphaning their own children.

Some will reply that this is just "the marketplace in action." But even if one accepts such libertarian notions, the contracting parties have such wildly disparate bargaining power that these "deals" are hardly "fair." In 50 to 60 percent of the cases, surrogate mothers and their husbands were illiterate or had primary education, meaning they had to rely on the brokers to explain the agreement they were signing:

> In most of the cases the hospitals/clinics/doctors [narrated] the content
> of the agreement to the surrogate mother before signing it [leaving] a
> wide scope for avoiding any unpleasant thing to be told to the surrogate
> mother by the hospitals/clinics/doctors which in [the] future could be
> used against her interest...., Since the surrogate mother is already four
> months pregnant at the time of contract signing, she has no option left
> other than sign the contract and agree to what has been explained to
> her by the hospitals/clinics/doctors, which leaves no chances for them
> to understand the medical jargon or complicated procedures that might
> affect the health and well-being of the surrogate mother.[48]

It is ironic: Apologists for commercial surrogacy in developing nations claim that the women make more money than they ever could otherwise. That may be true in the very short term, but think about it: that could also be said of workers exploited in sweatshops to make our running shoes and manufacture our smart phones. Exploiting desperate laborers has led to international calls for reform. In contrast, gestational serfdom of the kind seen in India causes few ripples of concern and not nearly the level of international umbrage. In the end, these women aren't deemed important as human beings but merely as a means to an end.

That is why exploiters of gestational capacities are often cheered and celebrated when they bring their babies home, while the fate of the surrogates is often forgotten. I saw this phenomenon up close on a visit to Israel in 2015 at the time of the catastrophic earthquake in Nepal. Apparently, Nepal was the country of choice for gay partners to have babies via surrogates—a strictly regulated practice in Israel only allowed to certain heterosexual married couples. When Israel rescued these fathers and they brought their new babies home, the *Jerusalem Post* celebrated the escape with a front-page story and accompanying editorial. I found it striking that neither story nor editorial seemed concerned for the women who, after birthing the new Israelis, were still trapped in a ruined country.[49]

The babies special ordered in these overseas surrogacy contracts can also become victims. Sometimes the buyers decide that they don't want the baby. Such was apparently the case in 2014 when an Australian couple rented a Thai woman's womb, and in due course, she delivered fraternal twins. But one of the babies had Down syndrome, which the surrogate had refused to abort, and that just wouldn't do. So they simply left "Gammy," their disabled son, behind with no means of support except the love given him by his surrogate mother. From the Associated Press story:

> A Thai surrogate mother said Sunday that she was not angry with the Australian biological parents who left behind a baby boy born with Down syndrome, and hoped that the family would take care of the boy's twin sister they took with them. Pattaramon Chanbua, a 21-year-old food vendor in Thailand's seaside town of Sri Racha, has had to take a break from her job to take care of her 7-month-old surrogate baby, named "Gammy," who also has a congenital heart condition. The boy, with blond hair and dark brown eyes, is now being treated in a hospital for infection in his lungs. Pattaramon said she met the Australian couple once when the babies were born and knew only that they lived in Western Australia state.[50]

The parents denied abandoning their son but have made no attempts to see or obtain custody of him for more than a year. When it was reported that the twins' biological father had served prison time for sexually molesting three prepubescent girls in the 1990s, any hope they had to gain the world's sympathy was lost.[51]

How to care for Gammy, who had challenging health issues with which to contend in addition to his developmental disability? Hands Across the Water,[52] an Australian charity that helps at-risk Thai children, raised hundreds of thousands in contributions for the family, money now used to pay a monthly stipend to help Chanbua care for Gammy.[53] One good thing resulted from this mess: In the wake of the scandal, Thailand outlawed commercial surrogacy contracts.[54]

Commercial surrogacy sometimes results in "stateless children." As reported by the *Berkeley Journal of International Law*, one Japanese infant was, for a time, a baby without a country when his father had a very difficult time bringing him from India to Japan.[55] Baby Manji had three potential mothers—none of whom wanted her. The surrogate was Indian. Manji's biological mother was an egg donor. The would-be adopting mother who, along with the biological father, had contracted for the baby walked away after she and her husband divorced. When the biological father tried to take her home, the Japanese embassy wouldn't issue a passport because the birth mother was Indian. When he tried to obtain an Indian passport, India wouldn't issue a passport because the biological mother was Japanese. When the father imaginatively tried to adopt his own child, India refused because of laws against single males adopting. What a mess.

Manji wasn't able to go home before the case went to the Indian Supreme Court, which referred her father to the National Commission for Protection of Child Rights. "After much legal wrangling, the state finally issued Baby Manji a certificate of identity, a legal document given to those who are stateless."[56] Such are the potential consequences and imbroglios caused when people pay foreign women to gestate.

A similar case of "stateless children" roiled the waters in Germany when Jan Balaz and Susan Lohle found they couldn't take their surrogate-birthed twins home because German nationality is determined by the citizenship of the birth mother—who, in this case, was Indian.[57] It took years to unravel the mess.

An even worse case left children born in India of a surrogate mother without known parents. A Canadian couple paid $7,000 for a surrogate birth. When they applied to take the twins home, DNA tests found that the babies were unrelated to either parent. In other words, the wrong embryos had been implanted.[58] The children—as have other babies born of Indian surrogates who, for various reasons, were rejected or unable to leave the country—were sent to an orphanage.

Domestic commercial surrogacy has become normalized, partly because it has become the rage among the celebrity set—Elton John, Nichole Kidman, Sarah Jessica Parker, the list could go on and on. But domestic surrogacy can also lead to life complications. Thus, when American television personality Sherri Shepherd contracted with an egg donor and surrogate to carry her husband's baby, the celebrity gossip media were abuzz. Ditto when Shepherd and her husband broke up; she decided she no longer wanted the baby and asked a judge to declare she had no parental rights—and one could also add financial responsibilities—toward the soon-to-be-born baby.[59] (The gambit failed. After months of expensive litigation, a judge ruled in 2015 that Shepherd is the legal mother.)[60]

The sordid story illustrates the culture of baby buying we are allowing to emerge because people will do *anything* to have a baby. If the surrogate gives birth and the baby is wanted, he or she is usually the purchaser's by right of contract, no matter how attached the birth mother might be to the child. But if the buyer or buyers change their mind, some believe the unwanted merchandise can simply be returned. And even if a court rules they are the legal parents, what kind of relationship can the special-ordered baby expect to have with a mother or father who tried to refuse delivery of the goods?

With such problems associated with surrogacy—and these stories are just the tip of the iceberg—one would think that the bioethics community would seek to apply the brakes to commercial surrogacy. But the international baby industry is huge—some $6 billion annually and growing.[61] That pays for a lot of baby-carrying storks! Moreover, the predominate view in bioethics sees procreation—by almost any means necessary, whether single or married, gay or straight, young or old—as a fundamental human right. For example, the bioethicist John A.

Robertson, a law professor at the University of Texas, Austin, also reflects the nearly "anything goes" attitudes that are rife throughout the bioethics establishment on these issues. In his book *Children of Choice*, Robertson asserts that women not only have an absolute right to terminate their pregnancies but, ironically, just as absolute a right to access whatever "non-coital technology" they require to bear children. Indeed, this right is so fundamental, Robertson believes, that it also includes the license to genetically engineer progeny—a process he crassly calls "quality control of offspring."[62]

Others, this author included, support outlawing all commercial surrogacy. A growing movement—such as Stop Surrogacy Now, a coalition of politically diverse individuals and organizations—would go further, outlawing all surrogacy as the "buying and selling of children."[63] Thus, Jennifer Lahl, president of the Center for Bioethics and Culture and a leading figure in the international anti-surrogacy movement, says:

> It is not just the moral argument about using women as a breeding
> class for the well off and ignoring the inherent good of maternal-child
> bonding that takes place during nine months of pregnancy, but we must
> recognize the risks of surrogacy to women and the children born of
> these more high-tech pregnancies are real and significant. These risks
> are present regardless of whether the woman is paid or not. In fact, one
> study on the outcomes of surrogate pregnancies in one hospital showed
> that women who gave birth to a singleton or twins had hospital charges
> 26 times of a normal natural delivery. Surrogate mothers who gave birth
> to triplets saw hospital charges increased 176 times. For these many
> reasons I oppose surrogacy in any fashion."[64,65]

At the moment, this is the minority view, but who knows what the future holds. India seems be awakening to the harm done to destitute women in the country by its surrogacy industry. In October 2015, the government ordered surrogacy clinics to stop serving foreigners, a preliminary step to legislative action that will hopefully end industrial surrogacy in India—at least involving customers from outside the country.[66] This much is sure: The question of biological colonialism and surrogacy will roil domestic discourse and international politics for decades to come.

EGGS FOR SALE

From this discussion, the reader might conclude that black-market organs are the world's most expensive biological products. They are pricey, to be sure. But ounce for ounce, the world's most precious commodity isn't a tissue-typed black-market human liver. It isn't diamonds, titanium, or, for that matter, cocaine. Rather, the world's most pricey commodity is also one of the tiniest: human eggs, a marketable item worth far more than its weight in gold.

Human eggs are purchased in the foreign market. But the really high-priced products are produced domestically, where young women at elite universities are solicited to sell their eggs—sometimes for tens of thousands of dollars if they exhibit certain eugenically approved characteristics, such as the beauty of Marilyn Monroe and the brains of Albert Einstein. One ad promised to pay $100,000 for the eggs of Harvard women who passed eugenic muster.[67]

These ubiquitous ads—which can be very enticing to college students whose knees are buckling under the pressure of student loans—don't mention the potentially lethal consequences of being mined for eggs. Egg harvesting is onerous—and can be dangerous. First, the supplier's ovaries are flooded with strong hormones to stimulate the release of twenty or so eggs in the next ovulation cycle instead of the normal one or two. The eggs are then extracted through an invasive procedure that requires anesthesia, in which the egg harvester inserts a needle through the vaginal wall to collect the eggs.

Most extractions are performed safely. But some women are wounded by significant complications requiring ready access to quality medical treatment. For example, one out of one hundred women experiences ovarian swelling that can enlarge her ovaries to the size of a grapefruit, a condition that often causes the belly to fill with fluid, requiring hospitalization. Some women even suffer ovarian rupture. A higher incidence of ovarian tumors in women who underwent egg extraction has also been reported. For example, a 2011 study published in the *Human Reproduction Journal Report* found that "The long-term risk for ovarian malignancies (ovarian cancer and borderline ovarian tumours) is twice as high among women who undergo ovarian stimulation for IVF compared with sub-fertile women not treated with IVF."[68] (This study apparently only looked at the subsequent health results of women who had IVF to get pregnant using their own eggs versus those who didn't. But surely the study is also pertinent to the issue of egg donors generally.) Other potential health hazards include infection, pulmonary and vascular complications (including life-threatening acute respiratory distress syndrome), blood clots, and future cancers. In rare cases, hyperovulation results in death.

The market for eggs for use in IVF is steady and strong. But the demand for eggs may soon reach a frenzied level with the first successful cloning of human embryos in 2013. Why? Human eggs are the essential ingredient for every act of human cloning.

But what exactly is meant by the term "human cloning"? There are several potential methods for cloning, such as embryo splitting. Somatic cell nuclear transfer (SCNT) is the most common option—the scientific term for the process that led to Dolly the sheep. Cloning is easy to explain but very difficult to perform in humans. Let's say a biotechnologist wanted to clone me—although, as my wife will quickly tell you, one Wesley is more than sufficient. Here is how she would do it:

1. First, take one of my skin or other cells and remove the nucleus;
2. Next, take an egg and remove its nucleus;
3. Place the skin cell nucleus where the egg nucleus used to be; and
4. Stimulate with an electric current or other means.

Once the SCNT process was completed, a one-celled embryo would come into existence and develop thereafter, like an embryo created through fertilization. This is sometimes called asexual reproduction because it is accomplished without using sperm and egg.

The question next becomes what to do with the nascent human life thereby created. If the cloned embryo is destroyed for stem cells or otherwise used in experiments, it is often called "therapeutic cloning." If the embryo is implanted in a uterus for gestation and birth, it is often called "reproductive cloning." But it is important to reemphasize that these distinctions describe *uses* made of the cloned embryo, not the actual act of cloning.

Cloning is an important bioethical controversy in and of itself—I have written about the issue at length elsewhere—so we won't deal with it here.[69] But it also has a potentially direct nexus with biological colonialism. Perfecting human cloning techniques—first for use in stem cell research and eventually, I have little doubt, to bring a cloned baby into the world—will be a very difficult and extended process requiring the use of an untold number of eggs. Dr. David A. Prentice, a cell biologist and adult stem cell researcher, is one of the world's foremost experts on the science and morality of human cloning. He worked for almost twenty years as a professor at Indiana State University and Indiana University School of Medicine; then he spent more than a decade as a science policy special-ist. He is currently vice president and research director at the Charlotte Lozier Institute. In an interview for my book on biotechnology issues, *Consumer's Guide to a Brave New World*, Prentice described the intense trial-and-error approach required to learn how to safely engage in clon-ing to produce children:

> Scientists would have to clone thousands of embryos and grow them to the blastocyst stage to ensure that part of the process leading up to transfer into a uterus could be "safe," monitoring and analyzing each embryo, destroying each one in the process. Next, cloned embryos would have to be transferred into the uteruses of women volunteers. The initial purpose would be analysis of development, not bringing the pregnancy to a live birth. Each of these clonal pregnancies would be terminated at various points of development, each fetus destroyed for scientific analysis. The surrogate mothers would also have to be closely monitored and tested, not only during the pregnancies but also for a substantial length of time after the abortions.... Finally, if these experi-ments demonstrated that it was probably safe to proceed, a few clonal pregnancies would be allowed to go to full term. Yet even then, the born cloned babies would have to be constantly monitored to determine whether any health problems develop. Each would have to be followed (and undergo a battery of tests both physical and psychological) for their entire lives, since there is no way to predict if problems [associ-ated with gene expression] might arise later in childhood, adolescence, adulthood, or even into the senior years.[70]

In preparation for this chapter, Prentice told me that the above quote "still applies today." But an unexpected discovery made concomitantly with the manufacture of human cloned embryos makes the threatened biotech egg stampede even more potentially frenzied. "Newer evidence," Prentice said, "indicates that only certain women produce eggs with suitable genetic characteristics for the successful creation of viable human clones. This means the research will require screening a huge number of women to find those with the desired genetic characteristics who can produce the prized eggs to create clones successfully."[71]

Prentice is referring to an unexpected finding of the successful cloning experiments that found that it wasn't the nucleus of the somatic cell donor that mattered in maintaining the cloned embryo beyond the initial stage of development but instead *the quality of the egg*. "SCNT reprogramming is dependent on human oocyte [egg] quality," the authors of the first successful human cloning experiment write. Indeed, most of the eggs the researchers used provided poor embryos, but the four highest-quality cloned embryos—those from which embryonic stem cells were derived—all grew from eggs supplied by the same donor. The authors conclude that "oocyte quality is ultimately linked to the genetic constitution of individual egg donors." This unexpected result, the paper says, "warrants further studies ... to elucidate the genetic and clinical parameters associated with optimal oocyte quality for human SCNT."[72]

Even in the unlikely event that attempts aren't eventually made to create cloned babies, in the nearer term there will be a concerted push to perfect cloning human embryos for use in biotechnological research. *There's money in them thar hills!*

For example, a 2013 article published in the *New England Journal of Medicine* called for the creation of a commodities market for "made-to-order" human embryos.[73] The authors, I. Glenn Cohen and Eli Y. Adashi—university professors, of course—treat embryos as the equivalent of a prize cattle herd. They note that sperm and eggs are already bought and sold for IVF and, further, that New York legalized buying eggs for use in biotechnological research a few years ago. Hence "it is not clear" (an oft-used phrase in bioethical advocacy that frees the author from actually having to prove a point) why we should not also allow companies to make "made-to-order embryos" for profit, since that activity would be "more similar to the sale of gametes than the sale of children."[74]

As a matter of basic biology, that isn't true: A human embryo is an organism, a nascent human being, while an egg or sperm is just a cell. But, hey, what's a little sophistry in the cause of deconstructing ethics? The authors engage in misdirection by focusing on special-order embryos as just another service to be offered in the already ethically wide-open infertility industry. But expanding IVF opportunities—which also requires one egg per try—isn't what their proposal is really about. Rather, the primary customers of a future embryo manufacturing industry would be biotech companies and their university affiliates, which would pay top dollar for merchandise possessing desired genetic traits, just as they now do for genetically engineered research mice.

But designing the human embryo product line will not be easy. Fertilization is an inexact process. Sure, some desired attributes—sex or certain genetic defects—could be obtained through using specifically selected or altered eggs or sperm and genetic testing of embryos to find those that possess the desired characteristics. But made-to-order embryos would be hit or miss, limiting the industry's growth potential.

And that brings us back to human eggs. Women are far less likely to risk hyperovulation to make cloned embryos for use in experiments than they are the sentimental endeavor of enabling an infertile couple to have a baby. Thus scientists are unlikely to be able to fill the demand for genetically designed research embryos unless they pay for a bounteous supply of eggs—unless other ethically questionable sources can be developed, such as taking them from aborted late-term female fetuses or morphing stem cells into usable eggs.

But these potential sources are probably many years away from being perfected, assuming they ever are. Thus, at least for the time being, the eggs needed for human cloning and biotechnological research will have to come from living women. Those lining up to be hyperovulated for pay are unlikely to be members of the professional class. Rather, they would primarily be the poor and/or unemployed—women in such dire financial need that they are willing to risk their health, fecundity, and lives for a relatively small stipend.

And if the supply provided locally proved insufficient, what would stop the bounteously funded biotech industry from exploiting women in very poor countries—just as what happens to poor women in India in the surrogacy industry. As with that business, the most money would be made by the brokers, not the women. But the risk? That would be exclusively that of the suppliers. And it even could be worse: In surrogacy, the industry has a financial interest in keeping pregnant women healthy during their pregnancy. That would not be true of egg buying. Once the eggs were harvested, the women would be of no further profit value to the harvesting companies—at least until the next egg extraction. Given that quality medical help could well be unavailable to women in developing countries experiencing dangerous side effects from hyperovulation, an international egg hunt could become dangerous indeed.

I began this chapter by briefly discussing a cultural factor that drives so much of my concerns discussed in this book, including biological colonialism. So how should society best continue the struggle against "the worst of evils?" Rather than a headlong neurotic flight from pain, difficulty, and disease that is coming to include killing the sick, exploiting the weak, and oppressing the powerless, we should instead refocus our cultural energies and emphases on more righteous approaches. By all means, ameliorate suffering, mitigate pain, support the sick, suffer with those in extremis—but do so *morally* and with due regard for the equal value of all human life. We'll get into some ideas about that in the next chapter.

CHAPTER 7

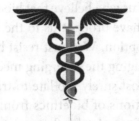

TOWARD A "HUMAN RIGHTS" BIOETHICS

"The theme of *Brave New World*," Aldous Huxley once wrote, "is not the advancement of science as such; it is the advancement of science as it affects human individuals."[1] While there are clearly significant differences between the dystopian future that Huxley feared when he published *Brave New World* in 1932 and the reality of today, we should not be sanguine. For us, a BNW may not have arrived yet, but it is on the delivery truck. Indeed, there can be no question that the "scientific caste system"[2] against which Huxley warned is just around the corner.

Consider: The mainstream bioethics movement actively pushes dehumanizing ideas and health policies that can fairly—if provocatively—be described as "medical cleansing": intentional dehydration of cognitively disabled people has become routine and normalized by the Terri Schiavo case; futile care theory (FCT) protocols empower physicians to refuse wanted end-of-life medical treatment in hospitals around the country; medical discrimination based on age or state of health and disability is promoted in the name of an alleged need for health care rationing in our most notable professional journals; euthanasia and assisted suicide are being redefined from crimes into a "medical treatment," while at the same time we see increased advocacy for redefining death to allow the harvesting of living human beings.

A POLICY OF CONTAINMENT

What to do? For those of us who believe that bioethics' advances—policy creep by policy creep—have brought us to the brink of a moral abyss, complacency is not an option. We must resist being remade in a crass utilitarian image by engaging the emerging medical culture of death at all levels. Since it is almost surely too late to transform the utilitarian, "quality of life" assumptions of bioethics from within the movement itself, a policy limiting the societal influence of bioethics appears to be the best strategy. Doing that will require increasing public awareness of what bioethics is, why it is important, what the movement generally stands for, and the societal and personal consequences of allowing the "new medicine" to become our effectuated reality.

But utilitarianism is an infectious moral pathogen that has already infested public perceptions and cultural attitudes. So, the question must be asked: Have we reached the point of no return? Not yet—but we are certainly closer to the chasm than when this book was first published. Here are some of the steps I believe can help us maintain our ethical moral footing.

Reform Hospice: Dying is not dead; it is a stage of living. The question thus becomes: How do we best care for those among us who have entered their final stage of life? It seems to me we have been forced by the events of recent years to a time of choosing: Will we improve care for people or authorize doctor-facilitated death? The choice we make is the difference between involvement and abandonment, caring and killing, true compassion (which means to "suffer with") and normalizing suicide or homicide deaths by which our loved ones put themselves, at least sometimes, out of *our* misery.

This is not to promote a cruel vitalism in which people are forced to remain alive beyond reason. But it is to say that we desperately need to improve our provision of end-of-life care, specifically by reforming hospice so that—instead of taking lethal actions— it becomes normalized as the true "death with dignity." Indeed, it seems to me that the spread of assisted suicide laws is, in some senses, a vote of "no confidence" in hospice as currently provided, or at least, as understood by the general public.

Changing these (perhaps unfair) perceptions will require both expanding the services one can receive while in hospice and improving the care that is provided by that sector. When this book came out, only 15 percent of dying people took advantage of the tremendous benefits hospice can provide. Numbers have risen dramatically since those bad old days, but they are still insufficient and mask a deeper problem. Too often, patients enter the program a mere day or three before they die—what hospice advocate Dr. Ira Byock cogently calls "brink of death care"—when it is too late for the patient and their families to receive hospice's full benefit.[3]

When I interviewed Dame Cecily Saunders for the first edition of this book in 1998, she warned me that the rules under which American hospices operate stifle its full potential. Saunders also believed that there was insufficient publicity given to hospice in the United States. I second the opinion. In my work against assisted suicide, I have seen how the killing message too often eclipses detailed discussions of all that hospice can do—and does—for dying people and their families—a damning-with-faint-praise phenomenon that has become more pronounced in recent years.

If you doubt me, take a good look at the startling contrast in media coverage around two young women who both tragically contracted terminal brain cancer in 2014. Brittany Maynard received explosive media attention of a kind usually reserved for rock stars, reality show megacelebrities, and the most connected politicians during a presidential campaign. For example, she and her family were the subjects of repeated cover stories in *People*, her obituary ran more than 1,100 words—huge by that magazine's standards—and the media breathlessly picked over the details of her last days, extolling her courage for choosing suicide.[4] Maynard was even named one of CNN's extraordinary people of 2014 *because* she killed herself and explicitly rejected hospice. In contrast, an even younger Lauren Hill, a college basketball player afflicted with the same cancer as Maynard, spoke out repeatedly on behalf of living until natural death. When her peaceful demise finally came, her death received distinctly mild coverage—only 196 words in *People*—mostly involving her determination to continue playing basketball until near the end.[5]

Why the contrasting coverage of two young women with the same disease? Blame our increasingly tabloid and culturally subversive media:

- Hill was not glammed up in stories about her circumstance. Photographs of her usually showed her as hot and sweaty on a basketball court. For want of a better description, she was presented as an everywoman.
- Maynard, in contrast, received the full movie star glamour treatment, with virtually every story including a photo of her holding a puppy with a beaming smile that lit up the page.
- Hill wasn't transgressive. She lived with cancer until she died, accepting hospice care, playing basketball, and raising money for research.
- Maynard used her remaining time to promote hastened death, backed by a sophisticated and expensive PR campaign sponsored by the assisted suicide advocacy group Compassion and Choices.
- Hill told the world that hospice allowed her to continue living with terminal illness, meaning that the timing of death was not hers to control.
- Maynard told the world that poison pills would provide her a dignified end on "my own terms."
- Hill pushed life with dignity.
- Maynard pushed death with dignity.

In the current nihilistic cultural milieu, the media knew which story would generate the most Internet clicks and published accordingly.

Hospice leaders are partially to blame for their sector's eclipse. Rather than defending hospice vigorously as the true "death with dignity" in the face of the assisted suicide threat to its philosophy, approach, and patients, most of the sector's leaders—excepted for Dr. Ira Byock—have tended to stay very quiet. Since movements with the most energy usually to carry the day, the hospice sector's general passivity subverted its own mission.

But a vigorous defense of hospice theory isn't enough. We need reform to eliminate the "cruel choice" currently required of those who enter hospice in the United States.

What do I mean? Unlike England and most other countries, under Medicare and most health insurance programs, hospice patients are forced to eschew all life-extending or potentially curative care. Saunders told me this was not only cruel but placed an obstacle in the path to expanding hospice's use. She told me: "More people are willing to go into hospice here [in England] because it is not a one-way street."[6] In other words, in the USA, hospice patients must give up that last ditch round of chemotherapy and all life-extending care. Some hospices even interpret the cruel choice as *requiring patients to forgo feeding tubes* when they can't swallow. I have heard from some readers who refused hospice because they see it as quasi-euthanasia. It most certainly isn't—when properly applied—but I understand the fear.

Happily, some of our most energetic end-of-life physicians are urging an end to the cruel choice. Byock, as just one example, has proposed a "Safe Dying Act" that would materially expand hospice services and generally improve care for the dying. He writes:

> Let's start by requiring medical schools to adequately train young doctors to assess and treat pain, listen to patients' concerns and collaborate with patients and families in making treatment decisions—and test for those skills before awarding medical degrees. Let's require nursing home companies to double staffing of nurses and aides, and the hours of care accorded each resident. Let's set minimum standards for palliative care teams within every hospital. Let's routinely publish meaningful quality ratings for hospitals, nursing homes, assisted living, home health and hospice programs for people to use in choosing care. And let's repeal the Medicare statute that forces incurably ill people to forgo disease treatments in order to receive hospice care.

But wouldn't that increase costs?

Probably not. Dr. Atul Gawande writes in his best-selling book, *Being Mortal*, that permitting "concurrent care"—e.g., both hospice and curative—is both humane and cost-effective: "A study conducted by Aetna Insurance permitting patients to access both hospice and life-extending treatments saw hospice participation rise from 26 to 70 percent." Moreover, many were so pleased with the hospice care they were receiving, they did not pursue painful last-ditch efforts, visiting "the emergency room half as often" compared to a control group in traditional hospice. Moreover, their admissions "into ICUs dropped by more than two-thirds. Overall costs fell by almost a quarter."[7] To deploy a cliché, that's a true win-win scenario.

There are positive signs that the US government understands that the "cruel choice" is not only heartless, but is also bad public policy. Beginning on January 1, 2016, a four-year pilot program will allow some Medicare beneficiaries in hospice to also receive curative and life-extending treatment to determine whether this reformed approach "can improve the quality of life and care received by Medicare beneficiaries, increase patient satisfaction, and reduce Medicare expenditures."[8] It is a shame that the bureaucratic approach to policy moves at the speed of glaciers. But at least we may be witnessing the beginning of the end for the "cruel choice."

Close the Door to Futile Care Theory: Aside from assisted suicide, FCT is the most immediate danger facing weak and vulnerable patients. If we are to stop medicine from becoming a culling process in which some people are given optimal care and others are neglected, FCT must not become a dishonored guest at the table of medical ethics discourse.

To prevent the stealth adoption of futile care protocols in our hospitals and among our medical societies—which, as noted earlier, can become a form of health care rationing—we will need to break through the intense secrecy in which these protocols are usually adopted. Court action may be necessary to overcome the *ad hoc* futility decisions that are already being imposed in some cases on patients and families just when they are at their most vulnerable and defenseless: during the throes of a crisis caused by catastrophic illness or injury when they are least able to stand up for their own values. In that regard, panels of doctors and lawyers willing to donate their time and talents for little or no pay to defeat FCT may have to be formed to ensure that embattled families have a fighting chance to stand against the superior financial resources of hospitals, insurance companies, and, potentially, the government.

Legislation also has a part to play to create a system that allows a doctor to transfer care he or she believes to be inappropriate. Such laws would permit doctors to find a replacement physician and allow the hospital to ask that the patient transfer elsewhere if it can be done without harming the patient's welfare. But doctors and hospitals should be legally prohibited from unilaterally terminating wanted end-of-life medical treatment when the refusal is based on quality of life or economic values rather than objective medical science. In this regard, Texas recently reformed its awful Advance Directives Act—which authorizes hospital bioethics committees to impose futile care impositions—to prohibit unilateral withdrawal of feeding tubes that served the wanted purpose of keeping the patient alive.[9] This still provides inadequate protection for vulnerable and devalued patients, but at least it is a start in the right direction.

Along these same lines, hospital ethics committees should be denied quasi-judicial authority to determine issues of life and death in such disputes. Such power would not only be corrupting but also shake the faith of people in the health care system. It is far better that ethics committees remain neutral mediating bodies that help people and their doctors reach agreement or find accommodation in difficult cases. In the few situations where no accord is possible, as reluctant as we should be to bring in the courts, it is better to resolve these matters in an open legal forum subject to rules of due process and appeal than in an internal Star Chamber-like process that breeds distrust and suspicion.

If patient autonomy is to be more than a one-way street, FCT must not be permitted. Physicians must not be allowed to abandon patients based on their personal opinions about the quality of their patients' lives. We must ensure that the love of a family never takes a backseat to the philosophy of strangers. At the same time, by allowing court intervention on truly intractable cases, we can assure transparency and the assurances provided by the rule of law.

Hold the Line in Dehydration Cases: Dehydrating the cognitively devastated on feeding tubes is legal in all fifty states, but this backdoor euthanasia should continue to be ethically and, where warranted, legally challenged. To state that an act is "legal" isn't the same thing as saying that it is morally right. Considering that dehydration results in an inevitable slow death, should we really be sanguine about viewing tube-feeding as no different ethically from giving aspirin or antibiotics? Indeed, before we dehydrate a cognitively disabled human being, should we not at least be ready to give the benefit of any doubt in the matter to life rather than death?

We can do this by assuring ourselves with clear and convincing evidence that the person both would not want to live as a cognitively disabled person and would rather die *by dehydration* than live with his or her disabilities. A written advance directive would provide such evidence, although too many people sign them blithely, unaware of what dehydration actually entails. Moreover, we must guard against bait-and-switch tactics in these dehydration cases: Withholding medically supplied food and water is being sold as a matter of "choice," but now some futility protocols provide that tube-feeding be withheld or withdrawn from those diagnosed as persistently unconscious. Moreover, a detailed report by the Robert Powell Center for Medical Ethics of the National Right to Life Committee found that there is a bias against life-extending treatment in many advance directives that "nudges" people toward refusing medically supplied sustenance without fully alerting them to the pain and suffering that being dehydrated to death can cause.[10] If these protocols multiply in the coming years, people with profound brain damage will indeed be reduced to a disposable caste of people.

Continue the Struggle over Abortion: When the issue of legalizing abortion was debated in the years just prior to *Roe v. Wade*, abortion opponents warned that once legalized, abortion would become "just another form of birth control" and would, sooner or later, open the door to legalized euthanasia. Those who wished to legalize abortion disagreed. They promised that few women would terminate their unplanned pregnancies and dismissed fears of the slippery slope from abortion to euthanasia as paranoid alarmism.

Forty-plus years—and tens of millions of dead fetuses later—and now we know which side had it more right. Each year more than 1 million pregnancies are terminated in United States, with far more than 50 million feticides since *Roe*. And while many euthanasia opponents also support abortion rights, bioethicists like Peter Singer and Jacob Appel— joined by many euthanasia advocates seeking to bootstrap mercy killing to abortion—explicitly link the right to abortion with proposals to permit infanticide and euthanasia. Whatever one thinks about the legality of abortion, that we have been affected culturally by abortion on demand is undeniable, which is why the pro-life movement continues to receive support from wide swaths of the American people.

In fact, anti-abortion successes in recent years—proposals for waiting periods, the outlawing of "partial-birth abortion," the mandatory use of ultrasounds to show the humanity of the fetus—have reduced abortion numbers, pushing some "pro-choice" advocated into a decidedly pro-abortion direction. Gone are the days when abortion rights supporters described pregnancy termination as an unfortunate necessity that should be "safe, legal, and rare." Increasingly, abortion is described as a positive good to the point that the old standby political identifier "pro-choice" is falling out of favor.[11] Moreover, some advocates have come out as explicitly pro-abortion. Thus, a former executive of Emily's List, an organization that financially boosts female abortion-supporting political candidates, wrote in the *Washington Post* that activists should stop "calling abortion a difficult decision":

> When the pro-choice community frames abortion as a difficult decision, it implies that women need help deciding, which opens the door to paternalistic and demeaning "informed consent" laws.... But there's a more pernicious result when pro-choice advocates use such language: It is a tacit acknowledgment that terminating a pregnancy is a moral issue requiring an ethical debate. To say that deciding to have an abortion is a "hard choice" implies a debate about whether the fetus should live, thereby endowing it with a status of being. It puts the focus on the fetus rather than the woman.[12]

At *Salon*, Mary Elizabeth Williams expressed a similar opinion approving Planned Parenthood's decision to downplay "pro-choice" as an advocacy meme. Asking, "So what if abortion ends a human life?" William announced her blunt premise—one perfectly consistent with mainstream bioethics views:

> All life is not equal. That's a difficult thing for liberals like me to talk about, lest we wind up looking like death-panel-loving, kill-your-grandma-and-your-precious-baby storm troopers. Yet a fetus can be a human life without having the same rights as the woman in whose body it resides. She's the boss. Her life and what is right for her circumstances and her health should automatically trump the rights of the non-autonomous entity inside of her. Always.[13]

Liberal jurists may have also turned in the "pro-abortion" direction. In *Planned Parenthood v. Bentley*, Alabama's law regulating abortion clinics was declared to be unconstitutional. That might not be surprising, but the reasoning in the decision certainly was. US District Judge Myron H. Thompson's equated *access* to abortion with the Second Amendment's enunciated right to keep and bear arms:

At its core, each protected right is held by the individual: the right to decide to have an abortion and the right to have and use firearms for self-defense. However, neither right can be fully exercised without the assistance of someone else. The right to abortion cannot be exercised without a medical professional, and the right to keep and bear arms means little if there is no one from whom to acquire the handgun or ammunition.[14]

That's a big step in an absolute-right-to-abortion direction—so notable, in fact, that the case was celebrated by *New York Times*'s openly pro-abortion legal reporter, Linda Greenhouse, as "remarkable" and "delicious."[15]

That's a notable shift. Rather than moderating, abortion-rights activists have embraced an advocacy model they once eschewed—being explicitly *pro-abortion*. In this new approach, *Roe v. Wade* is no longer a moment to celebrate. Rather, it must be overturned because it is *too restrictive* of what they believe should be an absolute right to terminate an unwanted pregnancy at any time for any reason.

The potent possibility of a "reverse reversal" (if you will) hit me while listening to pro-life lawyers discuss the current status of abortion litigation at a University Faculty for Life Association Convention at the University of San Francisco in 2013, at which I had been invited to speak about euthanasia. Not being involved with abortion jurisprudence, I was interested to hear about the current state of the law in this contentious field.

Roe and its progeny cases, such as *Planned Parenthood v. Casey*, left room for pro-life advocates to deploy subversive legislative and litigation strategies that have opened significant cracks in the once-unbreachable judicial wall around the abortion right. For example, court rulings have permitted the outlawing of most late-term abortions, a ban on "partial-birth abortion," mandatory waiting periods, ultrasound testing, and building code regulation of abortion facilities, all contributing to a substantial reduction in annual terminations.

Almost as an aside, one of the seminar presenters noted the implacable opposition of Supreme Court Justice Ruth Bader Ginsburg to this limited right to regulate the status quo. Ginsburg believes adamantly that women are denied "equal citizen stature" by boundaries placed around access to abortion. Not only that, but in an angry dissent to the 2007 Supreme Court ruling upholding the federal ban on partial-birth abortion, she (joined by Justice Breyer among the current justices) railed against the majority allowing "moral concerns" to "override fundamental rights."

That sounded to me as advocacy for an unfettered right to abortion. So I asked expert anti-abortion attorney Clarke D. Forsythe, the senior counsel for Americans United for Life, whether Ginsburg's view would abolish all abortion regulation. Yes, he told me: "If the right to an abortion were based on equal protection of the law," as opposed to other constitutional standards, it would "permit no regulations at any time," perhaps even "requiring [government] abortion funding."[16]

In other words, even though the most well-known anti-*Roe* efforts are aimed at overturning the case to permit greater state regulation, a significant—if quieter—counter-push seeks to (essentially) overturn *Roe* by making the abortion right virtually absolute. At the very least, it would repair those cracks in the protective wall.

As an article in the *UCLA Law Review* supportive of the equal protection standard put it, "Crucially, once the Supreme Court recognizes that people have a right to [abortion] by virtue of equal citizenship," the right would be "on a stronger legal and political footing," making it far less susceptible to the current pro-life strategy of "chipping away."[17] As if that weren't enough, I thought about how *Roe* had permitted some limits on abortion based on the "important and legitimate [state] interest in protecting the potentiality of human life," an interest that the court ruled becomes "compelling" at the point of fetal "viability."[18]

But as we have seen throughout this book, many powerful voices no longer consider "human life" to be a morally relevant category. For example, as we have seen, the mainstream bioethics movement argues that what matters morally isn't being "human," but rather value arises by possessing sufficient mental capacity to be considered a "person." According to this view, only persons have a right to life. Since a fetus does not possess personhood capacities at any time during gestation— contrary to *Roe*—the state has no interest in protecting fetal life, even after viability.

Now, add a third element to the equation: *Roe* was intended to settle the abortion issue once and for all. It clearly didn't do that. Many frustrated abortion supporters still dream of obliterating all impediments between a woman experiencing an unwanted pregnancy and termination on demand.

Pro-abortion ideas are beginning to be proposed for legal implementation. For example, in 2013, New York Governor Andrew Cuomo announced a plan to permit the termination of viable fetuses to protect the mother's "health."[19] That might seem properly restrictive. But the term "health" has been very broadly interpreted by the United States Supreme Court in *Doe v. Bolton*:

> The medical judgment [for a late-term abortion] may be exercised in the light of all factors—physical, emotional, psychological, familial, and the woman's age—relevant to the well-being of the patient. All these factors may relate to health. This allows the attending physician the room he needs to make his best medical judgment. And it is room that operates for the benefit, not the disadvantage, of the pregnant woman.[20]

Forsythe told me that a scheme like that proposed by Cuomo would harness *Doe's* limitless definition of "health," resulting in a virtually unlimited abortion license through the ninth month. Relevant to the overturning of *Roe* from the other direction, Forsythe says that, "As a matter of policy, Cuomo's bill would [have done] in New York what Ginsburg's judicial view would impose across the nation."[21]

Finally, assume a United States Supreme Court in which Justices Clarence Thomas and/or Antonin Scalia have been replaced by Ginsburg-thinking replacements. A new 5-4 or 6-3 majority could then exist to make equal protection the primary pillar supporting the abortion license, perhaps also installing "personhood" in place of "humanhood" as the relevant legal standard for applying a right to life. That could be the end of *Roe v. Wade*—but not in the way that pro-lifers hope.

Allowing an unlimited right to abortion that couldn't be struggled against would unleash a moral tsunami that would sweep away virtually all limits. If we are to have any chance of containing the culture of death in other areas discussed in these pages, the pro-life movement must continue to prick the consciences of people about the morality of abortion and the intrinsic importance of nascent human life, an important task regardless of the legality of abortion.

PREVENT "MEDICAL MARTYRDOM"

Doctors haven't taken the Hippocratic Oath for several decades. That shouldn't be surprising. The Oath's ethical proscriptions against doctors participating in abortion and assisted suicide cut against the contemporary moral grain, leading medical schools to dumb it down or remove the parts that offend contemporary sensibilities. Here's part of what the Hippocratic Oath stated:

> I will follow that system of regimen which, according to my ability and judgment, I consider for the benefit of my patients, and abstain from whatever is deleterious and mischievous. I will give no deadly medicine to anyone if asked, nor suggest any such counsel; and in like manner I will not give to a woman a pessary to produce abortion. With purity and with holiness I will pass my life and practice my Art. I will not cut persons laboring under the stone, but will leave this to be done by men who are practitioners of this work. Into whatever houses I enter, I will go into them for the benefit of the sick.[22]

And now here's Cornell Medical School's diluted substitute:

> That I will lead my life and practice my art with integrity and honor, using my power wisely.... That whatever house I enter, it shall be for the good of the sick; That I will maintain this sacred trust, holding myself far all of from wrong, from corrupting, from the tempting of others to vice; That above all else I will serve the highest interests of my patients through the practice of my science and my art; That I will be an advocate for patients in need and strive for justice in the care of the sick.[23]

What does that even mean? Contrary to the specificity of Hippocrates, the modern substitute contains bromides such as "wrong," "vice," "highest interests," and "justice," vague terms that can mean mirror opposites to different practitioners.

Be that as it may, many doctors—along with nurses, pharmacists, and other modern medical professionals—still want to practice their "science and art" in a traditionally Hippocratic manner, meaning to never intentionally kill or otherwise do a patient physical harm.

Until now, despite the changes in medical practice of the kinds described in this book and exemplified by modified Oaths, Hippocratic professionals could remain true to their consciences, ethics, and religious or moral values. But the space allowing moral heterodoxy is shrinking. Today, a concept known as "patient rights" prevails; the competent customer is always right and, hence, held to be entitled to receive virtually any legal procedure from every "service provider" for which payment can be made (unless, as discussed previously, it is rationed or deemed "futile")—be it abortion, assisted suicide, or, someday perhaps, embryonic stem cell therapies and products made from cloned and aborted human fetuses: no conscientious objection allowed.

Hippocratic-believing professionals are increasingly being pressured to practice medicine without regard to their personal faith or conscience beliefs. Not only that, but this moral intolerance is slowly being imbedded into law and/or the ethical canons of medical societies. Victoria, Australia, for example, *legally requires all doctors to perform—or be complicit in—abortions*: If a patient requests a legal termination and the doctor has moral qualms, he is required to refer her to a colleague who the doctor knows to be willing to do the deed.[24] At least one doctor has already been professionally sanctioned under the law for refusing to refer a couple for a sex-selection abortion.[25] Indeed, when I toured Australia in 2010 on a national speaking tour against euthanasia, I met doctors in Perth who had moved clear across the country to escape the clutches of Victoria's anti-conscience law—a distance akin to leaving New York for Los Angeles.

Canadian doctors may soon have to be similarly complicit in abortion and euthanasia as a condition of professional licensure. Quebec euthanasia legalization law, passed in 2014, allows no conscience exemptions, along the same general lines as Victoria's abortion law.[26] Later that same year, as we discussed in some detail earlier, Canada's Supreme Court made access to euthanasia a charter right for those with a diagnosable medical condition that causes "irremediable suffering," including "psychological" pain. Recognizing that some doctors will have moral qualms about "terminating life," the court gave Parliament twelve months to pass enabling legislation, stating that "the rights of patients and physicians will need to be reconciled" by law or left "in the hands of physicians' colleges."[27]

That doesn't bode well for medical conscience rights. The College of Physicians and Surgeons of Saskatchewan's ethics policy forces doctors morally opposed to providing "legally permissible and publicly-funded health services"—which now include euthanasia as well as abortion—to "make a timely referral to another health provider who is willing and able to … provide the service."[28] If no other doctor can be found, the dissenting physician will have to do the deed personally, "even in circumstances where the provision of health services conflicts with physicians' deeply held and considered moral or religious beliefs."[29]

Similarly, the Ontario College of Physicians and Surgeons favors forcing doctors with a conscience objection to legal procedures—abortion, assisted suicide/euthanasia, clearly included to participate in life ending through active referral to a physician they know will do the deed—even if a requesting person is not yet a patient:

> Where physicians are unwilling to provide certain elements of care due to their moral or religious beliefs, an effective referral to another health care provider must be provided to the patient. An effective referral means a referral made in good faith, to a non-objecting, available, and accessible physician or other health-care provider. The referral must be made in a timely manner to reduce the risk of adverse clinical outcomes. Physicians must not impede access to care for existing patients, or those seeking to become patients.[30]

The Dutch Medical Association (KNMG) takes a similar position on the only 14 percent of doctors in that country who would not consider euthanizing patients. From, "The Role of the Physician in Voluntary Termination of Life" position paper:

> Patients, too, often have difficulty telling a physician they have an authentic wish to die. Physicians, for their part, are under an obligation to take such requests seriously. *This also means that if a physician cannot or does not wish to honour a patient's request for euthanasia or assisted suicide he must give the patient a timely and clear explanation of why, and furthermore must then refer or transfer the patient to another physician in good time.*[31] (My emphasis.)

It is also worth noting that if a patient does not qualify for euthanasia, according to the KMNG position paper, a doctor *may refer him/her to how-to-commit-suicide literature*: "There is no punishment for physicians and other persons if they provide information about suicide. Physicians are also legally permitted to refer patients to information that is available on the Internet or to publications sold by book vendors, or provide these on loan, and to discuss this information with patients."[32]

So, let's recap: It is unprofessional for a doctor to refuse to kill or refer for that purpose when a patient asks for euthanasia. But it is okay to help patients learn how to commit suicide if they don't qualify for euthanasia under the law.

In the United States, doctors are currently protected against forced participation in abortion and assisted suicide (in the few jurisdictions where it is legal), although nurses and pharmacists generally may not receive the same explicit protection. But the medical establishment generally opposes these professional safeguards. As just one example, the American College of Obstetricians and Gynecologists (ACOG) published an ethics opinion in 2007, openly hostile to medical conscience in its intolerance of Hippocratic adherence:

> Conscientious refusals should be limited if they constitute an imposi-
> tion of religious and moral beliefs on patients.... Physicians and other
> healthcare providers have the duty to refer patients in a timely manner
> to other providers if they do not feel they can in conscience provide the
> standard reproductive services that patients request.... In an emergency
> in which referral is not possible or might negatively impact a patient's
> physical or mental health, providers have an obligation to provide
> medically indicated requested care.[33]

The "mental health" wording is the key, for it could mean (as in abortion jurisprudence) that the emotional anxiety of a woman denied an abortion could be enough to force the doctor's compliance, despite her moral objections.

Laws like Victoria's and ethical opinions such as those in Canada, the Netherlands, and some US medical associations are prescriptions for what I call "medical martyrdom," by which I mean doctors and other medical professionals being forced to choose between adhering to their faith or moral code and remaining in their chosen profession. If these trends continue, twenty years from now, those who feel called to a career in health care will face an agonizing dilemma: Either participate in acts of killing—a descriptive word meaning to end life—or stay out of medicine. Those who stay true to their consciences will be forced into the painful sacrifice of embracing martyrdom for their faith or conscience by facing the humiliation of professional discipline, litigation, leaving the practice of medicine—or not getting into it in the first place.

That's precisely what many in bioethics want. Canadian bioethicist Udo Schuklenk argued on his blog that doctors objecting to legal procedures—even those that kill—have no place in the profession:

> The very idea that we ought to countenance conscientious objection in any profession is objectionable. Nobody forces anyone to become a professional. It is a voluntary choice. A conscientious objector in medicine is not dissimilar to a taxi driver who joins a taxi company that runs a fleet of mostly combustion engine cars and who objects on grounds of conscience to drive those cars due to environmental concerns. Why did she become a taxi driver in the first place? Perhaps she should have opened a bicycle taxi company instead.[34]

The very idea that Schuklenk compares driving a taxi to practicing a medical profession and worries about pollution *to the active and intentional taking of human life* tells you so much about what has gone wrong in bioethics. Moreover, when today's doctors and nurses entered the profession, they weren't required to kill.

Oxford bioethicist Julian Savulescu is unequivocal in his opposition to permitting doctors freedom from participating in procedures to which their conscience or religious beliefs object. In the *British Medical Journal*, he writes:

- A doctor's conscience should not be allowed to interfere with medical care
- All doctors and medical students should be aware of their responsibility to provide all legal and beneficial care
- Conscientious objection may be permissible if sufficient doctors are willing to provide the service
- Conscientious objectors must ensure that their patients are aware of the care they are entitled to and refer them to another professional

- Conscientious objectors who compromise the care of their patients must be disciplined
- The place for expression and consideration of different values is at the level of policy relating to public medicine.[35]

So this is where we are heading: Kill or get out of medicine. Not willing to actively take human life? Then stay out of medicine in the first place. If you are an orthodox religious believer or philosophically opposed to abortion and euthanasia, you have no place in the healing arts. In short, we are coming to a time when the only people who will (or can) become doctors are those willing to, at least in some circumstances, kill—or, at the very least, be willingly complicit in the act. How frightening is that?

But it doesn't have to be that way. To preserve the current generally applying comity that permits Hippocratic physicians to practice according to their moral values, the rights of medical conscience need to be expanded and made explicit. With the understanding that there may be nuances in specific circumstances not discussed here, I suggest that the following general principles apply in crafting such protections:

- Conscience rights should be legally established.
- The rights of conscience should apply to medical facilities such as hospitals and nursing homes, as well as to individuals.
- Except in rare and compelling circumstances in which a patient's life is at stake, no medical professional should be compelled to perform or participate in procedures or treatments that take human life. (This is in contrast to FCT, when physicians object to keeping a patient alive.)
- It should be the *procedure* that is objectionable, not the patient. In this way, for example, physicians could not refuse to treat a lung cancer patient because the patient smoked, treat an AIDS patient because he is gay, or to maintain the life of a patient in a vegetative state because the physician believed that people with profound impairments do not have a life worth living.
- To avoid conflicts and respect patient autonomy, patients should be advised, whenever feasible, in advance of a professional's or facility's conscientious objection to performing or participating in legal medical procedures or treatments.

- The rights of conscience should be limited to bona fide medical facilities such as hospitals, skilled nursing centers, and hospices and to licensed medical professionals such as physicians, nurses, and pharmacists.

(There are also conscience issues dealing with elective procedures worthy of discussion, but they are beyond our scope here.)

It is a sad day when medical professionals and facilities have to be protected legally from coerced participation in life-terminating medical procedures. But there is no denying the direction in which the scientific and moral currents are flowing. The ethical views in society and medicine are growing increasingly polyglot. The sanctity of human life is increasingly under a cloud in the medical context. And, given the establishment's marked hostility toward medical professionals who adhere to the traditional Hippocratic maxims, legally enacted conscience protections may be the only shelter shielding traditional professionals from medical martyrdom.

BEWARE THE NEW EUGENICS[36]

Just as it is wrong to dehumanize, objectify, and disparage the lives of ill and disabled people, so too should we worry about transforming unborn human life into a malleable resource to be exploited for the benefit of the born and breathing in cellular procedures such as cloning, stem cell extraction, and genetic manipulation. Why is this important? Perhaps Dr. Leon R. Kass puts it best in an essay entitled "The Wisdom of Repugnance." Kass writes that the stakes at risk in these *Brave New World* issues are very high, asserting, "We are faced with having to decide nothing less than whether human procreation is going to remain human."[37]

One need only hark back to the writings of the bioethics patriarch Joseph Fletcher to understand the basis of Kass's alarm. To Fletcher, nothing in the natural way of life was sacrosanct. Indeed, he was such a wild-eyed radical that even basic biology did not prevent his advocating the most unnatural biological manipulation. For example, he positively swooned at the prospect of *males giving birth*:

[T]ransplant or replacement medicine foresees the day, after the automatic rejection of alien tissue is overcome, when a uterus can be implanted in a human male's body—his abdomen has spaces—and gestation started by artificial fertilization and egg transfer. Hypogonadism could be used to stimulate milk from the man's rudimentary breasts—men too have mammary glands. If surgery could not construct a cervical canal the delivery could be effected by a Caesarean section and the male or transsexualized mother could nurse his own baby.[38]

Hard as it is to believe, some doctors predict that we may only be a few years away from men becoming mothers. From a story in *Yahoo Health*:

> "My guess [men giving birth] is five, ten years away, maybe sooner," says Dr. Karine Chung, director of the fertility preservation program at the University of Southern California's Keck School of Medicine. Today, medical advances let transgender women adjust their biochemistry to suppress male and introduce female hormones, have breasts that can lactate, and obtain surgically constructed vaginas that include a "neoclitoris," which allows sensation. Until now, however, a place to carry the fetus—a womb of its own—was a major missing link. Uterus transplants could conceivably surmount that hurdle. "I'd bet just about every transgender person who is female will want to do it, if it were covered by insurance," says Dr. Christine McGinn, a New Hope, Pa., plastic surgeon who performs transgender surgeries on men and women and is a consultant to the new movie *The Danish Girl*, about one of the first recipients of sex reassignment surgery.[39]

Fletcher was also an unrepentant eugenicist, advocating genetic "quality control" aimed at "selecting for intelligence."[40] To identify "carriers" of "undesirable" genetic traits, Fletcher supported an idea first made by Linus Pauling: that genetic "carriers should wear a small tattoo on their foreheads as Indians wear caste marks."[41] Proving that he learned little from the horrors of the last century released by the eugenics enterprise, Fletcher also wrote:

> If we choose family size we should choose family health. This is what the controls of reproductive medicine make possible. Public health and sanitation have greatly reduced human ills; now the major ills have become genetic and congenital. They can be reduced by medical controls. We ought to protect our families from the emotional and

material burden of such diseased individuals, and from the misery of their simply "existing" (not living) in a nearby "warehouse" or public institution.[42]

Demonstrating that "choice" has never been the be-all and end-all of bioethics, Fletcher was no respecter of autonomy in these matters: "Testes and ovaries are social by nature," he opined, "and it would appear ethically that they should be controlled in the social interest."[43] How? Through the forced abortion of genetically defective children, if necessary, actions he justified with the ludicrous argument that the unborn are "fungible." "It could be right either voluntarily or coercively," he wrote, "to limit procreation by prevention either before or after conception—if and when specified genetic diseases or defects are predictable or at risk."[44]

If any reader still doubts the urgency of Kass's warning about the power of reproductive issues to distort our essential humanity, pay heed to this bit of truly nauseating Fletcher advocacy that could have been taken right out of the pages of *Brave New World* but with one crucial difference: Genetic manipulation that Huxley so urgently warned against in his great novel Fletcher wholeheartedly embraced:

> Chimeras [part human/part animal] or parahumans might legitimately
> be fashioned to do dangerous or demeaning jobs. As it is now, low grade
> work is shoved off on moronic and retarded individuals, the victims
> of uncontrolled reproduction. Should we not program such workers
> "thoughtfully" instead of accidentally, by means of hybridization? Cell
> fusion and putting human nuclei into animal tissues is possible (such
> hybrid tissue exists already as a matter of fact).... Hybrids could also
> be designed by sexual reproduction, as between apes and humans. If
> inter-specific coitus is too distasteful, then laboratory fertilization and
> implant could do it. If women are unwilling to gestate hybrids animal
> females could. Actually, the artificial womb would bypass all such
> repugnancies.[45]

How can one read these words and not be repulsed to the marrow of our bones? Is Kass not precisely on the mark when he writes, "Shallow are the souls that have forgotten how to shudder."[46]

Fletcher is far from alone among modern bioethics writers who embrace a new eugenics. Space does not permit a complete recitation, but Philip Kitcher's book *The Lives to Come: The Genetic Revolution and Human Possibilities* illustrates the point. In his chapter "Inescapable Eugenics," Kitcher foresees "laissez-faire eugenics" in which people will create their own versions of optimal human life—a prospect that Kitcher assures readers will work out just fine because there would also be "universally shared respect for difference."[47] Paradoxically, Kitcher admits, "individual choices are not made in a social vacuum"; instead, we "can anticipate that many future prospective parents ... will have to bow to social attitudes" by aborting their genetically inferior children "not to avoid suffering but to reflect a set of social values."[48] If infanticide ever becomes respectable, Fletcher's and Peter Singer's dreams of "post-birth abortions" might also become normalized, if perhaps not formally legalized, as in the Netherlands.

Since the first edition of this book was published, a new social movement/quasi-religion has appeared on the scene promoting these very ideas in the professional literature and popular media that can only be called a new eugenics. Transhumanism is a utopian social movement and philosophy that looks toward a massive breakthrough in technological prowess, known as "the singularity," that will open the door for transhumanists to "seize control of human evolution" and create a "post-human species" of near immortals. Don't roll your eyes. Transhumanists believe in their ageless post-human future with a desperate passion that borders on—and often serves as a substitute for—religious faith.[49]

Not only that, but the movement is receiving good press. For example, *Time* published a laudatory profile of transhumanist author and Google's in-house futurist Raymond Kurzweil's quest to live indefinitely under the serious title "2045: The Year Man Becomes Immortal."[50] Similarly, anti-aging researcher Aubrey de Gray seeks to defeat human aging, receiving much respectful media attention—even though I heard him give a speech in which he claimed his research should take precedence over funding health care aid to Africa, and indeed, that failing to fund his immortality project is akin to terrorism.[51]

Alas, when it comes to transhumanism, much attention is paid to immortality and quirky personalities, but little attention is given to transhumanism's poisonous core beliefs and goals. It isn't the unlikely singularity event or other fanciful technologies required to transform us into post-humans that make transhumanism so potentially destructive. Rather, it is the movement's explicitly eugenic and anti-human values that cause one's neck hair to stand on end.

So much has been written in recent years promoting transhumanism that an entire book could—and should—be written deconstructing the movement. But given our limited space, let's focus on just one article published in *Discover* magazine in 2011.[52] The author is Kyle Munkittrick, who is, as of this writing, the director of the Envisioning the Future program for transhumanist think tank Institute for Ethics and Emerging Technologies (IEET). (The IEET was cofounded by Oxford's Nick Bostrom and transhumanist bioethicist James Hughes. Its board of trustees includes bioethics luminaries such as Arthur Caplan and Glenn McGee.)[53]

Munkittrick's article is well worth studying because it reveals transhumanism's dark soul (if transhumanists, who are mostly stark materialists, will pardon the term). Munkittrick's article informs readers of what the age of transhumanism will look like. First, prosthetics will be preferred over natural limbs. A "key social indicator" of the arrival of transhumanism, he writes, will be when you "find yourself seriously considering having your birth-given hand lopped off and replaced with a cybernetic one."[54]

Again, don't roll your eyes. What could be called a right to radical self-creationism is already emerging, evidenced by the Bruce-to-Caitlyn Jenner media frenzy. It isn't just transgender advocates arguing that people should be aided medically to become who they self-identify as. Serious writers in notable bioethics journals have already advocated treating the mental illness body identity integrity disorder (BIID)—in which people anguish and obsess over becoming amputees or paralyzed as their "true" selves—by amputating healthy limbs or otherwise disabling themselves.[55] Indeed, trying to bootstrap off of the success of transgender rights advocacy, some are now calling people with BIID "transable."[56] Some have even advocated amputation as a proper treatment:

> When faced with a patient requesting the amputation of a healthy limb, clinicians should make a careful diagnostic assessment. If the patient is found to have body integrity identity disorder, amputation of the

healthy limb may be appropriate after a trial of selective serotonin reuptake inhibitors and after careful consideration of the risks, benefits, and unknowns of all possible treatment alternatives.... Sufferers of BIID might be relieved to know that members of the medical profession will take their concerns seriously, and that, after careful deliberation, elective amputation of their troubling limb is a real possibility.[57]

It's not just talk. While intentionally disabling a patient as a "treatment" is probably illegal, a few outlaw doctors and mental health professionals have already disabled their BIID patients. For example, one psychologist reportedly destroyed a woman's vision by administering toxic chemicals into her eyes because she identified as blind.[58]

Needless to say, transhumanists support brain implants and other measures taken to "improve" intelligence (not the ability to love, I notice), including the ludicrous notion of uploading individual human consciousnesses into computers. And, of course, in keeping with the transhumanism's desperate materialist yearning for a corporeal eternal life, Munkittrick says we will know we are in a transhumanist world when the average age exceeds 120.

Things go downhill steeply from there. Shades of *Brave New World* and *Gattaca*—transhumanism would remove intimacy from reproduction and female child bearing. Dripping with eugenics values, Munkittrick expects future children to come into being via IVF or cloning technologies that will permit "genetic modification, health screening, and, eventually synthetic wombs" to allow "the child with the best possibility of a good life to be born."[59] (Somewhere, Joseph Fletcher is smiling.)

At the same time, freedom to have children would be legally constrained. Rather than anyone being allowed to "accidentally spawn a whelp"[60]—the disgusting metaphor is not accidental—our future transhumanist masters would require "parental licensing" before one could cause a child to be brought into the world. Thus, state control and official permitting over human manufacturing—including custom design, special order, quality and inventory control—are core goals of the transhumanist social revolution.

Transhumanism foresees doctors as mere order takers and an anything-goes public morality around personal recreationalism (to borrow a term from Leon Kass) that would be sanctioned by the state. Munkittrick writes:

> Actions such as abortion, assisted suicide, voluntary amputation, gen-
> der reassignment, surrogate pregnancy, body modification, legal unions
> among adults of any number, and consenting sexual practices would be
> protected under law. One's genetic make-up, neurological composition,
> prosthetic augmentation, and other cybernetic modifications will be
> limited only by technology and one's own discretion. Transhumanism
> cannot happen without a legal structure that allows individuals to
> control their own bodies. When bodily freedom is as protected and
> sanctified as free speech, transhumanism will be free to develop.[61]

Needless to say, creating such a society foresees the destruction of human exceptionalism, which transhumanists disdain as limiting their genetic ambitions and re-establishing behavioral norms. Thus, being human in a transhumanist world would be morally irrelevant. Rather, Munkittrick writes, "Rights discourse will shift to personhood instead of common humanity."[62] Hello, Peter Singer!

In a transhuman milieu, the value of human life would become relative. "Animals (including humans)," Munkittrick writes—deploying yet another human-diminishing sentiment—"will be granted rights based on varying degrees of personhood.... When African grey parrots, gorillas, and dolphins have the same rights as a human toddler, a transhuman friendly rights system will be in place."[63]

Transhumanism is a long way from being attained, and the technology the movement envisions will bring in the post-human nirvana is still a long way off, if it ever can be developed. But that doesn't mean we won't become crassly transhumanist in our personal and societal values. If we are going to preserve a culture founded on the Judeo/Christian ideal of equal human dignity and the obligation for individual behavioral restraint, transhumanism must be resisted intellectually and rejected, both in our public policies and the ways in which we lead our personal lives.

Meanwhile, scientists are beginning to tinker seriously with genetic engineering of progeny, which is also a transhumanist goal. As we have already noted, the first human clones have been created. Meanwhile, scientists in China have successfully "edited" the genomic makeup of human embryos, a prelude to germline genetic engineering that would fix any changes down the generations.[64] The United Kingdom—and soon, perhaps, the USA—has authorized IVF using genetically modified eggs to create "three parent" embryos[65]—using health as the pretext but pointing toward the use of biotechnologies to engineer the human genome and enable the creation of novel family forms.

These nascent breakthroughs threaten a new eugenics, which, unlike the old form, will have sharp technological teeth. Which brings us back to the wisdom of Leon R. Kass. While "revulsion is not argument," he argues that in "crucial cases" repugnance is "the emotional expression of deep wisdom beyond reason's power to fully articulate it."[66]

Some reply that these technologies are "inevitable," that "resistance is futile." I reject such pessimism. We are not mere flotsam and jetsam floating on a troubled sea. We (still) have free will. We can decide the kind of future we want. That's part of what makes us human.

REMEMBER: WORDS MATTER

The lexicon we adopt and the terminology we employ not only reflect our values but help define them as well. For example, the use of pejoratives to describe racial minorities casts a bright light on the mind-set of the speaker or writer. When utilized in advocacy speech, words have even more power. That is why so much energy is spent in political debates attempting to define terms. Polemicists know that the side that sets the definitions generally wins the debate.

Words and phrases have power to diminish and degrade human dignity to the point that some people become a "them" rather than an "us." A classic example of this is the term "vegetable" to describe people with serious cognitive disability or persistent unconsciousness. No human being is a cucumber or a carrot. To describe defenseless human beings in that dismissive and disrespectful way is to remove them from their community and expose them to the worst forms of oppression and exploitation—as this book illustrates.

At the same time, it is important that our language be precise and descriptive, particularly when describing issues of life and death. Euphemisms have the power to suck truth out of debate and argument, to transform the odious into the commonplace. Thus, over the years, euthanasia advocates have searched for words and phrases that obscure rather than clarify the hard acts they propose to legalize, and organizations that once called themselves "euthanasia societies" renamed themselves to use soothing words, such as "compassion" or "dignity," and the language of rights, such as "choice," in their names and polemics. For example, the Euthanasia Society of America morphed into the Society for the Right to Die, finally becoming the now-defunct Choice in Dying. Assisted suicide is renamed "aid in dying," a vague misnomer that misappropriates the caring values of hospice rather than accurately describes the deadly ethics of Jack Kevorkian.

This truth is well known by people who promote death as an answer to medical difficulty. The Dutch euthanasia practitioner Dr. M. A. M. de Wachter, the ethicist/director for the Institute of Health in the Netherlands, made this point explicitly when he appeared at a 1990 international euthanasia society convention. "The definitions build the road to euthanasia," he stated. True, "euthanasia is the intentional ending of the life of another … it is always a question of terminating human life." But describing mercy killing even by the euphemism of euthanasia (good death) harms the cause because people naturally recoil from the killing act. Thus, de Wachter urged his audience to prevaricate and obfuscate, telling them, "Definitions are not neutral. They are not just the innocent tools that allow us to describe reality. Rather, they shape our perceptions of reality. They select. They emphasize. They embody a bias. Therefore, definitions constantly need redefinition."[67] This is precisely why the assisted suicide advocacy organization Compassion and Choices changed its name from the more honest Hemlock Society and deployed the euphemism "aid in dying" in its media and advocacy materials.

In these postmodern times, language as an accurate conveyor of ideas is under constant assault. Knowing this, we must strive to keep our language precise and descriptive, particularly when it comes to life and death. We should be vigilant against words that dehumanize weak and vulnerable people and, at the same time, we should be suspicious of rhetoric that masks a movement's goals behind a façade of euphemistic obfuscation. This is not a call for political correctness or a brief for censorship. It is a warning to be wary of the words that function as honey to make the hemlock go down.

LEARN FROM THE DISABLED COMMUNITY

Carol J. Gill, a psychologist and assistant professor in the Department of Disability and Human Development at the University of Illinois at Chicago, told me, "Disability culture has much to share with society."[68] Gill, who has studied disability culture for many years in her work with disability rights organizations and independent living centers, has identified what she calls the "core values" of disability culture.

Among those that Gill has identified are "an acceptance of human differences," a "matter-of-fact orientation toward helping other people," a recognition that "vulnerability is a part of life," and "a flexible, adaptive approach to tasks" with great emphasis on "creativity and untraditional modes of operating" to make up for limited resources and experience. And while disabled people are as diverse as the rest of society, according to Gill, disability culture has "developed a heritage that circumvents differences, encourages mutual support, and underscores our common values." In other words, the experiences that disabled people share often trump the conflicts that might otherwise be generated by differences in economic status, race, gender, sexual orientation, etc. (although Gill worries that there is insufficient racial diversity in some disability organizations).

Some people believe that the key ingredient that has forged disability culture is the discrimination that disabled people often face. However, Gill believes that far more is involved than a reaction to perceived oppression.

> I perceive that disability culture rose from our need to negotiate the vicissitudes of life differently than able-bodied people. Our strategies for surviving and thriving in difficult circumstances, the unique ways in which we interpret and transmit facts and ideas, the intense emotional connection we experience whenever we are able to come together, whether in hospital wards, special schools, charity camps, demonstrations, hotel corridors at disability conferences, or even in jail. All of this and more has resulted in our developing a remarkably unified worldview.[69]

Let's think deeply about what it might mean were the broader society to emulate the equality-of-life-enhancing values that are inherent in disability culture. Gone would be any implication or insinuation that people who need care are "burdens" or that there can ever be something as odious as a "duty to die." The bioethical hierarchy of human life would cease to exist: people would be judged upon the content of their character rather than by the supposed "quality" of their lives.

AFFIRM THE VALUE OF LIFE

In researching and writing this book—both in its first and present iterations—I have detected a subversive, if unstated, theme in bioethics' embrace of the quality-of-life ethic: Our love for each other as fellow human beings should be conditional. The constant message of the new "do harm" medicine is that some of us deserve greater care and concern than do others, that culling based physical, mental, and cognitive invidious distinctions is sometimes necessary, and that this need should be established in our health care policies, medical ethics, and moral expectations about family caregiving obligations.

There is little doubt that these attitudes are distorting public perceptions of our mutual interpersonal and community responsibilities. I recall being very disturbed more than twenty years ago by an article in the *Wall Street Journal* written by a woman named Lucette Lagnado, who reported on the difficulties she experienced when she brought her mother home to care for her during the last two years of the elder woman's life. It wasn't the travails and difficulties of caregiving that upset Lagnado; it was the negative reaction of her friends and her mother's doctors to her loving devotion. She wrote, "In the two years I cared for Mom at home, if friends didn't make me feel that I was somehow mishandling—even wasting—my life, then the professionals did.... Forced to rely on a battery of neurologists, cardiologists, gastroenterologists and pulmonologists ... I learned to steel myself for that cold look, the shake of the head that meant there wasn't much hope for her, so why bother?" One doctor even yelled at Lagnado. "What was I doing keeping a sick mother at home, he thundered. Posing a question as loaded as it was insidious, he asked: 'Is she really alive?'"[70]

What has happened to us that a daughter's loving kindness toward her elderly mother generates hostility and derision? Perhaps Lagnado's friends and doctors were truly worried that Lagnado was letting life pass her by. Maybe Lagnado's altruism made them feel guilty about family issues in their own lives. Or perhaps it reflected a growing ethos aided and abetted by mainstream bioethics—negative attitudes that I believe have worsened since she penned her lament—that people should not be expected to sacrifice for people with "poor" qualities of life. That burdensome people have a moral duty to die was certainly John Hardwig's thesis, a point he made quite explicit when discussing how my wife and I cared for my mother during her recuperation from hip replacement surgery. Hardwig agreed that was my moral responsibility because it was a short-term commitment. "But suppose your mother has Alzheimer's and wants you to take care of her for six years," Hardwig then said. "Could you drop what you are doing to accomplish that?"

"But she spent eighteen years raising me," I replied. "Don't I have an obligation to her?"

"Sure," he said. "But the question is, does she have an obligation to you? I would feel very strongly that if I were your mother, I would not want to ruin your life." He then explained his duty-to-die position further: "I don't think somebody has a duty to die so their family can go to Europe. But suppose your mother needed care in your home for six years, around the clock. She wanders, gets upset if strangers take care of her. That's the end of your consumer advocacy" [referring to my previous work with Ralph Nader]. "That's the end of your writing. You probably can't pick that up later. That's the end of your career. You could still work but probably not in the areas that really interest you. If I were your mother, I wouldn't want to do that to you."

"At that point, then, you are talking about assisted suicide or euthanasia?" I asked.

"Well, maybe an unassisted suicide," Hardwig replied.[71]

Now, nearly twenty years later, as I write these words, my mother is ninety-eight—with Alzheimer's. When I interviewed Hardwig, she was vital and independent. Today, she is frail, uses a walker, is very forgetful, has pronounced visual impairments, can barely hear, and *refuses* to use a hearing aid, requiring me to loudly repeat myself continually—very irritating. And while she is remarkably still able to live near me on her own—approved by the appropriate geriatric professionals that assessed her circumstances—she could not do so without our continual involvement in almost every decision and action she takes, supplemented by a wonderful senior caregiving service. It is true: I *have* curtailed some of my professional and recreational activities for her. There are fewer hours in the day for me to write. My wife and I take shorter vacations. Being with her on a continual and ongoing basis can be very tiring—and sometimes exhausting. As I write these words, matters look to be worsening. Moreover, she *would* want to die if she believed she was "ruining" my life. She's not, of course, and even if she were, I would never tell her. She's my mother! How selfish would I be to cast her needs aside so I could do more of what I wanted?

Hardwig and others, whose ideas underpin the culture of death, miss so much of the point of being human: Our individual worth is far greater than a mere measurement of the quantifiable measurements of our lives. Life is so much more than utilitarian rationalizations and outcome balancing tests. Providing loving care for people whom some regard as "burdens" may be the most humanly important endeavors we ever undertake.

That certainly is what my friend Tom Lorentzen discovered after he walked away from a very successful career in government in Washington, DC to care for his dying mother in California—the very act that bioethics utilitarian ideologues finds so abhorrent. In the first edition of this book, I asked Tom how his adventure in selfless love began. He replied,

I was visiting my mother over the Labor Day Weekend in September of 1991. I stayed with my mother, and as I was getting ready to leave for the airport, she stood out on the front porch and hugged me. I could tell that she was aging more rapidly and that her health was beginning to deteriorate. I knew she was having some early stages of kidney failure. I said, "Mom, I hope you are going to be okay." She said, "If I need you, I know you will know what to do." That was different than anything else she had ever said to me.... For the next few months, we would speak on the phone at least twice a week. Then came mid-November and Mother developed some bleeding in her stool. She became quite frightened. A friend came over and stayed with her because she was so afraid. I called her. She was so scared, she could hardly talk.... I spoke with some of my friends at the Small Business Administration [where I then worked as a political appointee]. One friend in particular came to see me, Aileen, and she told me, "Tom, you have to go. You only get one mother. If she needs you, you have to go." Another friend came in who a few years earlier had taken care of her brother who died of AIDS. She told me that there are things more important than work and if your mother needs you, you have to go…. Those two conversations made up my mind. I called the airport and made plans to fly out to mom the next morning.

This involved no small sacrifice. "I had a great run at the SBA," he recalls. "I had a girlfriend who I loved. I loved my dog. I was being paid better than I ever had in my life. I had a condominium with a great view of the Capitol." Still, Tom decided his mother needed him in California more than he needed his life in Washington, DC. He took a less remunerative and prestigious job in San Francisco and never looked back.

But why give up such a happy life? I inquired. Surely you could have paid someone to watch over your mom or brought her back to Washington. Tom said,

I knew she would hate that. And certain things were clicking with me. I had promised my dad before he died that I would always take care of my mother. Plus, my parents always dealt with people who were ill or dying in a very caring and responsible manner. It was a way of life. I remember my mother sitting with the wife of a friend of my father's, who was dying of cancer. And she would sit there with the lady and keep her company and hold her hand. And I remember my mother saying that she didn't know why the lady wanted my mother to visit because they were not close friends, but my mother said that it was important to do it because the lady was dying of cancer and she needed love.

"Was caring for your mother difficult?" I wanted to know. He said,

Very. I would sleep in the room next to her. She had real trouble sleeping and I was often up at night holding her and talking with her. When I got discouraged, I would think about when my mother took care of her mother: it took some of the best years out of her life, and I thought, now that she needs help, what if nobody responded? What an injustice that would be. I was the only one who could give her some justice and show her that there was caring and compassion and love for her. And I wanted to keep my promise to my dad. It was what I wanted to do because it was the right thing to do.

After his mother died, Tom's career was in tatters. I asked him whether he had any regrets. He replied,

> There are more important things than jobs and careers. The truly important things in life are doing what is right and one should not measure success by the outward appearances of money, jobs, fame. I can't imagine turning my back on my mother. I was fortunate that I could do it. It wasn't easy. In fact, it was real hard. But it was the right thing to do. I can't quite imagine what it would be like to turn my back on a loved one in need. I don't know how to address that in my mind.... After it was all over, I felt a peace and enrichment I had never experienced before in my life. As my mother was placed in the crypt next to my dad, I looked up at where he was and my mom now was, and I felt the type of peace that I will never feel again in my life. I was so grateful that I was able to do what I did. I was grateful for good parents and a good life. Those days changed me forever. They were very spiritual days.[72]

In the years since that interview, Tom and I have remained good friends and golfing buddies. His career was off the rails for several years; he was, for a time, a struggling entrepreneur in Las Vegas, and then he had a relatively unsuccessful run as a fundraiser for a nonprofit botanical center. But he closed strong, spending the last few years of President George W. Bush's presidency as the regional director of Region IX at the US Department of Health & Human Services.

Mostly retired, Tom is now a consultant on health care issues, serves on a couple of nonprofit boards, and does volunteer work. I asked him, "Looking back, knowing the uncertainty and the financial and social difficulties you endured—do you have any regrets?" His answer was unequivocal:

> None. Nor did I ever have any. It has been nearly twenty-five years since I left my home and career to take care of my ailing mother. I took care of her in the house she loved for seven months. It was not easy. She passed in my arms after a final conversation. I had done all I could do for her and kept my promise to my late father. The great sense of loss and total emptiness was replaced within minutes with a sense of

enrichment. During her final year I gave her love, loyalty, justice, and meaning. I was now emancipated and enriched—not financially or professionally, but as a person.

"But wasn't there a high cost?" I asked. He said,

Sure. After my mother passed it took a number of years for my life to come together again, both professionally and personally. Eventually, however, both did. My sixties have been the best decade of my life....
More importantly, however, is what I have felt inside. I feel very rich. Although I gave up a lot to take care of her, I received far more in return. Quite often I tell friends that I am a very rich man. Indeed, I think I am perhaps richer than Bill Gates. He has a lot of money, but I have a lot of wealth in terms of more important things that involve loyalty, love, gratitude, altruism, benevolence, and commitment. That is true wealth. I know who I am and what I have done and have absolutely no regrets. If I had to do it over again, even knowing the problems I had, I absolutely would.[73]

Love is not a perpetual motion machine. It needs constant renewal to retain its vitality and sometimes the commitment of extraordinary devotion and sacrifice of the kind demonstrated so beautifully and profoundly by Lucette Lagnado and Tom Lorentzen. And while it is true that most people would be unable to devote themselves so radically to caregiving, having other family responsibilities or financial concerns, shouldn't these examples of selflessness be the models we emulate—and toward which we strive—rather than the growing abandoning ethic of the overcrowded boat?

If we are to defeat the culture of death that has enshrouded our medical and moral worlds during the last generation, we need not be reactionaries striving to restore the old order. Rather, we must move confidently toward democratically steering society toward a better approach. Toward that end, we must create a vibrant, robust, and influential school of bioethics that can effectively challenge the utilitarian school in all venues in which it operates. Such a "human rights bioethics" would analyze and boldly propose public health care policies based upon the foundational belief that each of us is equal, wanted, and loved, that there is no such thing as "them"—only "us."

Under a revitalized Hippocratic tradition, doctors' exclusive loyalty would remain with each patient as individuals, not to patient groups, HMOs, or society. Our commitment to the "patient as a person" would prevent very ill and dying patients from being hooked up to machines against their will. The dead donor rule would be reemphasized to assure a wary public that organ donors will always be truly dead before their gifts of life are ever procured. The siren temptation to participate in assisted suicide as a medical professional or patient, or attending such a death as a family member or friend, would be resisted, and hospice would be reformed to further reduce or eliminate suffering without eliminating the *sufferer*. We would reject health care rationing while redoubling our efforts to make health care accessible to those who are currently under-served. In short, our public health care policies and medical protocols would be grounded in a granite-like adherence to the sanctity and equality of each human life.

Is such a system possible today? It won't be easy—and I am less optimistic than I was when this book was first published, but I remain convinced it can be done. The fog is lifting. People are beginning to clearly see the jagged shoals toward which we are steaming. It's not too late to change course. We are not—yet—beyond the point of no return.

Whatever our moral future—whether based on life's inherent equality or upon invidious judgments based on capacities or subjective notions of quality—that which we sow through our public policies and ethics protocols we surely shall reap in the way in which we and those we love are treated in our individual lives. We all age. We fall ill. We grow weak. We become disabled. As inevitably as the changing of the tides, a day comes when our need to receive from our fellows adds up to far more than our ability to give in return. When we reach that stage of life, will we still be loved, cared for, valued? Will we still be deemed persons entitled to equal protection under the law? These are the questions that will determine the medical morality of the rest of the twenty-first century and beyond.

ENDNOTES

CHAPTER 1

1 Wesley J. Smith, *A Rat Is a Pig Is a Dog Is a Boy: The Human Cost of the Animal Rights Movement* (New York: Encounter Books, 2010).
2 Wesley J. Smith, *Consumer's Guide to a Brave New World* (New York: Encounter Books, 2004).
3 John Campbell, interview with the author, April 29, 1999.
4 Sheryl Gay Stolberg, "Study Finds Elderly Receive Little Pain Treatment in Nursing Homes," *New York Times*, June 17, 1998.
5 Source: California Nurses Association.
6 Ted Robbins, "Arizona Budget Cuts Put Organ Transplants at Risk," National Public Radio, November 17, 2010.
7 Tom L. Beauchamp and James F. Childress, *The Principles of Biomedical Ethics*, 4th edition (New York: Oxford University Press, 1994), 3.
8 Joseph Fletcher, *Humanhood: Essays in Biomedical Ethics* (Buffalo, NY: Prometheus Books, 1979), 5.
9 "Bioethics and Its Implications Worldwide for Human Rights Protection," United Nations Educational Scientific and Cultural Organization (UNESCO), 93rd Inter-parliamentary Conference, Madrid, March 1995.
10 Gilbert C. Meilaender, *Body, Soul, and Bioethics* (Notre Dame, IN: University of Notre Dame Press), 7.
11 Albert R. Jonsen, *The Birth of Bioethics* (New York: Oxford University Press, 1998), 372.
12 See, for example, Matthew K. Wynia and Arthur Derse, "Culture of Death: The Assault on Medical Ethics in America," (book review), *Medscape*, September 4, 2001, http://www.medscape.com/viewarticle/408168.
13 Albert R. Jonsen, "The Birth of Bioethics," *Hastings Center Report* (Special Supplement) (Nov.-Dec. 1993): S8 S4.
14 Alexander M. Capron, "Lessons from Ethics," Ethics, Equity, and Health for All, CIOMS Twenty-ninth Conference, Geneva, 1997.
15 Capron, "Lessons from Ethics," S1.
16 Daniel Callahan, "Why America Accepted Bioethics," *Hastings Center Report* (Special Supplement) (Nov.–Dec. 1993): S8.
17 Leon R. Kass, MD, interview with the author, February 9, 1999.

18 Renée C. Fox, PhD, interview with the author, January 5, 1999.
19 *Human Lives: Critical Essays on Consequentialist Bioethics*, eds. David S. Oderberg and Jacqueline A. Laing (New York: St. Martin's Press, 1997), 2.
20 Renée C. Fox and Judith P. Swazey, "Medical Morality Is Not Bioethics," *Bioethics: An Introduction to the History, Methods, and Practice*, eds. Nancy S. Jecker, Albert R. Jonsen, Robert A. Pearlman (Sudbury, MA: Jones and Bartlett Publishers, 1997), 249–250.
21 Howard L. Kaye, *The Social Meaning of Modern Biology: From Social Darwinism to Sociobiology*, 2nd edition (New Brunswick, NY: Transaction Publishers, 1997).
22 Howard L. Kaye, PhD, interview with the author, January 23, 1999.
23 Chris Mooney, "Irrationalist in Chief," *The American Prospect* 12, no. 17 (Sept. 24, 2001).
24 Glenn McGee, "The Wisdom of Leon Kass," *American Journal of Bioethics* 3, no. 3 (2003): vii–viii.
25 Fox interview.
26 Richard John Neuhaus, "The Return of Eugenics," *Commentary* (Apr. 1988): 19.
27 For example, see *Cruzan v. Director, Missouri Department of Health*, 110 Supreme Court, 2841, 1990.
28 For example, see Robert D. Truog et al., "The Dead-Donor Rule and the Future of Organ Donation," *New England Journal of Medicine* 369 (Oct. 3, 2013): 1287–1289, www.nejm.org/doi/full/10.1056/NEJMp1307220.
29 Kass interview.
30 "A New Ethic for Medicine and Society," editorial, *California Medicine* 113, no. 3 (Sept. 1970): 67–68.
31 Fletcher, *Humanhood*, from the introduction by Thomas H. Hunter, MD, xii, first published in *Hastings Center Report* (Hastings on Hudson, New York: Institute of Society, Ethics, and Life Sciences, 1973), 47–58.
32 "'O Brave New World': Rationality in Reproduction," in *Birth to Death: Science and Bioethics*, eds. Albert R. Jonsen, David C. Thomasma and Thomasine Kushner, 50.
33 Fletcher, *Humanhood*, 85.
34 Ibid., 11.
35 Ibid., 12.
36 Ibid., 12.
37 Ibid., 12–16.
38 Ibid., 16–17.
39 Ibid., 16–17.
40 Joseph Fletcher, "Being Happy, Being Human," *Humanist* 35, no. 1 (Jan. 1975): 47–58, as republished in *Humanhood*.
41 Fletcher, "Being Happy," 22.
42 Ibid., 20.
43 Joseph Fletcher, "Infanticide and the Ethics of Loving Concern," *Infanticide and the Value of Life*, ed. Marvin Kohl (Buffalo, NY: Prometheus Books, 1978), 13–22, as republished in *Humanhood*, 144.
44 Joseph Fletcher, "New Definitions of Death," *Prism*, American Medical Association (Jan. 1974): 13–14, 36, as republished in *Humanhood*, 159–165.
45 Joseph Fletcher, "Fetal Research, an Ethical Appraisal," in Appendix: Research on the Fetus (Washington, DC: National Commission for the Protection of

Health, Education and Welfare Publication No (OS) 76-1888, 1975), 3-1-3-14, as republished in *Humanhood*.

46 Joseph Fletcher, "The Ethical Aspects of Genetic Controls," *New England Journal of Medicine* (Sept. 30, 1971): 776–783, republished in *Humanhood*, 85.

47 Paul Ramsey, "Preface to the Patient as a Person," as published in eds. William Werpehowski and Stephen D. Crocco, *The Essential Paul Ramsey: A Collection* (New Haven, CT: Yale University Press, 1994), 170.

48 From the essay "Justice and Equal Treatment," as published in *The Essential Ramsey*, 250.

49 Ibid., 248.

50 Meilaender, *Body, Soul, and Bioethics*, 44.

51 Peter Singer, *Practical Ethics*, 2nd edition (Cambridge, UK: Cambridge University Press, 1993), 87.

52 Singer, *Practical Ethics*, 132.

53 Peter Singer, *Rethinking Life and Death: The Collapse of Our Traditional Ethics* (New York: St. Martin's Press, 1994), 220.

54 Bettina Schone-Seifert and Klaus-Peter Rippe, "Silencing the Singer: Antibioethics in Germany" (Nov.–Dec. 1991): 20–26.

55 John Harris, "The Concept of the Person and the Value of Life," *Kennedy Institute of Ethics Journal* 9, no. 4 (Dec. 1999): 304, 307.

56 Tom Beauchamp, "The Failure of Theories of Personhood," *Kennedy Institute of Ethics Journal* 9 (1999): 309–324, 320.

57 Alasdair Cochrane, "Undignified Bioethics," *Bioethics* (Dec. 2009): 234–241, 236, http://onlinelibrary.wiley.com/doi/10.1111/j.1467-8519.2009.01781.x/pdf.

58 Cochrane, "Undignified Bioethics," 237.

59 Ibid., 241.

60 Ronald Dworkin, *Life's Dominion: An Argument about Abortion, Euthanasia, and Individual Freedom* (New York: Vintage Books, 1993).

61 Dworkin, *Life's Dominion*, 238.

62 Ibid., 93.

63 Ibid., 87.

64 Leon R. Kass, MD, "Death with Dignity and the Sanctity of Life," *Commentary* (Mar. 1990): 35.

65 Meilaender, *Body, Soul, and Bioethics*, 5.

66 "The Hippocratic Oath: Text, Translation and Interpretation." *Bulletin of the History of Medicine*, S1, (Baltimore, MD: Johns Hopkins Press, 1943), as published on the University of Chicago website, Chicago, IL.

67 Dianne N. Irving, PhD, interview with the author, May 7, 1999.

68 H. Tristram Englehardt, Jr. "Bioethics in the Third Millennium: Some Critical Anticipations," *Kennedy Institute of Ethics Journal* 9, no. 3 (Sept. 1999): 227.

69 Robert D. Orr, MD, Norman Pang, MD, Edmund D. Pellegrino, MD, and Mark Siegler, MD, "Use of the Hippocratic Oath: A Review of Twentieth-century Practice and a Content Analysis of Oaths Administered in Medical Schools in the US and Canada in 1993," *Journal of Clinical Ethics* 8, no. 4 (Winter 1997): 377–387.

70 Orr et al., "Use of the Hippocratic Oath," 385.

71 Sherwin Nuland, "Physician-Assisted Suicide and Euthanasia in Practice," *New England Journal of Medicine* (Feb. 24, 2000).

72 Edmund D. Pellegrino, "The Metamorphosis of Medical Ethics: A Thirty-Year Retrospective," *Journal of the American Medical Association* (Mar. 3, 1993): 1159.

73 Pellegrino, "The Metamorphosis of Medical Ethics," 1159.

74 Beauchamp and Childress, *Principles*, 25.

75 Ibid., 189.

76 Fletcher, *Humanhood*, 18.

77 Callahan, "Why America Accepted Bioethics," S8.

78 Dan Block, "Voluntary Active Euthanasia," *Hastings Center Report*, 19.

79 Beauchamp and Childress, *Principles*, 62.

80 Patricia O'Brien, "Cold Look at Right to Die Gives Off Ghastly Chill," *St. Paul Sunday Pioneer Press*, August 28, 1993.

81 James W. Walters, *What Is a Person?: An Ethical Exploration* (Chicago: University of Illinois Press, 1997), 10.

82 Dame Cicely Saunders, interview with the author, December 8, 1998.

83 Saunders interview.

84 David Clark, "Originating a Movement: Cicely Saunders and the Development of St. Christopher's Hospice, 1957–1967," *Mortality* 3, no. 1 (1998): 46.

85 Sheryl Gay Stolberg, "Dame Cicely Saunders: Reflections on a Life of Treating the Dying," *New York Times*, May 11, 1999.

86 Stolberg, "Dame Cecily Saunders."

87 Clark, "Originating a Movement," 48.

88 Ibid.

89 Ibid.

90 Saunders interview.

91 Jeremiah A. Barondess, MD, "Care of the Medical Ethos: Reflections on Social Darwinism, Racial Hygiene, and the Holocaust," *Annals of Internal Medicine* (Dec. 1, 1998): 896.

92 Renée C. Fox and Judith P. Swazey, "Medical Morality Is Not Bioethics—Medical Ethics in China and the United States," *Perspectives in Biology and Medicine* (Spring 1984): 355.

93 Fox interview.

94 Kass interview.

95 Daniel Callahan, "Bioethics: Private Choice and Common Good," *Hastings Center Report* (May–June 1994): 28.

96 Callahan, "Bioethics: Private Choice," 31.

97 Anne Maclean, *The Elimination of Morality: Reflections on Utilitarianism and Bioethics* (London: Rutledge, 1993), 9.

98 Keown interview.

99 Fox and Swazey, "Medical Morality Is Not Bioethics," 356.

100 Wikipedia, "Utilitarian Bioethics," http://en.wikipedia.org/wiki/Utilitarian_bioethics.

101 Maclean, *Elimination of Morality*, 10.

102 Fletcher, *Humanhood*, 24.

103 Singer, *Practical Ethics*, 14.

104 Ibid.

105 Maclean, *The Elimination of Morality*.

106 Ibid., 99, quoting John Harris, "The Survival Lottery," in ed. Peter Singer's, *Applied Ethics* (Oxford, UK: Oxford University Press, 1986).

107 Jonsen et al., *Clinical Ethics*, 108.

108 Peter Singer, *Rethinking Life and Death*, 191.

109 Diane Coleman, interview with the author, February 16, 1999.

110 Ibid.

111 Peter J. Neumann and Milton C. Weinstein, "Legislating against Use of Cost-Effectiveness Information," *New England Journal of Medicine* 010, no. 363 (Oct. 14, 2010): 1495–1497, http://www.nejm.org/doi/full/10.1056/NEJMp1007168?ssource=hcrc.

112 Pellegrino, "Metamorphosis," 1160.

113 Beauchamp and Childress, *Principles*, 38.

114 Ibid.

115 Ibid.

116 K. K. Fung, "Dying for Money: Overcoming Moral Hazard in Terminal Illnesses through Compensated Physician-assisted Death," *American Journal of Economics and Sociobiology* 52, no. 3 (July 1993): 285.

117 Fung, "Dying for Money," 287.

118 Maclean, *The Elimination of Morality*, 3.

CHAPTER 2

1 *Buck v. Bell*, 274 US 200 (1927), 207.

2 Daniel V. Kelves, *In the Name of Eugenics: Genetics and the Uses of Human Heredity* (Cambridge, MA: Harvard University Press, 1985), 110.

3 Kelves, *In the Name of Eugenics*, 112.

4 "Three Generations of Imbeciles Is Enough," editorial, *Detroit News*, December 16, 1992.

5 Statement of the Board of Directors of the American Society of Human Genetics: Eugenics and the Misuse of Genetic Information to Restrict Reproductive Freedom, October 1998.

6 See, for example, Wesley J. Smith, "Transhumanism's Eugenic Authoritarianism," *Human Exceptionalism* (blog), *National Review Online*, August 15, 2014, http://www.nationalreview.com/human-exceptionalism/385496/transhumanisms-eugenics-authoritarianism-wesley-j-smith.

7 Kelves, *In the Name of Eugenics*, 4.

8 Ibid., xii.

9 Ibid., 10.

10 Kelves, *In the Name of Eugenics*, 89.

11 Diane B. Paul, *Controlling Human Heredity, 1865 to the Present* (Atlantic Highlands, NJ: Humanities Press International, Inc., 1995), 11.

12 Paul, *Controlling Human Heredity*, 8.

13 Kelves, *In the Name of Eugenics*, 77.

14 Ibid., 83.

15 Paul, *Controlling Human Heredity*, 14.

16 Ibid., 88.

17 Ibid., 81, citing A. J. Ochsner, "Surgical Treatment of Habitual Criminals," *Journal of the American Medical Association* (Apr. 1899).

18 Paul, *Controlling Human Heredity*, 81–82.

19 Howard L. Kaye, *The Social Meaning of Modern Biology: From Social Darwinism to Sociobiology* (New Brunswick, NY: Transaction Publishers, 1986, 1997), 12.

20 C. W. Hufeland, "Die Verhaltnisse des Artes," *Journal der Praktishen*

Azznykunde und Wundarzneykunst (1806), 23, as cited in Michael Burleigh, *Death and Deliverance: Euthanasia in Germany, 1900–1945* (New York: Cambridge University Press, 1994), 12.

21 Michael Franzblau, interview with the author, January 20, 1999.

22 Ibid.

23 Karl Binding and Alfred Hoche, "Permitting the Destruction of Life Unworthy of Life: Its Extent and Form" (Leipzig, Germany: Felix Meiner Verlag, 1920), as reprinted in *Issues in Law and Medicine* 8, no. 2 (1992): 231–265.

24 Robert Jay Lifton, *The Nazi Doctors: Medical Killing and the Psychology of Genocide* (New York: Basic Books, 1986), 46.

25 Binding and Hoche, "Permitting the Destruction of Life," as published in *Issues*, 247.

26 Ibid., 260–261.

27 Ibid., 249.

28 Dominick Wilkinson and Julian Savulescu, "Should We Allow Organ Donation Euthanasia? Alternatives for Maximizing the Number of Quality Organs for Donation," *Bioethics* 26, no. 1 (2010): 32–48, http://onlinelibrary.wiley.com/doi/10.1111/j.1467-8519.2010.01811.x/full.

29 Burleigh, *Death and Deliverance, Supra.*, 22–23.

30 *New York Times*, October 3, 1933, as cited by Hugh Gregory Gallagher, *By Trust Betrayed: Physicians and the License to Kill in the Third Reich* (Arlington, VA: Vandamere Press, 1995), 62.

31 Ibid., 27.

32 Dick Sobsey, Anne Donnellan, and Gregor Wolbring, "Reflection on the Holocaust: Where Did It Begin and Has It Really Ended?" *Developmental Disabilities Journal* 22, no. 2 (1994).

33 Richard Sobsey, EdD, interview with the author, January 27, 1999.

34 As quoted in Sobsey et al., "Reflection on the Holocaust, " *Developmental Disabilities Journal, Supra.*

35 "MS Woman Wins Right-to-Die Fight," *BBC*, July 30, 2009, http://news.bbc.co.uk/2/hi/health/8176713.stm.

36 "Debbie Purdy: Right to Die Campaigner, Dies," *BBC*, December 29, 2014, http://www.bbc.com/news/uk-england-leeds-25741005.

37 Franzblau interview.

38 Ibid.

39 As quoted in Lifton, *Nazi Doctors*, 63.

40 Burleigh, *Death and Deliverance*, 125.

41 Ibid., 200.

42 Ibid., 200.

43 Hugh Gregory Gallagher, interview with the author, May 21, 1996.

44 Sobsey et al., "Reflection on the Holocaust."

45 Ibid., 100.

46 Franzblau interview.

47 Michael Franzblau, MD, "Investigate Nazi Ties of German Doctor," *San Francisco Chronicle*, December 29, 1993.

48 Lifton, *Nazi Doctors*, 18.

49 Ibid., 267–414.

50 Michael Franzblau, speech, "German Medicine and Nazism: Lessons for American Physicians?"

51 Lifton, *Nazi Doctors*, 46.
52 Franzblau interview.
53 Leo Alexander, MD, "Medical Science Under Dictatorship," (reprint), *New England Journal of Medicine* (July 14, 1949): 9.
54 Alexander, "Medical Science," 11.
55 Paul Wilkes, "When Do We Have the Right to Die?" *Life*, January 14, 1972.
56 Interview with James D. Watson, "Children From the Laboratory," *Prism* (May 1973): 13.
57 As reported by Pacifica New Service, 1978.
58 C. Everett Koop, "Life and Death and the Handicapped Newborn," *Issues in Law and Medicine* 5, no. 1 (1989), 110.
59 As reported in Peter Singer, *Rethinking Life and Death*, 121–123.
60 As quoted in Koop, "Life and Death," 107.
61 Peter Singer, *Rethinking Life and Death*, 118.
62 C. Mansfield et al., "Termination Rates After Prenatal Diagnosis of Down Syndrome, Spina Bifida, Anencephaly, and Turner and Klinefelter Syndromes: A Systematic Literature Review," *Prenatal Diagnosis*, 19, no. 9 (Sept. 1999): 808–812.
63 Koop, "Life and Death," 112.
64 Joseph Fletcher, "Infanticide," published in *Infanticide and the Ethics of Loving Concern*, (Buffalo, NY: Prometheus Books, 1978), as republished in Fletcher, *Humanhood*, 144.
65 Ibid., 146.
66 Kathryn Federici Greenwood, "Dangerous Words," *Princeton Alumni Weekly*, January 26, 2000.
67 Singer, *Practical Ethics*, 186.
68 Ibid.
69 Singer, *Rethinking Life and Death*, 213–214.
70 Ibid., 215.
71 Lifton, *Nazi Doctors*, 51.
72 Ibid., 115.
73 "Open Minds, Open Hearts, and Fair-Minded Words," A Conference on Life and Choice in the Abortion Debate, Princeton University (panel), October 15–16, 2010, http://uchv.princeton.edu/Life_Choice; Panel II, October 15, from the author's transcription.
74 Jonathan Glover, *Causing Death and Saving Lives* (New York: Penguin Books, 1977), 159.
75 Glover, *Causing Death*, 159.
76 Ibid., 156–158.
77 Udo Schuklenk, "Physicians Can Justifiably Euthanize Certain Severely Impaired Infants," *Journal of Thoracic and Cardiovascular Surgery* S0022-5223, no. 14 (Oct. 12, 2014): ii, http://www.jtcvsonline.org/article/S0022-5223(14)01532-3/abstract.
78 Ibid.
79 Ibid.
80 Alberto Giubilini and Francesca Minerva, "After-Birth Abortion: Why Should the Baby Live?" *Journal of Medical Ethics*, 10.1136/medethics-2011-100411, http://jme.bmj.com/content/early/2012/03/01/medethics-2011-100411.full#aff-3.
81 Ibid.

82 Alberto Giubilini and Francesca Minerva, "An Open Letter from Giubilini and Minerva," *Journal of Medical Ethics Blog*, March 12, 2012, http://blogs.bmj.com/medical-ethics/2012/03/02/an-open-letter-from-giubilini-and-minerva/.

83 Ibid.

84 Agnes van der Heide, Paul J. van der Maas, Gerrit van der Wal, Carmen L. M. de Graaf, John G. Kester, Louis A. A. Koilee, Richard de Leeuw, and Robert A. Holl, "Medical End-of-Life Decisions Made for Neonates and Infants in the Netherlands," *The Lancet*, 350 (July 26, 1997): 251.

85 Astrid M. Vrakking, Agnes van der Heide, et al., "Medical End-of-Life Decisions Made for Neonates and Infants in the Netherlands, 1995-2001," *The Lancet*, 365 (Apr. 9, 2005): 1329–1331.

86 van der Heide, "Medical End-of-Life Decisions," 253.

87 Ibid., 251.

88 Ibid., 253.

89 Ibid., 254.

90 Ibid., 255.

91 Eugene Sutorius, interview with the author, October 17, 1995, as quoted in Wesley J. Smith, *Forced Exit: Euthanasia, Assisted Suicide, and the New Duty to Die* (New York: Encounter Books, 2006), 105.

92 "Dutch Court Says Baby's Euthanasia Justifiable," Reuters, April 26, 1995.

93 "Report of the Dutch Royal Society of Medicine: Life Terminating Actions with Incompetent Patients," Part I, "Severely Handicapped Newborns," *Issues in Law and Medicine* 8, no. 2 (1992).

94 Ibid., 173.

95 Groningen Hospital press release, December 10, 2004.

96 Eduard Verhagen and Pieter J. J. Sauer, "The Groningen Protocol: Euthanasia in Severely Ill Newborns," *New England Journal of Medicine* 352 (Mar. 10, 2005): 959–962.

97 Hilde Lindemann and Marian Verkerk, "Ending the Life of a Newborn: The Groningen Protocol," *Hastings Center Report* (Jan.-Feb. 2008): 43, 42–51.

98 United Nations, "The Universal Declaration of Human Rights," December 10, 1948, http://www.un.org/en/documents/udhr/.

99 "Position of the American Academy of Neurology on Certain Aspects of the Care and Management of the Persistent Vegetative State Patient," *Neurology* 39 (1989).

100 Daniel Callahan, "On Feeding the Dying," *Hastings Center Report* (Oct. 1983): 22.

101 Jonsen, *The Birth of Bioethics*, 259.

102 Fred Rosner, "Withdrawing Fluids and Nutrition: An Alternate View," *New York State Journal of Medicine* (Nov. 1987): 591.

103 *Barber v. Superior Court* (1983), 147 Cal. App. 3d, 1006.

104 *Conservatorship of Drabick* (1988), 200 Cal App. 3d, 185.

105 American Medical Association Council on Ethical and Judicial Affairs, "Opinion 2.15," 1986.

106 *Nancy Beth Cruzan v. Robert Harmon et al.* (1988), 760 SW 2nd 408.

107 Patricia Wen, "Girl With Damage to Brain is Sent to Rehab Center, *Boston Globe*, January 27, 2006.

108 Patricia Wen, "Missed Warning Signs Nearly Killed Haleigh Poutre," *Boston Globe*, July 6, 2008.

109 Patricia Wen, "New Life for Haleigh," *Boston Globe*, August 3, 2014.
110 "The Larry King Show," *CNN*, October 27, 2003.
111 Wesley J. Smith, "The Interview That Wasn't," *Weekly Standard* (blog), October 28, 2003, http://www.weeklystandard.com/Content/Public/Articles/000/000/003/306hhsrh.asp.
112 Some of the following material first appeared in Smith, *Forced Exit*, 65–76.
113 In the Circuit Court of Pinellas County, Florida, Probate Division, *In re Guardianship of Theresa Schiavo, an Incapacitated Person*, Case No. 90-2908BGD-003, Report of Guardian *Ad Litem*, Richard L. Pearse, December 29, 1998 (hereafter Trial Court Case).
114 Trial Court Case, Report of Guardian *Ad Litem*.
115 Ibid.
116 Ibid.
117 Trial Court Case, Order of Court, February 11, 2000: "The court is mystified as to how these present tense verbs would have been used some six years after the death of Karen Ann Quinlan."
118 Florida Statutes, Chapter 2003-418.
119 Jay Wolfson, Ph.D., J.D. "A Report to Governor Jeb Bush and the Sixth Judicial Circuit in the Matter of Theresa Marie Schiavo, December 1, 2003, 31.
120 There is a widespread impression that Governor Jeb Bush appointed Wolfson as Terri's guardian. He did not. Under Terri's Law, the guardian was to be court appointed.
121 *Bush v. Schiavo*, Supreme Court of Florida, Case No. SC04-925, September 23, 2004.
122 Terri Schiavo Incapacitated Protection Bill, filed March 25 2005, https://www.govtrack.us/congress/bills/109/s686/text.
123 https://www.govtrack.us/congress/votes/109-2005/h90.
124 Theresa Marie Schiavo et al., vs. Michael Schiavo et al., "Order," Case Number 8:05-CV-530-T-27TBM, March 22, 2005.
125 Bobby Schindler, interview with the author, February 25, 2015.
126 Jon R. Thogmartin, MD, "In re Theresa Marie Schiavo, deceased," medical examiner case number 5050439, June 8, 2005.
127 Lenny Bernstein, "What It's Like to Die of Thirst," *Washington Post*, August 7, 2014, http://www.washingtonpost.com/news/to-your-health/wp/2014/08/07/what-its-like-to-die-of-thirst/.
128 Many wonder what happened to the participants who lived through such an agonizing drama. Schiavo married the mother of his children and now lives quietly with his family in Florida. Bob Schindler never recovered from the death of his daughter. His blood pressure soared in its aftermath, and he died from complications of a stroke in 2009. Mary, Bobby, and sister Suzanne created the Terri Schiavo Life and Hope Network, a nonprofit organization centered in Philadelphia that assists families in the throes of the kind of awful legal and media crucibles they experienced.
129 William F. Stone, interview with the author, August 27, 1996.
130 In the Guardianship of Edna M.F., (1997) 210 Wis. 2d, 557: 556.
131 Medical records of Michael Martin, New Medico Neurological Center of Michigan, "Augmentation Evaluation Summary," April 19, 1992.
132 Ibid.
133 Dr. Kreitsch medical report, October 13, 1992.

134   Ibid.

135   Andrew J. Broder and Ronald E. Cranford, "'Mary, Mary, Quite Contrary, How Was I to Know?' Michael Martin, Absolute Prescience, and the Right to Die in Michigan," *University of Detroit Mercy Law Review* 72 (1995): 756–852.

136   *In re Michael Martin*, 538 N.W. 2d 399 (Mich. 1995).

137   *In re the Conservatorship of Robert Wendland*, Superior Court of California, County of San Joaquin, Case No. 65669, testimony of Rose Wendland.

138   Ibid.

139   Ibid., testimony of Dr. Ernest Bryant.

140   *In re the Conservatorship of Robert Wendland*, Court of Appeal of the State of California, Third Appellate District, Case No. Civil C-029439, "Appellant Robert Wendland's Opening Brief," 30.

141   *Wendland*, Superior Court, Trial Record.

142   Gillian Graig, MD, FRCP, "Palliative Care from the Perspective of a Consultant Geriatrician: The Dangers of Withholding Hydration," *Ethics and Medicine* 15, no. 1 (1999): 16.

143   William J. Burke, interview with the author, 1996, as quoted in Wesley J. Smith, *Forced Exit: Euthanasia, Assisted Suicide, and the New Duty to Die* (New York: Encounter Books, 1996), 75.

144   *Wendland*, Testimony of Dr. Ronald Cranford.

145   Ibid.

146   *Wendland*, "Bifurcated Decision: Findings of Fact and Conclusions of Law."

147   "Conservatorship of Robert Wendland," California Supreme Court, 26 Cal. 4th 522.

148   Thaddeus Mason Pope and Amanda West, "Legal Briefing: Voluntary Stop Eating and Drinking," *Journal of Clinical Ethics* 25, no. 1, Spring 2014, 68–80, 77.

149   Paul T. Menzel and M. Colette Chandler-Cramer, "Advance Directives, Dementia, and Withholding Food and Water by Mouth," *Hastings Center Report* (May–June 2014), http://www.thehastingscenter.org/Publications/HCR/Detail.aspx?id=6876.

CHAPTER 3

1   Ramsey, *The Essential Ramsey*, preface.

2   Jonsen, *The Birth of Bioethics*, 50.

3   Ramsey, *The Essential Ramsey*, 218.

4   Ibid., 210–211.

5   *Bouvia v. Superior Court* (1986), 179 Cal App. 3d 1127.

6   Robert M. Veatch, "Which Grounds for Overriding Autonomy Are Legitimate?" *Hastings Center Report* (Nov.-Dec. 1996): 42.

7   Paul Longmore, interview with the author, July 27, 1999.

8   Arthur Caplan, "System Messed Up, Hands Down," *Oakland Tribune*, May 31, 1996.

9   Juan P. Suarez, "Doctors Didn't Fail Georgette Smith," *Orlando Sentinel*, May 26, 1999.

10   Coleman interview.

11   Joseph Shapiro, *No Pity: People with Disabilities Forging a New Civil Rights Movement* (New York: Random House, 1993), 259.

12   Veatch, "Overriding Autonomy," 42.

13   Beauchamp and Childress, *Principles*, 216.

14 Rita Marker, "Advance Directive: Protecting Yourself and Your Family," Patients Rights Council, http://www.patientsrightscouncil.org/site/advance-directive-protecting-yourself-and-your-family-part-two/.

15 For more information on the National Institute on Health and Clinical Excellence, see http://www.liv.ac.uk/media/livacuk/mcpcil/migrated-files/liverpool-care-pathway/updatedlcppdfs/What_is_the_LCP_-_Healthcare_Professionals_-_April_2010.pdf.

16 Michael P. Hahn, "Review of Palliative Sedation and Its Distinction from Euthanasia and Lethal Injection," *Journal of Pain & Palliative Care Pharmacotherapy* 26 (2012): 30–39.

17 Ibid., 31.

18 Ibid.

19 Marie Curie Palliative Care Institute, "What Is the Liverpool Pathway for the Dying Patient?: Information for Health Care Professionals," (April 2010): 2, http://www.liv.ac.uk/media/livacuk/mcpcil/migrated-files/liverpool-care-pathway/updatedlcppdfs/What_is_the_LCP_-_Healthcare_Professionals_-_April_2010.pdf.

20 P. H. Millard et al., "A Group of Experts Who Care for the Terminally Ill Claim That Some Patients Are Being Wrongly Judged as Close to Death," *Telegraph*, September 3, 2009.

21 Kate Devlin, "Sentenced to Death on the NHS," *Telegraph*, September 2, 2009.

22 Chris Irvine and Kate Devlin, "Daughter Claims Father Wrongly Placed on Controversial NHS End of Life Scheme," *Telegraph*, September 8, 2009.

23 Sarah-Kate Templeton, "Daughter Saves Mother, 80, Left by Doctors to Starve," *Sunday Times*, October 11, 2009.

24 James Tozer, "My Husband Had Beaten Cancer, Then Doctors WRONGLY Told Him It Had Returned and Sent Him to a Hospice Who Let Him Die," *Daily Mail*, October 14, 2009, http://www.mailonsunday.co.uk/news/article-1219853/My-husband-beaten-cancer-doctors-wrongly-told-returned-let-die.html.

25 Laura Donnelly, "Half of Those on Liverpool Pathway Never Told," *Telegraph*, December 1, 2012, http://www.telegraph.co.uk/health/healthnews/9716418/Half-of-those-on-Liverpool-Care-Pathway-never-told.html.

26 United Kingdom Department of Health, "Overhaul of End of Life Care System," July 15, 2013, https://www.gov.uk/government/news/overhaul-of-end-of-life-care-system.

27 American Foundation for Suicide Prevention, "Facts and Figures," accessed on March 13, 2015, https://www.afsp.org/understanding-suicide/facts-and-figures.

28 Roger Dobson, "Internet Sites May Encourage Suicide," *British Medical Journal* (Aug. 7, 1999).

29 Right to Die Network of Canada, "Exit Bag" promotional advertisement.

30 HBO, *You Don't Know Jack*, 2010, http://www.hbo.com/movies/you-dont-know-jack/index.html#/.

31 Beauchamp and Childress, *Principles*, 287.

32 *Contemporary Perspectives on Rational Suicide*, ed. James L. Werth, Jr. (Philadelphia: Taylor and Francis, 1999), 5.

33 Werth, *Contemporary Perspectives*, 6.

34 Robin Marantz Henig, "Is There Such a Thing as 'Rational Suicide'?" *Psychology Today* (blog), April 7, 2014, https://www.psychologytoday.com/blog/cusp/201404/is-suicide-ever-rational.

35   Arthur Caplan, "Physician Assisted Suicide Only as a Last Resort," *Medscape*,
     September 24, 2014, http://ww w.medscape.com/viewarticle/831314.
36   Jack Kevorkian, *Prescription Medicide*, (Buffalo, NY: Prometheus Books, 1991),
     214.
37   Kevorkian, *Prescription Medicide*, 243.
38   Nichole Weisensee Egan, "Terminally Ill Brittany Maynard: Why I'm Ending
     My Life in Three Weeks," *People*, October 15, 2014, http://www.people.com/
     article/brittany-maynard-brain-cancer-death-with-dignity-suicide.
39   "11 Extraordinary People of 2014," *CNN*, December 5, 2014, http://www.cnn.
     com/2014/12/05/living/extraordinary-people/.
40   Brittany Maynard, "My Right to Death with Dignity at Age 29," *CNN*,
     November 2, 2014.
41   NBC Health News, "Maynard Slams Doctor's Remarks on Her Decision
     to Die," October 23, 2014, http://www.nbcnews.com/health/health-news/
     brittany-maynard-slams-doctors-remarks-her-decision-die-n232576.
42   Brittany Maynard, "My Name Is Brittany Maynard, and I Am Choosing to
     Die with Dignity," *Elite Daily*, October 15, 2014, http://elitedaily.com/life/
     brittany-maynard-death-exclusive/798957/.
43   Lisa Belkin, "There's No Such Thing as a Simple Suicide," *New York Times*
     magazine, November 14, 1994.
44   CBS, *60 Minutes*, November 22, 1998.
45   Saunders interview.
46   Walter R. Hunter, interview with the author, November 30, 1998.
47   World Health Organization, "Preventing Suicides: A Resource for Media
     Professionals," Geneva, 2000.
48   George Delury, *Countdown: A Daily Log of Myrna's Mental State and View
     Toward Death*, entry dated February 27, 1995.
49   Delury, *Countdown*, entry dated May 1, 1995.
50   Susan Cheever, "An Act of Mercy?" *New York Times Book Review*, July 20, 1997.
51   George Delury, *But What If She Wants to Die?* (Buffalo, NY: Prometheus Books,
     1997).
52   Beverly Sloane, interview with the author, August 3, 1999.
53   Transcript of taped conversation between Susan Reynolds and John Bement,
     July 31, 1996.
54   Susan Randall, interview with the author, July 30, 1999.
55   Rita Marker, interview with the author, August 4, 1999.
56   Eric Chevlen, MD, interview with the author, July 22, 1996.
57   Belkin, "Simple Suicide."
58   Compassion in Dying of Washington, undated letter signed by Kirk Robinson,
     fundraising chair, and Rev. Fr. Michael Bonacci, executive director, received by
     my source in December 1997.
59   Faye Girsh, "Compassionate Act Is Not a Crime," *USA Today*, March 29, 1999.
60   World Federation of Right to Die Societies, "The Zurich Declaration on
     Assisted Dying," 1998, http://www.worldrtd.org/zurichdecl.html.
61   *Carter v. Canada (Attorney General)*, 2015 SCC 5, February 6, 2015, http://scc-
     csc.lexum.com/scc-csc/scc-csc/en/item/14637/index.do.
62   Henk Jochemsen and John Keown, "Voluntary Euthanasia Under Control?
     Further Empirical Evidence from the Netherlands," *Journal of Medical Ethics* 25
     (1999): 16.

63 "Choosing Death," *Health Care Quarterly*, WGBH Boston, first aired March 23, 1993.

64 Gene Kaufman, "State v Chabot: A Euthanasia Case Note," *Ohio Northern University Law Review* 20, no. 3 (1994): 817.

65 Eugene Sutorius, interview with the author, October 17, 1995.

66 *tijdschrift voor psychiatrie* 53 (2011): 8. (Google translation.)

67 Simon Caldwell, "Number of Mentally Ill Patients Euthanized in the Netherlands Trebles," *Daily Mail*, October 3, 2014, http://www.dailymail. co.uk/news/article-2779624/Number-mentally-ill-patients-killed-euthanasia-Holland-trebles-year-doctors-warn-assisted-suicide-control.html.

68 Tony Sheldon, "Euthanasia Endorsed in Dutch Patient with Dementia," *British Medical Journal*, July 10, 1999.

69 Royal Dutch Medical Association, *Vision of Euthanasia (1986)*, 14.

70 J. Remmelink et al., *Medical Decisions about the End of Life* Vol. II: 58, Table 7.2.

71 *Washington v. Glucksberg* (1997), 117 S. Ct. 2258.

72 Statline Statistics Netherlands, "Deaths by End of Life Decision Making," July 11, 2012, http://statline.cbs.nl/StatWeb/publication/?VW=T&DM=SLen&PA=81655ENG&LA=en.

73 Andrew Osborn, "Belgian Outcry Over First Mercy Killing Under New Law," *The Guardian*, October 8, 2002. http://www.theguardian.com/world/2002/oct/09/andrewosborn.

74 Wesley J. Smith, "Elderly Belgian Couple Euthanized Together," *National Review*, Human Exceptionalism (blog), March 31, 2011, http://www.nationalreview.com/human-exceptionalism/322963/culture-death-elderly-belgian-couple-euthanized-together-wesley-j-smith.

75 "Elderly Belgian Couple Euthanized Together," *Huffington Post*, June 26, 2013, http://www.huffingtonpost.com/2013/06/26/leopold-dauwe-paula-raman-euthanized_n_3504348.html?utm_hp_ref=world.

76 Simon Caldwell, "Elderly Couple to Die Together by Assisted Suicide Even Though They Are Not Ill," *Daily Mail*, September 25, 2014, http://www.dailymail.co.uk/news/article-2770249/Healthy-OAP-couple-die-assisted-suicide-Husband-wife-support-three-children.html.

77 Bruno Waterfield, "Belgian Identical Twins in a Unique Mercy Killing," *Telegraph*, January 13, 2013, http://www.telegraph.co.uk/news/worldnews/europe/belgium/9798778/Belgian-identical-twins-in-unique-mercy-killing.html.

78 Michael Cook, "Another Speedbump for Belgian Euthanasia," *Bioedge*, February 8, 2013, http://www.bioedge.org/bioethics/bioethics_article/10388.

79 Damien Gayle, "Transexual, 44, Elects to Die by Euthanasia After Botched Sex Change Operation," *Daily Mail*, October 1, 2013, http://www.dailymail.co.uk/news/article-2440086/Belgian-transsexual-Nathan-Verhelst-44-elects-die-euthanasia-botched-sex-change-operation.html.

80 "Annual 50 Times Euthanasia for Mental Illness," *Humo*, March 20, 2015, (Google translation), http://www.humo.be/actua/326521/jaarlijks-vijftig-keer-euthanasie-om-psychiatrische-redenen.

81 "Belgium Passes Law Extending Euthanasia to Children of All Ages," *Associated Press*, February 13, 2014.

82 Theo Boer, "Assisted Suicide: Don't Go There," Euthanasia Prevention Coalition, July 16, 2014, http://alexschadenberg.blogspot.ca/2014/07/dutch-ethicist-assisted-suicide-dont-go.html.

83 Erin Hoover Barnett, "Man with ALS Makes Up His Mind to Die," *The Oregonian*, March 11, 1999.

84 Erin Hoover Barnett, "Is Mom Capable of Choosing to Die?" *The Oregonian*, October 17, 1999.

85 Arthur Chin et al., "Legalized Physician-Assisted Suicide in Oregon—The First Year's Experience," *New England Journal of Medicine* (February 18, 1999): 577–583; Amy D. Sullivan et al., "Legalized Physician-Assisted Suicide in Oregon—The Second Year," *New England Journal of Medicine* (February 23, 2000): 588–604.

86 Timothy E. Quill, MD, *Death and Dignity: Making Choices and Taking Charge* (New York: W. W. Norton & Company, 1994), 162.

87 Oregon Division of Public Health, "Oregon's Death with Dignity Act 2013," https://public.health.oregon.gov/ProviderPartnerResources/EvaluationResearch/DeathwithDignityAct/Documents/year16.pdf.

88 Herbert Hendin and Kathleen Foley, "Physician-Assisted Suicide in Oregon: A Medical Perspective," *Michigan Law Review* 106 (June 2008): 1613, 1622, https://docs.google.com/file/d/0BwDPETL1NPnAMmFjZTNjNzctOGU4NSooMTUwLTgxZjAtM2I4NDhlMjA2OTFj/edit?hl=en.

89 Hendin and Foley, "Physician-Assisted Suicide," 1623–1624, https://docs.google.com/file/d/0BwDPETL1NPnAMmFjZTNjNzctOGU4NSooMTUwLTgxZjAtM2I4NDhlMjA2OTFj/edit?hl=en.

90 Ibid., 1613.

91 Oregon Public Health Division, "Prioritized Health Tables," February 14, 2014, 102. http://www.oregon.gov/oha/herc/PrioritizedList/4-1-2014%20Prioritized%20List%20of%20Health%20Services.pdf.

92 Susan Donaldson James, "Death Drugs Cause Uproar in Oregon," August 6, 2008, http://abcnews.go.com/Health/story?id=5517492.

93 Dan Springer, "Assisted Suicide Instead of Medical Care," Fox News, July 28, 2008, http://www.foxnews.com/story/2008/07/28/oregon-offers-terminal-patients-doctor-assisted-suicide-instead-medical-care/.

94 Ezekiel J. Emanuel, MD, PhD, and Margaret P. Battin, PhD, "What Are the Potential Cost Savings from Legalizing Physician-Assisted Suicide?" *New England Journal of Medicine* 339 (July 16, 1998): 167–171.

95 Margaret P. Battin, "Can Suicide Be Rational? Yes, Sometimes," in ed. Werth, *Contemporary Perspectives*, 21.

96 Wesley J. Smith, "Suicide Pays," *First Things* (June/July 1999): 14–15.

97 *Compassion in Dying v. Washington*, Ninth Circuit Court of Appeals, en banc.

98 Derek Humphry and Mary Clement, *Freedom to Die: People, Politics, and the Right-to-Die Movement* (New York: St. Martin's Press, 1998), 333.

99 Derek Humphry, "Oregon's Assisted Suicide Law Gives No Sure Comfort to Dying," Letter to the Editor, *New York Times*, December 3, 1994.

100 Ezekiel J. Emanuel et al., "The Practice of Euthanasia and Physician Assisted Suicide in the United States," *Journal of the American Medical Association* (August 12, 1998): 512.

101 Johanna H. Groenewoud et al., "Clinical Problems with the Performance of Euthanasia and Physician-Assisted Suicide in the Netherlands," *New England Journal of Medicine* (February 24, 2000).

102 Sherwin Nuland, "Physician-Assisted Suicide and Euthanasia in Practice," *New England Journal of Medicine* (February 24, 2000): 583–584.

103 Bert Keizer, *Dancing with Mister D: Notes on Life and Death* (New York: Doubleday, 1996), 37.

104 Keizer, *Dancing with Mister D*, 39.

105 Ibid., 94.

106 Ibid., 61.

107 Compassion and Choices, https://www.compassionandchoices.org/.

108 Compassion and Choices, "VSED: Voluntary Stop Eating and Drinking," https://www.compassionandchoices.org/userfiles/2011-VSEDBook.pdf.

CHAPTER 4

1 Washington Department of Child Protective Services, *Intake Summary Report for Referral*, dated November 23, 1994.

2 *In re Ryan Nguyen*, Case No. 94-06074-5. State of Washington Superior Court, Sacred Heart Medical Center Brief.

3 Maggie Schneider and Sabriya Rice, "'Baby Joseph,' Focus of Treatment Dispute, Dies in His Sleep," CNN, September 29, 2011. http://www.cnn.com/2011/09/28/health/baby-joseph/?hpt=he_c2.

4 Peter Singer, "Attempted Rescue of Baby Joseph Maraachli, Pro-life Poster Child, Is Deeply Misguided," *Daily News*, March 18, 2011, http://www.nydailynews.com/opinion/attempted-rescue-baby-joseph-maraachli-pro-life-poster-child-deeply-misguided-article-1.121912.

5 Susan Fox Buchanan, interview with the author, April 10, 1998.

6 Marcia Angell, "After Quinlan: The Dilemma of the Vegetative State," *New England Journal of Medicine* 330 (May 1994): 1524.

7 Daniel Callahan, *The Troubled Dream of Life* (New York: Simon and Schuster, 1993), 201–202.

8 American Thoracic Society Position Paper, "Withholding and Withdrawing Life-Sustaining Therapy," *Annals of Internal Medicine* (September 15, 1991): 481.

9 Michael P. Panicola and Ron Hamel, "A Third Generation Approach to Medical Futility," *Health Care Ethics* 20, no. 1 (Winter 2012): 21, http://www.chausa.org/docs/default-source/general-files/0925c03b0025465aa70b8b1547e6a5c51-pdf.pdf?sfvrsn=0.

10 Stuart J. Youngner, "Applying Futility: Saying No Is Not Enough," *Journal of the American Geriatric Society* 42 (August 1994): 887.

11 Edmund D. Pellegrino, "Autonomy, Beneficence, and the Experimental Subject's Consent: A Response to Jay Katz," *Saint Louis University Law Journal* 38 (1993): 58.

12 Margaret L. Eaton, "Tough Choices," *California Lawyer* (September 1998): 46.

13 Eaton, "Tough Choices," 48.

14 Ibid.

15 Ibid., 82.

16 "Foregoing Life-Sustaining Treatment," *Mayo Clinic* 71 (May 1996): 513.

17 http://badcripple.blogspot.com/.

18 William J. Peace, "Comfort Care as Denial of Personhood," *Hastings Center Report* 42, no. 4 (2012): 14–17, 15.

19 Peace, "Comfort Care", 14–17, 15.

20 Ibid., 16.

21 Ibid., 17.

22 Robert W. Wachter, "The Hospitalist Movement: Issues to Consider," *Hospital Practice* (February 15, 1999): 103.

23 Wachter, "The Hospitalist Movement," 104.

24 Thaddeus Mason Pope, "Unilateral 'Do-Not-Attempt-Resuscitation' Orders at Massachusetts General Hospital," (quoting a presentation made to the 2014 American Thoracic Society International Conference), May 11, 2014, http://medicalfutility.blogspot.com/2014/05/unilateral-do-not-attempt-resuscitation.html.

25 For example, the unsuccessful Texas S. 303, filed in 2013 provided in pertinent part (my emphasis): (c) Before placing a do-not-resuscitate (DNR) order in a patient 's medical record, the physician or the facility's personnel shall *make a reasonably diligent effort to contact or cause to be contacted the surrogate.* The facility shall establish a policy regarding the notification required under this section. The policy may authorize the notification to be given verbally by a physician or facility personnel. (d) *The DNR order takes effect at the time it is written in the patient's chart* or otherwise placed in the patient's medical record. (e) *If the patient or surrogate disagrees* with the DNR order being placed in or removed from the medical record, the patient or surrogate *may request a second opinion at the patient's or surrogate's expense.*

26 Gabriel T. Bosslet, Thaddeus M. Pope, et al., "An Official ATS/AACN/ACCP/ESICM/SCCM Policy Statement: Responding to Requests for Potentially Inappropriate Treatments in Intensive Care Units," *American Journal of Respiratory and Critical Care Medicine* 191, no. 11 (June 1, 2015): 1318–1330, 1319, http://www.atsjournals.org/doi/abs/10.1164/rccm.201505-0924ST#.VVoQc_lVhBc.

27 Bosslet, Pope, et al., "An Official ATS/ASCN/ACCP/ESICM/SCCM Policy Statement," 1318–1330, 1319.

28 Ibid.

29 Ronald E. Cranford, "Medical Futility: Transforming a Clinical Concept into Legal and Social Policies," *Journal of the American Geriatric Society* 42 (August 1994): 897.

30 Steven Miles, interview with the author, February 9, 1999.

31 State of Minnesota District Court, Probate Division, County of Hennepin, *In re Helga Wanglie,* "Findings of Fact, Conclusions of Law, and Order," July 1, 1991.

32 *In re Terry Achtabowski, Jr.,* Docket No. 93-1247-AV, Michigan Court of Appeals, 1994, Appellee's Brief, 2.

33 George Krausz, interview with the author, February 15, 1999.

34 Campbell Clark, "Was Herman Krausz Willing to Die?" *National Post,* February 11, 1999.

35 Clark, "Was Herman Krausz Willing to Die?"

36 Lynn Moore, "Man's Consent Not Needed to Remove Respirator, Inquest Hears," *National Post,* February 12, 1999.

37 Krausz interview.

38 Alexander Morgan Capron, "Abandoning a Waning Life," *Hastings Center Report* (July-Aug. 1995): 24.

39 Capron, "Abandoning," 24.

40 *Sawatzky and Riverview Health Centre, Inc.* Docket: C198-01-10245, [1998] M.J. No. 506.

41 Dominic Lawson, "The Death of Medicine," *Sunday London Telegraph,* April 25, 1999.

42 Policy Perspectives "A Multi-institution Collaborative Policy on Medical Futility," *Journal of the American Medical Association* (August 21, 1996): 571–574.

43 Texas Health and Safety Code 166.046, http://www.statutes.legis.state.tx.us/Docs/HS/htm/HS.166.htm#166.046.

44 Melanie Childer, "Killing My Sister—We Are Protesting—Help Us," *Democratic Underground* (blog), April 21, 2006, http://www.democraticunderground.com/discuss/duboard.php?az=show_mesg&forum=364&topic_id=986779&mesg_id=986779.

45 Wesley J. Smith, "Death by Ethics Committee," *National Review*, April 27, 2006. http://www.nationalreview.com/article/217472/death-ethics-committee-wesley-j-smith.

46 Melanie Childers, "Andrea Clarke Passed Away Today," *Democratic Underground* (blog), May 7, 2006, http://www.democraticunderground.com/discuss/duboard.php?az=view_all&address=364x1128570.

47 Wesley J. Smith, "The Deadly Ethics of 'Futile Care Theory,'" *Weekly Standard* (December 7, 1998): 32–35.

48 Correspondence from Daniel Callahan to Wesley J. Smith, March 23, 1999.

49 Charles L. Sprung, "Is The Patient's Right to Die Evolving into a Duty to Die?: Medical Decision Making and Ethical Evaluations in Health Care," *Journal of Evaluation in Clinical Practice* 3 (1997): 71.

50 Veatch, "Overriding Autonomy," 42–43.

51 Robert M. Veatch, "Why Physicians Cannot Determine If Care Is Futile," *Journal of the American Geriatric Society* 42 (1994): 872–873.

52 Donald J. Murphy, "New Do-Not-Resuscitate Policies: A First Step in Cost Control," *Archives of Internal Medicine* 153: 1641.

53 "Consensus Statement of the Society of Critical Care Medicine's Ethics Committee Regarding Futile and Other Possible Inadvisable Treatments," *Critical Care Medicine* 25, no. 5 (1997): 890.

54 Steven H. Miles, "Informed Demand for 'Non-Beneficial' Medical Treatment," *New England Journal of Medicine* (August 15, 1991): 515.

55 Miles interview.

56 Steven H. Miles, "Medical Futility," *Law, Medicine, and Health Care* 20 (1992): 313.

57 Thanh N. Huynh et al., "The Opportunity Cost of Futile Treatment in the ICU," *Critical Care Medicine* 42, no. 9 (September 2014): 1977–1982.

58 Al Lewis, "Go Gently in the Night," *San Francisco Chronicle*, September 28, 2009, http://www.sfgate.com/health/article/Go-gently-in-the-night-3216830.php.

59 Norman G. Levinsky, "The Doctor's Master," *New England Journal of Medicine* 311 (December 13, 1984): 1574.

60 Donald J. Murphy, MD, interview with the author, July 3, 1996.

61 Ezekiel K. Emanuel and Linda L. Emanuel, "The Economics of Dying," *New England Journal of Medicine* 330 (February 1994): 543.

62 Ezekiel J. Emanuel, "Cost Savings at the End of Life; What Do the Data Show?" *Journal of the American Medical Association* 275 (June 1996): 1907–1914.

63 Ezekiel Emanuel, "Better, If Not Cheaper, Care," *New York Times*, January 3, 2013, http://opinionator.blogs.nytimes.com/2013/01/03/better-if-not-cheaper-care/.

64 National Institute for Health Care Management, "NIHCM Data Brief: The

Concentration of Health Care Spending," July 2012, http://www.nihcm.org/pdf/DataBrief3%20Final.pdf.

65 United States Senate Finance Committee Hearings, "Advance Directives and Care at the End of Life," testimony of Joann Lynn, MD, MA, May 5, 1994.

66 C. Everett Koop, MD, interview with the author, August 19, 1999.

67 Sarah Palin, "Statement on the Current Healthcare Debate," Facebook, August 7, 2009, https://www.facebook.com/note.php?note_id=113851103434.

68 Angie Drobnic Holan, "Politifact's Lie of the Year: 'Death Panels,'" *Tampa Bay Times* concerning *Politifact.com*, December 19, 2009, http://www.politifact.com/truth-o-meter/article/2009/dec/18/politifact-lie-year-death-panels/.

69 Richard Lamm, interview with the author, November 19, 1998.

70 Robert M. Veatch, "Healthcare Rationing Through Global Budgeting: The Ethical Choices," *Journal of Clinical Ethics* 5 (Winter 1994): 291–296.

71 Daniel Callahan, *False Hopes: Why America's Quest for Perfect Health Is a Recipe for Failure* (New York: Simon and Schuster, 1998), 38.

72 Callahan, *False Hopes*, 204.

73 Ibid., 245.

74 Ibid., 41.

75 Ibid., 196.

76 Ibid., 198.

77 Ibid., 255.

78 Ibid., 256.

79 Ibid., 205.

80 Ibid.

81 Ibid., 245.

82 Ibid., 252.

83 Ibid., 245.

84 Ezekiel J. Emanuel, "Where Civic Republicanism and Deliberative Democracy Meet," *Hastings Center Report* (Nov.-Dec. 1996): 12–13, http://www.ncpa.org/pdfs/Where_Civic_Republicanism_and_Deliberative_Democracy_Meet.pdf.

85 Steven Rattner, "Beyond Obamacare," *New York Times*, September 16, 2012, http://www.nytimes.com/2012/09/17/opinion/health-care-reform-beyond-obamacare.html?_r=0.

86 Peter J. Neumann and Milton C. Weinstein, "Legislating against Use of Cost-Effectiveness Information," *New England Journal of Medicine*, 363 (October 14, 2010): 1495–1497. http://www.nejm.org/doi/full/10.1056/NEJMp1007168?ssource=hcrc.

87 Howard Brody, "From an Ethic of Rationing to an Ethic of Waste Avoidance," *New England Journal of Medicine* 366 (2012): 1949–1951.

88 Brody, "Ethic of Rationing," 1951.

89 Ibid.

90 Normal Levinsky, "Care for Alice," *The Lancet*: 1850.

91 Editorial, "A Duty to Die?" *Boston Globe*, April 8, 1984.

92 Leon R. Kass, *Toward a More Natural Science: Biology and Human Affairs*, (New York: The Free Press, 1985), 307, originally published as "The Case for Mortality," *The American Scholar* 52 (Spring 1983).

93 Kass, *Toward a More Natural Science*, 316.

94 Leon Kass, MD, interview with the author, August 24, 1999.

95 John Hardwig, "What About the Family?" *Hastings Center Report* (Mar.-Apr. 1990): 5.

96 Hardwig, "What About the Family?" 5–6.

97 Ibid., 7.

98 Ibid., 8.

99 John Hardwig, "Is There a Duty to Die?" *Hastings Center Report* (Mar.–Apr. 1997): 37–38.

100 "Letters to the Editor," Letter of Donald G. Flory, *Hastings Center Report* (Nov.-Dec. 1997): 6.

101 John Hardwig, interview with the author, October 22, 1998.

102 "Letters," *Hastings Center Report*, 5.

103 "Letters," *Hastings Center Report*, 7.

104 Caldwell, "Number of Mentally Ill Patients Euthanized."

105 Matthew Weaver, "British Conductor Dies with Wife at Assisted Suicide Clinic," *The Guardian*, July 14, 2009, http://www.theguardian.com/society/2009/jul/14/assisted-suicide-conductor-edward-downes.

106 Editorial, "Offering a Choice to the Terminally Ill," *New York Times*, March 14, 2015, http://www.nytimes.com/2015/03/15/opinion/sunday/offering-a-choice-to-the-terminally-ill.html?smid=tw-share&_r=3.

107 Hardwig interview.

CHAPTER 5

1 Correspondence from Ohio State Board of Pharmacy to Cuyahoga County Prosecutor's Office, January 7, 1997.

2 Ohio State Board of Pharmacy, Memorandum to Ohio Medical Board, January 13, 1997.

3 James L. Bernat, MD, interview with the author, December 28, 1998.

4 Proposed "Non-Heart-Beating Protocol," undated, and Jeffrey I. Frank, MD, interview with the author, February 9, 1999.

5 Frank interview.

6 Michael J. Goldstein and Dana Lustbader, "Organ Donation after Cardiac Death," Center for Advanced Palliative Care, Fast Fact #242, https://www.capc.org/fast-facts/242-rgan-donation-after-cardiac-death/.

7 R. F. Saidi and S. K. Jejasii Kenari, "Challenges of Organ Shortage for Transplantation: Solutions and Opportunities," *International Journal of Organ Transplantation Medicine* 5, no. 3 (2014): 87–96.

8 Michael A. DeVita et al., "Procuring Organs from a Non-Heart-Beating Cadaver: A Case Report," *Kennedy Institute of Ethics Journal* 3, no. 4 (1993): 381.

9 K. Hornby et al., "A Systematic Review of Autoresuscitation after Cardiac Arrest," *Critical Care Medicine* 38, no. 5 (May 2010): 1246–1253.

10 Rob Stein, "Changes in Controversial Organ Method Stir Fears," *Washington Post*, September 19, 2011, http://www.washingtonpost.com/national/health-science/changes-in-controversial-organ-donation-method-stir-fears/2011/09/15/gIQAlY9agK_story.html.

11 Stuart J. Youngner, interview with the author, November 15, 1998.

12 Stuart J. Youngner and Robert M. Arnold for the Working Group on Ethical, Psychosocial, and Public Policy Implications of Procuring Organs from Non-Heart-Beating Cadaver Donors, *Journal of the American Medical Association* 269 (June 2, 1993): 2773.

13 Yong W. Cho et al., "Transplantation of Kidneys from Donors Whose Hearts

Have Stopped Beating," *New England Journal of Medicine* 338 (Jan. 22, 1998): 221.

14 R. M. Arnold and S. J. Youngner, "Time Is of the Essence: The Pressing Need for Comprehensive Non-Heart-Beating Cadaveric Donation Policies," *Transplantation Proceedings* 27, no. 5, (Oct. 1995): 2918.

15 Frank interview.

16 Electronic correspondence from Dr. Alan Shewmon to the author, October 4, 1999.

17 Lindsey Tanner, "Study: Take Donor Organs Before Brain Death," Associated Press, June 2, 1998, as published in the *Philadelphia Inquirer*.

18 Erin Allday, "Doctor Charged with Hastening Death of Donor," *San Francisco Chronicle*, July 31, 2007.

19 Tracy Weber and Charles Ornstein, "Death in San Luis Obispo Organ Donor Case Is Ruled Natural," *Los Angeles Times*, March 9, 2007.

20 Youngner and Arnold, "Ethical, Psychosocial, and Public Policy Implications," 2771.

21 Louise Lears, "Obtaining Organs from Non-Heart-Beating Donors," *Ethical Issues in Health Care*, Saint Louis University Health Sciences Center, February 1996.

22 Michael DeVita and James Snyder, "Reflections on Non-Heart-Beating Organ Donation: How Three Years of Experience Affected the University of Pittsburgh's Ethics Committee's Actions," *Cambridge Quarterly of Healthcare Ethics* 5 (1996): 286.

23 Frank Koughan and Walt Bogdanich, "*60 Minutes* Sets the Record Straight," *Cambridge Health Care Quarterly* 8 (1999): 514–517.

24 Stephen P. Wall, Carolyn Plunkett, and Arthur Caplan, "A Potential Solution to the Shortage of Solid Organs for Transplantation," *Journal of the American Medical Association* (May 11, 2015), http://jama.jamanetwork.com/article. aspx?articleid=2293309.

25 Michael A. DeVita and James V. Snyder, "Development of the University of Pittsburgh Medical Center Policy for the Care of Terminally Ill Patients Who May Become Organ Donors after Death following the Removal of Life Support," in *Procuring Organs for Transplant*, eds. Robert M. Arnold et al. (Baltimore, MD: Johns Hopkins University Press, 1995), 58.

26 Diane Coleman, interview with the author, February 16, 1999.

27 Some of the following material first appeared in Wesley J. Smith, "Total Brain Failure Is Death," Human Life Review, Spring 2014, http://www. humanlifereview.com/total-brain-failure-death/.

28 Carolyn Jones and Bob Egelko, "Judge Rules against Brain-Dead Girl's Family," *San Francisco Chronicle*, December 24, 2013, http://www.sfgate.com/news/article/Jahi-McMath-is-brain-dead-doctor-testifies-5091298.php.

29 *California Health and Safety Code* section 7180. "An individual who has sustained either (1) irreversible cessation of circulatory and respiratory functions, or (2) irreversible cessation of all functions of the entire brain, including the brain stem, is dead. A determination of death must be made in accordance with accepted medical standards." See also section 1254.4.

30 Henry K. Lee, "Hospital Agrees to Let Jahi McMath Family Take Girl," *San Francisco Chronicle*, January 3, 2014, http://www.sfgate.com/bayarea/article/

Hospital-agrees-to-let-Jahi-McMath-family-take-5111584.php?cmpid.

31 *Natasha Nailah, et al. v. Frederick S. Rosen, MD, et. al.*, Superior Court of California for the County of Alameda, Case No. R615760730.

32 Texas Health and Safety Code Section 166.049.

33 *Munoz v. John Peter Smith Hospital*, District Court of Tarrant County, Texas, Cause number 096-270080-14, Judgment, January 24, 2014, http://www.scribd.com/doc/202053415/Judges-Order-on-Munoz-Matter.

34 Kristina Jananovski, "Baby Born to a Brain Dead Mother," *Daily Mail*, November 13, 2013, http://www.dailymail.co.uk/health/article-2506281/Baby-born-brain-dead-mother-foetus-survives-15-27-weeks.html.

35 James L. Bernat, "A Defense of the Whole-Brain Concept of Death," *Hastings Center Report* (March–April 1998): 15.

36 Bernat, "Whole-Brain Concept," 20.

37 See, for example, Mohamed R. Rady et al., "Organ Procurement after Cardiocirculatory Death: A Critical Analysis," *Journal of Intensive Care Medicine* 23 (2008): 303, http://jic.sagepub.com/content/23/5/303.full.pdf.

38 Uniform Determination of Death Act, 1980, http://pntb.org/wordpress/wp-content/uploads/Uniform-Determination-of-Death-1980_5c.pdf.

39 The American Academy of Neurology, "Practice Parameters for Determining Brain Death in Adults," November 1994.

40 Ronald W. H. Verer et al., "Cells in Human Postmortem Brain Tissue Slices Remain Alive for Several Weeks in Culture," *Federation of American Societies for Experimental Biology Journal* (Sept. 12, 2001), http://www.fasebj.org/content/16/1/54.long.

41 President's Council on Bioethics, "Controversies in the Determination of Death" (Dec. 2008): 17, https://bioethicsarchive.georgetown.edu/pcbe/reports/death/.

42 Ibid.

43 Ibid., 17–18.

44 President's Council, *Controversies*, 19.

45 Eelco F. M. Wijdicks, MD, PhD, et al., "Evidence-based Guideline Update: Determining Brain Death in Adults," *Neurology*, June 8, 2010, https://www.aan.com/PressRoom/Home/GetDigitalAsset/8470.

46 Paul A. Byrne, "A Living Human Person until Death," *Renew America*, February 11, 2015, http://www.renewamerica.com/columns/byrne/130211.

47 Ibid.

48 Dictionary.com, http://dictionary.reference.com/browse/respiration.

49 Lecia Bushak, "'Organ Care System,' Medical Device, Allows Lungs to 'Breathe' Outside Body Before Transplant," *Medical Daily*, February 11, 2014, http://www.medicaldaily.com/organ-care-system-medical-device-allows-lungs-breathe-outside-body-transplant-269099.

50 D. Alan Shewmon, "Chronic 'Brain Death': Meta-Analysis and Conceptual Consequences," *Neurology* 51 (December 1998): 1542. Electronic correspondence to author, October 5, 1999.

51 President's Council, "Controversies," 90–91.

52 Frank interview.

53 National Catholic Bioethics Center, "FAQ on 'Brain Death,'" http://www.ncbcenter.org/page.aspx?pid=1285.

54 *Court TV.com Talk*, March 24, 2005, as quoted in Wesley J. Smith, "Human Non Person," *National Review Online*, March 29, 2005, http://www.nationalreview.com/article/214019/human-non-person-wesley-j-smith.

55 Norman Fost, MD, "The Unimportance of Death," in *The Definition of Death: Contemporary Controversies*, eds. Stuart J. Youngner, Robert M. Arnold, and Renie Schapiro (Baltimore, MD: Johns Hopkins University Press), 172–173.

56 Walter Sinnott-Armstrong and Franklin G. Miller, "What Makes Killing Wrong?" *Journal of Medical Ethics* (January 19, 2012): http://jme.bmj.com/content/early/2012/01/19/medethics-2011-100351.full.

57 Ibid.

58 Walter Glannon, "The Moral Insignificance of Death in Organ Donation," *Cambridge Quarterly of Healthcare Ethics* 22, no. 2 (April 2013): 192–202.

59 Robert D. Truog, MD, and Franklin G. Miller, PhD, "The Dead Donor Rule and Organ Transplantation," *New England Journal of Medicine* 359 (August 14, 2008): 674–675.

60 Joshua Mesrich and Joseph Scalea, "As They Lay Dying," *The Atlantic*, April 2015, http://www.theatlantic.com/magazine/archive/2015/04/as-they-lay-dying/386273/.

61 For more details on Frances's suicide and my reaction to it, see Wesley J. Smith, *Forced Exit: Euthanasia, Assisted Suicide and the New Duty to Die* (New York: Encounter Books, 2006), originally published 1997.

62 Wesley J. Smith, "The Whispers of Strangers," *Newsweek*, June 28, 1993, http://www.newsweek.com/whispers-strangers-193804.

63 Ron French, "'Slaughterhouse,' Coroner Says of Way Kidneys Taken," *Detroit News*, June 9, 1998; see also Randi Goldberg, "Kidneys from Man Who Died in Kevorkian's Presence Unused," June 9, 1998, Associated Press.

64 Brian Murphy, "Kevorkian to Harvest Patients' Organs," *Detroit Free Press*, October 23, 1997.

65 Jane Daugherty et al., "Experts Denounce Kevorkian's Organ Donor Proposal," *Detroit News*, October 24, 1997.

66 David Goodman, "Kevorkian Gives Organs from Suicide," Associated Press, as published in the *Washington Post*, June 7, 1998.

67 Oliver Detry et al., "Organ Harvesting after Physician Assisted Death," *Transplant International*, 29, no. 9 (September 2008): 915, http://onlinelibrary.wiley.com/doi/10.1111/j.1432-2277.2008.00701.x/full.

68 D. Van Raemdonck et al., "Initial Experience with Transplantation of Lungs Recovered from Donors after Euthanasia," *Applied Cardiopulmonary Pathophysiology* 15 (2011): 38–48, http://www.applied-cardiopulmonary-pathophysiology.com/fileadmin/downloads/acp-2011-1_20110329/05_vanraemdonck.pdf.

69 Janine Van Jaarsveldt, "Euthanasia Should Lead to Organ Donation: Health Minister," *New York Times*, November 26, 2014.

70 See for example, Sharon Kirkey, "Doctors Worry How Organ Donation Will Be Affected by Assisted Suicide Ruling," *Ottawa Citizen*, March 16, 2015, http://www.ottawacitizen.com/health/Doctors+worry+organ+donations+will+affected+Supreme+Court+ruling/10897506/story.html.

71 Robert M. Arnold and Stuart J. Youngner, "The Dead Donor Rule: Should We Stretch It, Bend It, or Abandon It?" *Kennedy Institute of Ethics Journal* (1993): 270.

72 Arnold and Youngner, "Dead Donor Rule," 270.

73 Robert M. Arnold, interview with the author, January 27, 1999.

74 Youngner interview.

75 Renée C. Fox, "An Ignoble Form of Cannibalism: Reflections on the Pittsburgh Protocol for Procuring Organs from Non-Heart-Beating Cadavers," chapter in *Procuring Organs for Transplant*, 156.

76 Bernat interview.

77 Arthur Caplan, "Going Too Extreme," *Bioethica Forum* 3, no. 2 (2010): 30–31.

78 Arnold and Youngner, "Dead Donor Rule," 271–272.

CHAPTER 6

1 Yuval Levin, *Imagining the Future: Science and American Democracy* (New York: Encounter Books, 2008), 10.

2 Levin, *Imagining the Future*, 10.

3 Reuters, "Kidney Sales Worth Study, Ethicists Say," as published in the *Detroit Free Press*, June 27, 1998.

4 ABC News, "The Organ Trade," *Primetime*, July 1, 1998.

5 Bruce Johnston, "Alert over Trade in Children's Organs," *The Telegraph*, July 18, 1997.

6 http://www.humantrafficking.org/.

7 Arthur L. Caplan, *Am I My Brother's Keeper: The Ethical Frontiers of Biomedicine* (Bloomington, IN: University of Indiana Press, 1997), 95–97.

8 Renée Fox, interview with the author, February 11, 1999.

9 Caplan, *Brother's Keeper*, 100.

10 Gary S. Becker and Julio J. Elias, "Cash for Kidneys? The Case for a Market for Organs," *Wall Street Journal*, January 18, 2014, http://www.wsj.com/news/articles/SB10001424052702304149045793225660004817176?mod=WSJ_hpp_MIDDLENexttoWhatsNewsFifth&mg=reno64-wsj&url=http%3A%2F%2Fonline.wsj.com%2Farticle%2FSB10001424052702304149045793225660004817176.html%3Fmod%3DWSJ_hpp_MIDDLENexttoWhatsNewsFifth.

11 Ibid.

12 Sue Rabbitt Roff, "We Should Consider Paying Kidney Donors," *British Medical Journal* (August 6, 2011): 321.

13 Sally Satel, "Why People Don't Donate Their Kidneys," *New York Times*, May 3, 2014, http://www.nytimes.com/2014/05/04/opinion/sunday/why-people-dont-donate-their-kidneys.html?hp&rref=opinion.

14 Arthur L. Caplan, "Organ Transplantation," in *Bioethics Briefing Book* (Garrison, NY: Hastings Center, 2008), 131, http://www.thehastingscenter.org/uploadedFiles/Publications/Briefing_Book/organ%20transplantation%20chapter.pdf.

15 Arthur L. Caplan, interview with the author (email), March 14, 2015.

16 Sigrid Fry-Revere, *The Kidney Sellers: A Journey of Discovery in Iran* (Durham, NC: Academic Press, 2014), 205–208.

17 "Ministry of Health Concerned Over Sale of Iranian Kidneys," *Payvand News*, July 26, 2014. http://www.payvand.com/news/14/jul/1157.html.

18 Ibid.

19 John Bonifield and Elizabeth Cohen, "Kidney Donor Deaths Linked to Surgical

Clips Raise Issues of Alerts, Warnings," *CNN*, June 21, 2012, http://www.cnn.com/2012/06/20/health/kidney-clips/.

20 Michael Smith, "Desperate Americans Buy Kidneys from Peru Poor in Fatal Trade," Bloomberg, May 12, 2011, http://www.bloomberg.com/news/articles/2011-05-12/desperate-americans-buy-kidneys-from-peru-poor-in-fatal-trade.

21 Ibid.

22 Daniel Asa Rose, *Larry's Kidney: Being the True Story of How I Found Myself in China with My Black Sheep Cousin and His Mail-Order Bride, Skirting the Law to Get Him a Transplant—and Save His Life* (New York: William Morrow, 2009).

23 David Matas and David Kilgour, "Report into Allegations of Organ Harvesting of Falun Gong Practitioners in China," July 6, 2006, http://www.david-kilgour.com/2006/Kilgour-Matas-organ-harvesting-rpt-July6-eng.pdf.

24 Matas and Kilgour, "Organ Harvesting of Falun Gong Practitioners," 39.

25 Ibid., 16.

26 Ibid., 24.

27 Ibid., 24–25.

28 Ibid., 25.

29 Ibid., 26.

30 Ibid.

31 Ibid., 28.

32 Ibid., 27.

33 http://www.dafoh.org/.

34 A. Sharif et al., "Organ Procurement from Executed Prisoners in China," *American Journal of Transplantation* 14 (2014): 2246–2252.

35 "Bangladesh Busts Kidney Trafficking Gang," *Herald-Sun* (Melbourne, Australia), August 30, 2011, http://www.heraldsun.com.au/news/breaking-news/bangladesh-busts-kidney-trafficking-gang/story-e6frf7jx-1226125853362.

36 "Philippines Claims Success on Organ Trafficking," *Phys.org*, July 28, 2010, http://phys.org/news/2010-07-philippines-success-trafficking.html.

37 Kim Tae-jong, "Organ Trafficking Increasing," *Korea Times*, September 16, 2011, http://www.koreatimes.co.kr/www/news/nation/2011/09/117_94910.html.

38 Mel Evans, "'Black Market' Cash-for-Kidneys Trader Rosenbaum Gets Two-and-a-Half Years in Prison," from Associated Press, July 12, 2012, http://usnews.nbcnews.com/_news/2012/07/12/12695621-black-market-cash-for-kidneys-trader-rosenbaum-gets-2-12-years-in-prison?lite.

39 Dennis Campbell and Nicola Davison, "Illegal Kidney Trade Booms as New Organ Is Sold Every Hour," *Guardian*, May 27, 2012, http://www.theguardian.com/world/2012/may/27/kidney-trade-illegal-operations-who.

40 Participants in the International Summit on Transplant Tourism and Organ Trafficking, "The Declaration of Istanbul," May 2, 2008.

41 Gabriel M. Danovitch and Mustafa Al-Mousawi, "The Declaration of Istanbul—Early Impact and Future Potential," *Nature Reviews Nephrology* 8 (June 2012): 358–361.

42 "Surrogate Mother Dies of Complications," *Times of India*, May 17, 2012, http://timesofindia.indiatimes.com/city/ahmedabad/Surrogate-mother-dies-of-complications/articleshow/13181592.cms.

43 "Surrogate Mom Sees Her Premature Son, Dies Soon After,"
    DNA India, May 18, 2012, http://www.dnaindia.com/ahmedabad/
    report-surrogate-mom-sees-her-premature-son-dies-soon-after-1690532.
44 Richard Orange, "Surrogate Death Husband May Sue Norway,"
    The Local.NO, August 1, 2013, http://www.thelocal.no/20130801/
    surrogate-death-husband-may-sue-norway.
45 Stephanie M. Lee, "Outsourcing a Life," *San Francisco Chronicle*, October 2,
    2013, http://www.sfgate.com/local/bayarea/item/India-surrogacy-Chapter-
    One-23858.php.
46 Centre for Social Research, "Surrogate Motherhood: Ethical or Commercial?"
    March 2012, http://www.womenleadership.in/Csr/SurrogacyReport.pdf.
47 Centre for Social Research, "Surrogate Motherhood," 60.
48 Ibid., 42.
49 "Surrogacy Challenge," *Jerusalem Post*, April 28, 2015.
50 Papitchaya Boonngok and Thanyarat Doksone, "Thai Surrogate
    Forgives Australian Parents of Deserted Baby," from the Associated
    Press, August 4, 2014, http://www.theglobeandmail.com/news/world/
    thai-surrogate-forgives-australian-parents-of-deserted-baby/article19905680/.
51 Bridey Jabour and Brendan Foster, "Child Abuse Convictions
    of Gammy's Father Prompt Investigation," *Guardian*, August
    5, 2014, http://www.theguardian.com/world/2014/aug/05/
    gammy-father-child-abuse-convictions-investigation.
52 http://handsacrossthewater.org.au/.
53 Tracy Vo, "'Leave Us Alone': Baby Gammy's Surrogate Mother Slams
    His Biological Parents' Attempts to Access Charity Money," 9News.com.
    au, May 20, 2015, http://www.9news.com.au/national/2015/05/20/19/27/
    baby-gammys-biological-parents-want-charity-money.
54 Abby Phillip, "A Shocking Scandal Let Thailand to Ban Surrogacy for Hire,"
    Washington Post, February 20, 2015, http://www.washingtonpost.com/
    blogs/worldviews/wp/2015/02/20/a-shocking-scandal-led-thailand-to-ban-
    commercial-surrogacy-for-hire/.
55 Seema Mohapatra, "Stateless Babies and Adoption Scams: A Bioethical
    Analysis of International Commercial Surrogacy," *Berkeley Journal of
    International Law* 30, no. 2 (2012): 412–450, http://scholarship.law.berkeley.edu/
    cgi/viewcontent.cgi?article=1420&context=bjil.
56 Ibid., 9.
57 Matt Wade, "Babies Left in Limbo as India Struggles with Demand for
    Surrogacy," *Brisbane Times*, May 1, 2010, http://www.brisbanetimes.com.au/
    world/babies-left-in-limbo-as-india-struggles-with-demand-for-surrogacy-
    20100430-tzbl.html.
58 Rick Westhead, "Troubling Questions Surround Surrogate-Born Children in
    India," *Toronto Star*, April 26, 2010.
59 Julie Moult, "Sherri Shepherd Wants Nothing to Do with Unborn Surrogate
    Baby," *Daily Mail*, July 5, 2014, http://www.dailymail.co.uk/tvshowbiz/
    article-2681628/Sherri-Shepherd-wants-unborn-surrogate-baby-reports-
    emerge-used-egg-donor-conceive.html.
60 Emily Strohm and Diane Herbst, "Inside Sherri Shepherd's Surrogacy Ruling:
    What Happens Next?" *People*, April 22, 2015, http://www.people.com/article/
    sherri-shepherd-legal-mother-surrogate-baby-lamar-sally.

61　Usha Regarchary Smerdon, "Crossing Bodies, Crossing Borders: The Emerging Global Market for Patients and the Evolution of Modern Health Care," *IND. L. J.* 83 (2008): 71, 79.

62　John A. Robinson, *Children of Choice: Freedom and the New Reproductive Technologies* (Princeton, NJ: Princeton University Press, 1994), 150.

63　http://www.stopsurrogacynow.com/#sthash.UhgpoQIz.dpbs.

64　Jennifer Lahl, interview with the author, November 18, 2015.

65　The study referenced by Lahl is: Yona Nicolau et al., "Outcomes of Surrogate Pregnancies in California and Hospital Economics of Surrogate Maternity and Newborn Care," *World Journal of Obstetrics and Gynecology* 4, no. 4 (Nov. 10, 2015).

66　Joanna Sugden, "India Restricts Foreigners' Access to Surrogate Mothers," *Wall Street Journal*, October 29, 2015.

67　Jennifer Adaeze Anyaegbunam, "Ivy League Women Get Offers for Their Eggs," *CNN*, August 12, 2009, http://thechart.blogs.cnn.com/2009/08/12/ivy-league-women-get-offers-for-their-eggs/comment-page-1/.

68　FE van Leeuwen et al., "Risk of Borderline and Invasive Ovarian Tumours after Ovarian Stimulation for In Vitro Fertilization in a Large Dutch Cohort," *Human Reproduction*, December 26, 2011, http://www.medscape.com/viewarticle/753755.

69　I discuss the ethics and science of human cloning at length in Wesley J. Smith, *Consumer's Guide to a Brave New World* (New York: Encounter Books, 2004).

70　David A. Prentice, interview with the author, May 16, 2003.

71　David A. Prentice, interview with the author (email), May 21, 2015.

72　Masahito Tachibana et al., "Human Embryonic Stem Cells Derived by Somatic Cell Nuclear Transfer," *Cell* 153 (June 6, 2013): 1228–1238, http://www.ncbi.nlm.nih.gov/pmc/articles/PMC3772789/.

73　I. Glenn Cohen and Eli Y. Adashi, "Made to Order Embryos for Sale—a Brave New World?" *New England Journal of Medicine* 368 (June 27, 2013): 2517–2519.

74　Ibid., 2518.

CHAPTER 7

1　Aldous Huxley, "Forward," *Brave New World* (New York: Perennial Classics/HarperCollins, 1998), xi.

2　Huxley, "Forward," *Brave New World*, xvi.

3　Arthur Caplan and Wesley J. Smith, "Assisted Suicide Compromise," *USA Today*, November 13, 2014, http://www.usatoday.com/story/opinion/2014/11/13/assisted-suicide-compromise-hospice-hope-treatment-column/18994071/.

4　Nicole Weisensee Egan, "Terminally Ill Woman Brittany Maynard Has Ended Her Own Life," *People*, November 2, 2014, http://www.people.com/article/brittany-maynard-died-terminal-brain-cancer.

5　Caitlin Keating, "Terminally Ill Basketball Player Lauren Hill, Who Played at NCAA, Dies," *People* April 10, 2015, http://www.people.com/article/lauren-hill-dies-terminally-ill-college-basketball-player.

6　Dame Cicely Saunders, interview with the author, December 8, 1998.

7　Atul Gawande, *Being Mortal: Medicine and What Matters in the End* (New York: Metropolitan Books, 2014), 176.

8　"Medicare Care Choices Model," *CMS.gov*, October 5, 2015, https://innovation.cms.gov/initiatives/Medicare-Care-Choices/.

9   HB 3074, 2015.

10 Robert Powell Center for Medical Ethics at the National Right to Life
    Committee, "The Bias against Life-Preserving Treatment in Advance Care
    Planning," *National Right to Life Committee*, March 19, 2015, http://www.nrlc.
    org/uploads/advancecareplanning/advanceplanningbias2015.pdf.

11 Jacki Calmes, "Advocates Shun 'Pro Choice' to Expand Message,"
    New York Times, July 28, 2014, http://www.nytimes.com/2014/07/29/
    us/politics/advocates-shun-pro-choice-to-expand-message.
    html?partner=rss&emc=rss&_r=2.

12 Janet Harris, "Stop Calling Abortion a 'Difficult Decision,'" *Washington
    Post*, August 15, 2014, http://www.washingtonpost.com/opinions/stop-
    calling-abortion-a-difficult-decision/2014/08/15/e61fa09a-17fd-11e4-9349-
    84d4a85be981_story.html.

13 Mary Elizabeth Williams, "So What If Abortion Ends Life?" *Salon*, January 23,
    2013, http://www.salon.com/2013/01/23/so_what_if_abortion_ends_life.

14 *Planned Parenthood Southeast v. Strange*, 9 F. Supp 3d., 1272 (2014).

15 Linda Greenhouse, "A Right Like Any Other," *New York Times*, August 6, 2014,
    http://www.nytimes.com/2014/08/07/opinion/new-judicial-approaches-to-
    abortion-rights.html?ref=international&_r=1.

16 This material first appeared in Wesley J. Smith, "A 'Pro-Abortion'
    Reversal of Roe?" *First Things*, June 14, 2013, http://www.firstthings.com/
    web-exclusives/2013/06/a-pro-abortion-reversal-of-roe.

17 Neil S. Siegel and Reva B. Siegel, "Equality Arguments for Abortion Rights," 60
    UCLA L. Rev. Disc. 160.

18 *Roe v. Wade*, 410 US 113 (1973).

19 Thomas Kaplan, "Cuomo Bucks Tide with Bill to Ease Limits on
    Abortion," *New York Times*, February 17, 2013, http://www.nytimes.
    com/2013/02/17/nyregion/cuomo-bucks-tide-with-bill-to-lift-abortion-limits.
    html?pagewanted=all&_r=0.

20 *Doe v. Bolton*, 410 US 179 (Jan. 22, 1973).

21 Smith, "Reversal of Roe."

22 Hippocratic Oath: http://www.britannica.com/EBchecked/topic/266652/
    Hippocratic-oath.

23 Melissa Hantman, "Revised Oath Resonates with Students," *Cornell
    Chronicle*, June 22, 2005, http://www.news.cornell.edu/stories/2005/06/
    revised-hippocratic-oath-resonates-graduates.

24 Section 8 of the Abortion Law Reform Act 2008.

25 Protection of Conscience Project, "Victorian Premier and Opposition Leader
    Pledge to Allow Conscience Vote on Forcing Doctors to Participate in
    Abortion," September 24, 2014, http://consciencelaws.org/blog/?p=6029.

26 Quebec Act Respecting End of Life Care, Section 30.

27 *Carter v. Canada (Attorney General)*, 2015 SCC 5, February 6, 2015.

28 "Policy, Conscientious Refusal," *College of Physicians and Surgeons of
    Saskatchewan*, http://www.cps.sk.ca/Documents/Council/2015%201%2019%20
    Conscientious%20Objection%20policy%20approved%20in%20principle%20
    by%20Council.pdf.

29 Ibid.

30 The College of Physicians and Surgeons of Ontario, "Professional Obligations
    and Human Rights," http://www.policyconsult.cpso.on.ca/wp-content/
    uploads/2014/12/Draft-Professional-Obligations-and-Human-Rights.pdf.

31 KNMG, "Position Paper: The Role of the Physician in Voluntary Termination of Life," 2011, http://knmg.artsennet.nl/Publicaties/KNMGpublicatie/100696/Position-paper-The-role-of-the-physician-in-the-voluntary-termination-of-life-2011.htm.

32 Ibid.

33 ACOG Committee Opinion: http://www.acog.org/Resources-And-Publications/Committee-Opinions/Committee-on-Ethics/The-Limits-of-Conscientious-Refusal-in-Reproductive-Medicine.

34 Udo Schuklenk, "Conscientious Objection in Medicine: Private Ideological Convictions Must Not Supersede Public Service Obligations," *Udo Schuklenk's Ethx Blog*, March 26, 2015, http://ethxblog.blogspot.com.au/2015/03/conscientious-objection-in-medicine.html.

35 Julian Savulescu, "Conscientious Objection in Medicine," *British Medical Journal*, 332(7536): 294–297, February 4, 2006, http://www.ncbi.nlm.nih.gov/pmc/articles/PMC1360408/.

36 I believe the term "new eugenics" was coined by Fr. Richard John Neuhaus.

37 Leon R. Kass, "The Wisdom of Repugnance," in Leon R. Kass and James Q. Wilson, *The Ethics of Human Cloning* (Washington, D.C.: AEI Press, 1998), 12.

38 Kass and Wilson, *Human Cloning*, 45.

39 Lisa Kaplan Gordon, "Surgery Could Give Men Wombs of Their Own in Five Years," *Yahoo Health*, November 17, 2015, https://www.yahoo.com/health/surgery-could-give-men-wombs-1302360099545142.html?soc_src=social-sh&soc_trk=tw.

40 Ibid., 75.

41 Ibid., 61.

42 Ibid., 157.

43 Joseph Fletcher, *Humanhood: Essays in Biomedical Ethics* (Buffalo, NY: Prometheus Books, 1979), 118.

44 Fletcher, *Humanhood*, 119.

45 Ibid., 173.

46 Ibid., 19.

47 Philip Kitcher, *The Lives to Come: The Genetic Revolution and Human Possibilities* (New York: Touchstone, 1997), 202.

48 Kitcher, *Genetic Revolution*, 199.

49 For example, see Hannah Osborne, "Humans to Become God-Like Cyborgs within 200 Years as They Upgrade Themselves," *International Business Times*, May 25, 2015, http://www.ibtimes.co.uk/humans-become-god-like-cyborgs-within-200-years-they-upgrade-themselves-1502841.

50 Lev Grossman, "2045: The Year Man Becomes Immortal," *Time*, February 10, 2011, http://content.time.com/time/magazine/article/0,9171,2048299,00.html.

51 Wesley J. Smith, "The Catman Cometh," *Weekly Standard*, June 26, 2006, http://www.weeklystandard.com/Content/Protected/Articles/000/000/012/346czohh.asp.

52 Kyle Munkittrick, "When Will We Be Transhuman?" *Discover*, July 16, 2011, http://blogs.discovermagazine.com/sciencenotfiction/2011/07/16/when-will-we-be-transhuman-seven-conditions-for-attaining-transhumanism/#.VWd_f89VhBc.

53 http://ieet.org/.

54 Munkittrick, "Transhuman."

55 Tim Bayne and Neil Levy, "Amputees by Choice: Body Integrity Identity Disorder and the Ethics of Amputation," *Journal of Applied Philosophy* 22, no. 1 (March 2005): 75–86.

56 Sarah Boesveld, "Becoming Disabled by Choice, not Chance," *National Post*, June 3, 2015, http://news.nationalpost.com/news/canada/becoming-disabled-by-choice-not-chance-transabled-people-feel-like-impostors-in-their-fully-working-bodies#__federated=1.

57 Christopher James Ryan, "Out on a Limb: The Ethical Management of Body Integrity Identity Disorder," *Neuroethics* 2 (2009): 21–33.

58 "Woman Desperate to Be Blind Poured Drain Cleaner in Eyes, Now Happier than Ever," *Tribune Media Wire*, October 1, 2015, http://fox4kc.com/2015/10/01/woman-desperate-to-be-blind-had-drain-cleaner-poured-in-eyes-now-happier-than-ever/.

59 Munkittrick, "Transhumanism."

60 Ibid.

61 Ibid.

62 Ibid.

63 Ibid.

64 Sarah Knapton, "China Shocks World by Genetically Engineering Human Embryos," *Telegraph*, April 23, 2015, http://www.telegraph.co.uk/news/science/11558305/China-shocks-world-by-genetically-engineering-human-embryos.html.

65 Catherine Paddock, "Three-Parent Embryos Approved in UK," *Medical News Today*, February 4, 2015, http://www.medicalnewstoday.com/articles/288943.php.

66 Kass, "Wisdom of Repugnance," 18–19.

67 Rita L. Marker and Wesley J. Smith, "The Art of Verbal Engineering," *Duquesne Law Review* 35, no. 1 (Fall 1996): 83–84.

68 Carol J. Gill, interview with the author, April 17–18, 2000.

69 Gill interview.

70 Lucette Lagnado, "Mercy Living," *Wall Street Journal*, January 10, 1995.

71 John Hardwig, interview with the author, October 22, 1998.

72 Tom Lorentzen, interview with the author, March 7, 1999.

73 Ibid.

Index

Page numbers followed by n indicate notes.

9 781594 038556